TARDIVE DYSKINESIA

Research & Treatment

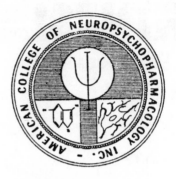

Published under the Imprimatur
of the
American College of Neuropsychopharmacology

TARDIVE DYSKINESIA

Research & Treatment

Edited by

William E. Fann, M.D.
Baylor College of Medicine
Houston, Texas

Robert C. Smith, M.D.
Texas Research Institute of Mental Sciences
Houston, Texas

John M. Davis, M.D.
Illinois State Psychiatric Institute
Chicago, Illinois

and

Edward F. Domino, M.D.
University of Michigan
Ann Arbor, Michigan

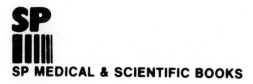

SP

SP MEDICAL & SCIENTIFIC BOOKS

New York • London

SPECTRUM PUBLICATIONS, INC.
175-20 Wexford Terrace, Jamaica, N.Y. 11432

Library of Congress Cataloging in Publication Data

Tardive dyskinesia.

  Includes index.
    1. Tardive dyskinesia.   2. Tardive dyskinesia—Chemotherapy.   3. Parasympatho-
mimetic agents.   4. Psychotropic drugs—Side effects.   5. Tardive dyskinesia—Animal
models.   I. Davis, John M., 1933-   [DNLM: Dyskinesia, Drug-induced.   2. Tranquilizing agents—Adverse effects.   WL390 T183]
RC394.T37T37   616.8'3   79-4468
ISBN 0-89335-076-1

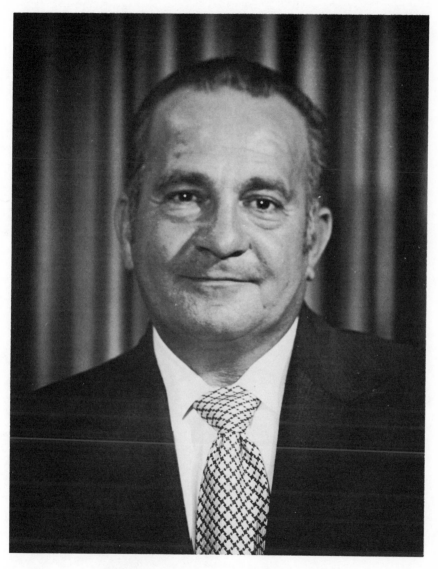

The editors dedicate this volume
to the memory of our respected colleague
Alberto DiMascio, Ph.D. (1928–1978).

CONTRIBUTORS

Murray Alpert, Ph.D.
Millhauser Laboratories
Department of Psychiatry
New York University School of
  Medicine
New York, New York

Ross J. Baldessarini, M.D.
Department of Psychiatry, Harvard
  Medical School
Mailman Laboratories for
  Psychiatric Research
McLean Division of Massachusetts
  General Hospital
Belmont, Massachusetts

Sven Bárány, M.D.
Psychiatric Research Center
Uppsala, Sweden

Phillip A. Berger, M.D.
Assistant Professor of Psychiatry
Director, Psychiatric Clinical
  Research Center
Stanford University School of
  Medicine
Stanford University
Stanford, California

Kenneth Bonnet, Ph.D.
Millhauser Laboratories
Department of Psychiatry
New York University School of
  Medicine
New York, New York

Kristin R. Carlson, Ph.D.
Department of Pharmacology
University of Massachusetts
  Medical School
Worcester, Massachusetts

Paul Carvey
Departments of Neurological
  Sciences and Pharmacology
Rush Medical Center
Chicago, Illinois

Caryle H. Chan, M.D.
Department of Psychiatry
University of Chicago
  and
Yale University School of Medicine
New Haven, Connecticut

Ching-piao Chien, M.D.
Professor of Psychiatry
UCLA School of Medicine
Brentwood Veterans Administration
  Hospital
Los Angeles, California

Anne Vibeke Christensen
Department of Pharmacology and
  Toxicology
H. Lundbeck & Co. A/S
Ottiliavej 7-9
DK 2500 Copenhagen-Valby
Denmark

Jonathan O. Cole, M.D.
Chief, Psychopharmacology
  Program
McLean Hospital
Belmont, Massachusetts

Maria Collora
Department of Psychiatry
Neuropsychopharmacology
  Research Unit
New York University Medical
  Center
New York, New York

George E. Crane, M.D.
817 Valley Avenue
Solana Beach, California

John W. Crayton, M.D.
Assistant Professor of Psychiatry
Department of Psychiatry
University of Chicago
Chicago, Illinois

Ian Cresse, Ph.D.
Department of Neuroscience
University of California Medical
    School
LaJolla, California

John M. Davis, M.D.
Director of Research
Illinois State Psychiatric Institute
and Professor of Psychiatry
    University of Chicago
Chicago, Illinois

Kenneth L. Davis, M.D.
Assistant Director, Psychiatric
    Clinical Research Center
Stanford University Associate
Veterans Administration Hospital
Palo Alto, California

Edward F. Domino, M.D.
Professor of Pharmacology
University of Michigan
Ann Arbor, Michigan

Maureen Donnelly, A.B.
The Albany Medical College of
    Union University
Albany, New York

David M. Engelhardt, M.D.
Professor of Psychiatry
Downstate Medical Center
Brooklyn, New York

William E. Fann, M.D.
Professor of Psychiatry
Associate Professor of
    Pharmacology
Baylor College of Medicine
    and
Chief, Psychiatry Service
Director, Psychotropics Research
    Laboratory
Veterans Administration Hospital
Houston, Texas

Arild Faurbye, M.D.
Sct. Hans Hospital, Dept. D
Roskilde, Denmark

Rasmus Fog, M.D.
Psychopharmacological Laboratory
St. Hans Mental Hospital
Roskilde
    and
Laboratory of Neurohistology
Hvidovre Hospital
Copenhagen, Denmark

Arnold J. Friedhoff, M.D.
Millhauser Laboratories
Department of Psychiatry
New York University School of
    Medicine
New York, New York

Eitan Friedman, Ph.D.
Millhauser Laboratories
    and
Neuropsychopharmacology
    Research Unit
New York University School of
    Medicine
New York, New York

Lawrence A. Frohman, M.D.
Department of Medicine
Michael Reese Hospital
Chicago, Illinois

George Gardos, M.D.
Director
Institute for Research and
    Rehabilitation
Boston State Hospital
Boston, Massachusetts

Lou Gerbino, M.D.
Department of Psychiatry
Neuropsychopharmacology
    Research Unit
New York University Medical
    Center
New York, New York

Jes Gerlach, M.D.
Section Hans Hospital,
    Department H
Roskilde, Denmark

Gerald Gianutsos, Ph.D.
Department of Pharmacology
St. John's University
College of Pharmacy
Jamaica, New York
    and
Department of Pharmacology and
    Toxicology
University of Rhode Island
Kingston, Rhode Island

**Alan C. Gibson, M.A., M.B.,
F.R.C.P., F.R.C. Psych.**

East Dorset Group of Hospitals
Bournemouth, Dorset, England

Robert P. Granacher, M.D.
Veterans Administration Hospital
    and
Assistant Professor of Psychiatry
University of Kentucky College of
    Medicine
Lexington, Kentucky

John W. Growdon, M.D.
Assistant Professor of Neurology
Tufts University Medical School
Boston, Massachusetts
    and
Research Associate
Massachusetts Institute of
    Technology
Cambridge, Massachusetts

Lars-M. Gunne, M.D.
Psychiatric Research Center
Uppsala, Sweden

Ana Hitri, Ph.D.
Department of Neurological
    Sciences and Pharmacology
Rush Medical Center
Chicago, Illinois

Leo E. Hollister, M.D.
Veterans Administration Hospital
Palo Alto, California

Koock Jung, M.D.
Department of Psychiatry: Research
The Albany Medical College of
    Union University
Albany, New York

David Klass, M.D.
Department of Mental Health
State of Illinois
Chicago, Illinois
    and
Department of Psychiatry
University of Chicago
Chicago, Illinois

Harold L. Klawans, M.D.
Department of Neurological
    Sciences and Pharmacology
Rush Medical Center
Chicago, Illinois

Beverly Kovacic
Department of Pharmacology
The University of Michigan
Ann Arbor, Michigan

Palle Kristjansen, M.D.
Sec. Hans Hospital, Department H
Roskilde, Denmark

Richard A. LaBrie
Institute of Research and
  Rehabilitation
Boston State Hospital
Boston, Massachusetts

Harbans Lal, Ph.D.
Department of Pharmacology and
  Toxicology
University of Rhode Island
Kingston, Rhode Island

Doddamane E. Leelavathi, Ph.D.
Research Specialist
Section of Behavioral
  Neurochemistry
Texas Research Institute of Mental
  Sciences
Houston, Texas

Emanuel Meller, Ph.D.
Millhauser Laboratories
Department of Psychiatry
New York University School of
  Medicine
New York, New York

Fathy S. Messiha, Ph.D.
Department of Pathology and
  Psychopharmacology Laboratory
Department of Psychiatry
Texas Tech University School of
  Medicine
Lubbock, Texas

Pavel Muller, Ph.D.
Department of Pharmacology
University of Toronto
Toronto, Canada M5S 1A8

Paul A. Nausieda, M.D.
Departments of Neurological
  Sciences and Pharmacology
Rush Medical Center
Chicago, Illinois

I. Møller Nielsen
Department of Pharmacology and
  Toxicology
H. Lundbeck & Company A/S
Copenhagen, Denmark

Henning Pakkenberg, M.D.
Laboratory of Neurology
Hvidovre Hospital
2650 Hvidovre, Denmark

Ghanshyam Pandey, Ph.D.
Research Department
Illinois State Psychiatric Institute
Chicago, Illinois

Polizoes Polizos, M.D.
Assistant Professor of Psychiatry
Downstate Medical Center
Brooklyn, New York

Ken Reed, Ph.D., M.D.
Clinical Fellow
Behavioral Neurochemistry Section
Texas Research Institute of Mental
  Sciences
Houston, Texas

Helen Rosengarten, M.D.
Millhauser Laboratories
Department of Psychiatry
New York University School of
  Medicine
New York, New York

Torkil Rye
Section Hans Hospital,
Department H
Roskilde, Denmark

Phillip Seeman, M.D.
Department of Pharmacology
University of Toronto
Toronto, Canada

Baron Shopsin, M.D.
Associate Professor of Psychiatry
Chief, Unit for the Study and
Treatment of Affective Disorders
Neuropsychopharmacology
Research Section
New York University Medical
Center
New York, New York

George Simpson, M.D.
Professor of Psychiatry
University of Southern California
and
Director,
USC-MSH Psychopharmacology
Service
Metropolitan State Hospital
Norwalk, California

Robert C. Smith, M.D., Ph.D.
Chief, Behavioral Neurochemistry
Texas Research Institute of Mental
Sciences
Houston, Texas
and
Research Assistant Professor of
Pharmacology
Baylor College of Medicine

Robert E. Smith
Clinical Research Division
Warner Lambert/Parke Davis
Ann Arbor, Michigan

Celia M. Sniffin, B.A.
Research Associate,
Psychopharmacology
McLean Hospital
Belmont, Massachusetts

Solomon H. Snyder, M.D.
Department of Pharmacology and
Experimental Therapeutics and
Psychiatry and Behavioral
Sciences
Johns Hopkins University School of
Medicine
Baltimore, Maryland

Michael Strizich
Manteno Mental Health Center
Manteno, Illinois
and
University of Chicago
Chicago, Illinois

Carol Tamminga, M.D.
Department of Psychiatry
University of Chicago
Chicago, Illinois
and
Visiting Scientist
National Institute of Mental Health
Bethesda, Maryland

Daniel Tarsy, M.D.
Department of Neurology
Boston Veterans Administration
Hospital and
Boston University School of
Medicine
and
Division of Neurology, Department
of Medicine
New England Deaconess Hospital
and Harvard Medical School
Boston, Massachusetts

CONTRIBUTORS

Anita Ross-Townsend, Ph.D.
Department of Psychiatry: Research
The Albany Medical College of
   Union University
Albany, New York

Isabelle Trenholm, R.N., M.S.
McLean Hospital
Belmont, Massachusetts

Bessel VanderKolk, M.D.
Institute of Research and
   Rehabilitation
Boston State Hospital
Boston, Massachusetts

Adela L. Vento, B.A.
Veterans Administration Hospital
Palo Alto, California

William J. Weiner, M.D.
Department of Neurological
   Sciences and Pharmacology
Rush Medical Center
Chicago, Illinois

Richard J. Wurtman, M.D.
Professor of Endocrinology and
   Metabolism
Massachusetts Institute of
   Technology
Cambridge, Massachusetts

PREFACE

In the late 1960's I summarized the literature on tardive dyskinesia and found about forty-five papers on this disorder; when I reviewed this topic 4 years later there were fifty additional communications. It was hardly an impressive number of reports and certainly small by comparison to the prolific output of psychopharmacologists in other areas. Yet there was sufficient information to be concerned about this new and unexpected complication. The majority of psychiatrists either ignored the existence of the problem or made futile efforts to prove that these motor abnormalities were clinically insignificant or unrelated to drug therapy. In the meantime the number of patients affected by tardive dyskinesia increased and the symptoms became worse in those already afflicted by this condition. In the last 5 years papers on long-term neurologic side effects have become so numerous that one seldom finds an issue of a major psychiatric journal that does not contain at least one communication on tardive dyskinesia. Furthermore, many scientific meetings, national and international, have devoted symposia and workshops to this topic in recent years.

There are several reasons why the profession has become so interested in the neurologic effects of neuroleptics. First, there are few investigators or clinicians who still have doubts about the iatrogenic nature of tardive dyskinesia. Second, the number of patients exhibiting motor abnormalities is increasing alarmingly, due to the cumulative effects of neuroleptics. Third, much progress has been made in the understanding of the biochemistry of the basal ganglia. Finally, recent reports have indicated that certain motor abnormalities are reversible when immediate remedial action is taken. This discovery imposes new responsibilities on the physician, who can no longer accept the fact that tardive dyskinesia is a necessary evil.

A book that summarizes and coordinates the multidisciplinary endeavors of many clinicians and basic scientists answers an important need of the psychiatric community. The great variety of reports included in this volume bears testimony not only to the advances that have been made in the last decade, but also to the complexity of the problem. It is evident that the more one learns about the toxic effects of neuroleptics on the central nervous system, the more one sees an urgent need to modify our current practices of drug use. It is unfortunate that many practitioners continue to prescribe psychotropics in excessive amounts, and that a considerable number of mental institutions have not yet developed a policy regarding the management and prevention of tardive dyskinesia. If this book, which reflects the opinions of the experts in this field, can make a dent in the complacency of many psychiatrists, it will be no small accomplishment.

George E. Crane
Solana Beach, California

INTRODUCTION

The aim of this book is to review research over the past 15 years of the current etiology and treatment of tardive dyskinesia. Our aim has been to produce a work that can serve as a reference source for several years, and that summarizes data that has been collected in most of the major areas of basic and clinical research relevant to this disorder. Consequently, although many of the papers contain data that is new and has not been presented previously, they also contain work that may have been previously presented or published in other forms, but is summarized or reinterpreted with new findings in this volume. We have tried to include the research and opinions of most of the clinicians and scientists who have done important work relevant to tardive dyskinesia over the last 15 years; by necessity we could not include contributions of every researcher or clinician without making the volume twice its size. Most of the chapters present findings of the work of a specific research group rather than a general review of all the work in a specific area relevant to tardive dyskinesia. Although this approach may lead to some overlap in chapter contents and to some differences in results or their interpretations, we believe that this more detailed presentation of each researcher's data will give the reader greater opportunity to evaluate the findings himself and draw his own conclusions. Since research in tardive dyskinesia is still in its "early adolescence," we feel that such an approach is more valuable at this time than a few highly condensed "review chapters" by a single author.

The first part of this book deals with the basic and animal models relevant to tardive dyskinesia. This will also serve as a review of the biochemical and behavioral pharmacology of chronic neuroleptic administration to animals. The second part of the book deals with tardive dyskinesia in man—its prevalence, possible etiology, and current approaches to treatment and management. Several of the currently utilized scales for rating tardive dyskinesia in man are included in the book. Some of the characteristics or applications of the scales are reviewed in other chapters in Part II. The use of these quantitative rating scales can help both the clinician and the researcher in diagnosing and following the development of dyskinetic symptoms in a standardized way. The editors and the authors have agreed that the scales can be reproduced for scientific and clinical use if reference is made to the scale and its published source.

Although at this time no single prescription can be made for the prevention or management of tardive dyskinesia, the clinician who uses the information contained in this book concerning the possible etiologies and treatment of tardive dyskinesia, and who modifies this clinical practice to conform with some of the suggestions made by these clinical experts, may help minimize the risks of tardive dyskinesia in the patients under his care who require treatment with neuroleptic drugs for their psychiatric or neurological diseases.

William E. Fann
Robert C. Smith
John M. Davis
Edward F. Domino

ACKNOWLEDGMENTS

The original ideas for a volume reviewing the current status of research in and treatment of tardive dyskinesia came from Ed Fann and John Davis. At a later stage Robert Smith and Ed Domino became coeditors. Because Drs. Fann and Davis were overburdened with other editorial and professional obligations, Dr. Smith eventually took up a major part of the burden of recruiting and organizing the manuscripts for the book.

Many of the contributions in the book were first presented at a symposium on basic and clinical research in tardive dyskinesia sponsored by the American College of Neuropsychopharmacology at their annual meeting in San Juan, Puerto Rico, in December 1977. Drs. Domino and Smith chaired the symposium on basic research relevant to tardive dyskinesia, and Drs. Fann and Alberto DiMascio chaired the session on clinical research. In addition to the presenters at the ACNP symposium, we also invited a number of other scientists and clinicians—who could not be at the meeting, but who had made important contributions to research in tardive dyskinesia over the past 15 years—to write chapters for the book. Because of the leading role the American College of Neuropsychopharmacology has played in promoting the interests of psychopharmacology in the United States and all over the world, and the interest it has taken in the side effects, as well as the therapeutic effects, of psychotropic drugs, the volume is being sponsored under the imprimatur of the ACNP, and proceeds from the sale of the book will aid the college with its future work.

In addition to the editors, several other people have substantially helped to get this large volume organized and edited. Bruce Richman and Ken Reed helped out in some of these tasks. Maurice Ancharoff and his staff at Spectrum provided help throughout the preparation of the book.

The secretarial burden for the correspondence, typing, and retyping, and final organization of the manuscripts fell on Carol Twidwell, whose efficiency and organizational ability greatly aided in recruiting the manuscripts and getting the final version to the publisher. Carol Hahn helped her in these tasks during the final months of the book's preparation.

The Editors

CONTENTS

Part II—Studies in Man and Pharmacology of Drugs Used in Treatment of Tardive Dyskinesia

Clinical Phenomenology and Measurement

Epidemiology

Drug History and Other Factors Related to Etiology

Part I

Basic Studies: Animal Models of Dyskinesia and Pharmacology of Chronic Neuroleptic Drugs

1

A Primate Model for Tardive Dyskinesia

LARS-M. GUNNE
and SVEN BÁRÁNY

Although several attempts have been made to create a primate model for tardive dyskinesia, a careful study of the literature shows that only the papers of Bédard (1,2) and ourselves (3) report on longstanding dyskinetic movements resulting from chronic administration of a neuroleptic (haloperidol) in monkeys. Many reports (4) have described a dyskinetic syndrome precipitated by each administration of the neuroleptic, lasting only for hours and reversible by administration of anticholinergics. This latter kind of reaction closely resembles acute dystonia as seen in the clinic. In our experience both the acute dystonia and the tardive or persistent type of dyskinesia may occur in the same animals.

In order to describe and study the occurrence and development of these phenomena, we have constructed 3 rating scales: one for coordinated motor activity (in order to record what we have called *sedation*, meaning reduction and slowing of spontaneous activity together with reduced response to standardized signals); one scale for acute dystonia and parkinsonism (measuring rigidity of movements, tremor and uncoordinated tonic and clonic muscle contractions); and one scale for tardive dyskinesia (measuring tongue protrusion, grimacing, chewing, and chorealike movements of the limbs and trunk).

We have also developed a technique for chronic cerebrospinal fluid (CSF) drainage in unanaesthetized, nearly unrestrained monkeys. To set up this method we have utilized experiences from Deneau *et al.* (5), who have used unrestrained monkeys self-administering drugs through in-dwelling i.v. catheters, and Gordon *et al.* (6), who have applied chronic CSF drainage in restrained monkeys (5,6). In our version a metal cannula is inserted in the left ventricle of a monkey's brain and connected with a plastic catheter through which CSF is delivered constantly via a pump (450 μl/3 h), into a fraction collector placed in a refrigerator. There is also one or two catheters in the venous system of the monkey, which allows blood sampling at convenient intervals, as well as i.v. injections or infusions with little disturbance of the experimental animal.

In our long-term experiments haloperidol 0.5 mg/kg/day was administered orally, dissolved in fruit juice to 6 Cebus appella monkeys. In some animals the dose had to be reduced half a year later due to severe attacks of acute dystonia; the anticholinergic biperiden, 0.07–0.14 mg/kg/day, was then added to the daily haloperidol dose. On experimental days when the ratings were performed, haloperidol was injected alone (i.m.) in doses specified for each experiment. Behavior ratings were performed by aid of videotaped recordings for 2 minutes before, and 1/2, 1, 2, 4, 6, 8, and 24 hours after haloperidol administration. Two independent raters showed a high interrater agreement (96%–100% for 9 different subscales).

THE TARDIVE DYSKINESIA SYNDROME (TD)

Two animals developed marked and persistent symptoms of TD, whereas one had only slight and transient signs. All 6 monkeys have shown various degrees of parkinsonism and acute dystonia (AD). Figure 1 shows the typical ratings during 24 hours in one animal with marked TD symptoms within the bucco-lingual region (tongue protrusion and grimacing) before the daily haloperidol administration. These TD signs disappeared for 4 hours after haloperidol, but instead, the monkey had increased rigidity of movements, followed by outbursts of widespread tonic and clonic contractions of the limbs and trunk. Between these outbursts there were intervals when coordinated motor activity was rated as reduced in amount and speed while the animal appeared drowsy and had a lowered reaction to knocking signals. Some months later the behavior became dominated by the dystonic abnormal movements, and coordinated motor activity could no longer be recorded.

Figure 2 shows that the intensity of the AD reaction was dose-dependent, and Figure 3 that the reduction of TD signs also appeared in a dose-dependent manner. Figure 4 shows the development of these movement abnormalities during monthly ratings in one animal during long-term administration of haloperidol. In all animals there were signs of tolerance to the sedative effect of the neuroleptic. (The reduction of coordinated activity, which was maximal during the first month, gradually became smaller.) Parkinsonism (broken lines) and later acute dystonia (open circles) developed in all animals (measured as area under curve for 8 hours during monthly recordings of behavior after 0.1 mg/kg haloperidol i.m.). TD signs (at 24 hours after haloperidol) did

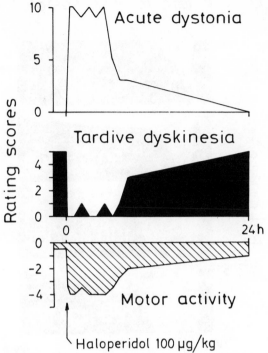

Figure 1.   Twenty-four hour ratings of acute dystonia, tardive dyskinesia, and motor activity in Cebus (3/75) after about 4 months of daily haloperidol administration.

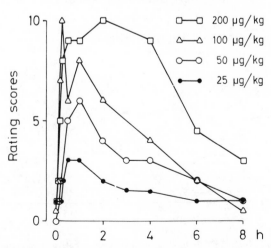

Figure 2.   Twenty-four hour ratings of acute dystonia following 25, 50, 100, and 200 μg/kg of haloperidol.

Tardive dyskinesia

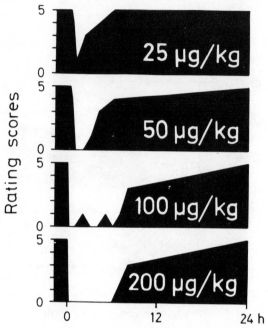

Figure 3.   Twenty-four hour ratings of tardive dyskinesia following 25, 50, 100, and 200 μg/kg of haloperidol.

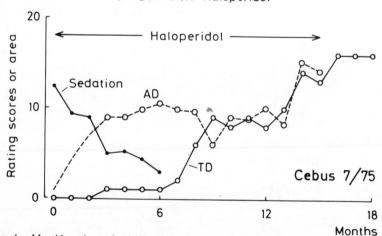

Figure 4.   Monthly ratings of sedation (area under curve of negative motor activity ratings for 8 hours), acute dystonia and parkinsonism (area under curve for 8 hours), and tardive dyskinesia (before daily administration) during long-term treatment with haloperidol.

not become evident until 4–6 months after the start of treatment. In animal (3/75) two withdrawal experiments resulted in abolishment of reduction of TD signs. In the first experiment after 5 months of haloperidol the TD signs disappeared after 2 weeks (Fig. 5), whereas in the second withdrawal experiment a year later there was only a reduction of TD signs, but some protrusion of the tongue persisted even after 200 days (Fig. 6). A single injection of 50

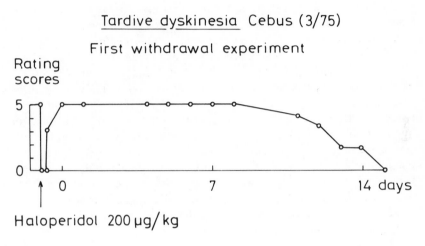

Figure 5.   TD ratings during first withdrawal experiment in cebus (3/75).

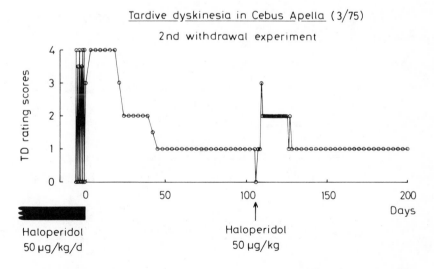

Figure 6.   TD ratings during the last few days of regular haloperidol administration (left, when each dose suppresses symptoms down to 0), and during the second withdrawal experiment in cebus (3/75). Note the effect of a single haloperidol dose on day 106 after withdrawal.

μg/kg haloperidol caused an immediate abolishment of symptoms, followed 2 days later by a deterioration lasting for 3 weeks. A similar rebound deterioration was seen after chlorpromazine, whereas clozapine (which does not seem to induce TD in humans) gave no such reaction. This indicates that the observed phenomenon might be a test for TD liability in neuroleptic drugs.

Soon after the first withdrawal experiment in Cebus (3/75), when the daily haloperidol administration was reinstated we tried to analyze the development of AD signs by an intensified schedule of ratings, 5 days weekly, during stepwise increases of the haloperidol dose every sixteenth day (Fig. 7). Each dose increase caused an accentuation of AD symptoms for a few days, followed by a return to lower levels as a sign of tolerance to this effect.

When other neuroleptics were substituted for haloperidol, the AD response was much smaller or absent, whereas the alleviation of TD was sometimes marked, for instance, after chlorpromazine, 1 mg/kg (Fig. 8). The area above the curve was used as a measure of TD reduction (together with maximal effect) in Tables 1–4. These tables illustrate various attempts to modify the TD signs, using drugs active on the catecholamine receptors (Table 1), the GABA system (Table 2), the serotonin system (Table 3), and the cholinergic system (Table 4). The effects recorded so far confirm various clinical reports on therapeutic effects and can be regarded as a validation of our primate model. We became particularly impressed with the dose-dependent TD alleviating effect of clonazepam.

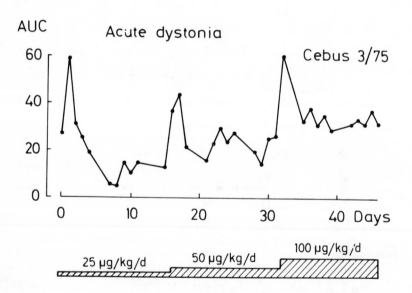

Figure 7.   AD ratings (AUC) in cebus (3/75) when haloperidol was reinstated in stepwise increasing doses after first withdrawal experiment.

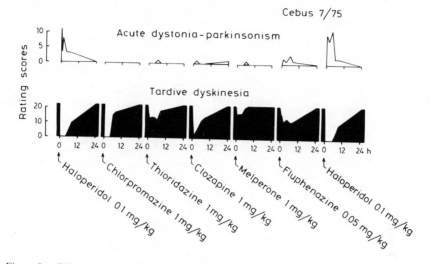

Figure 8. Effect on AD ratings (above) and TD ratings (below) when other neuroleptics were substituted for haloperidol.

Table 1

Effect on TD ratings (max. eff. and area above curve, AAC) of drugs active within the catecholaminergic system.

	Dose mg/kg	Effect %	
		max	AAC
saline		17	2
haloperidol	.05	100	89
chlorpromazine	.50	32	16
–"–	1	100	71
thioridazine	1	5	5
–"–	2	40	31
clozapine	1	90	57
fluphenazine	.05	46	38
thiethylperazine	.20	100	82
melperone	1	27	10
apomorphine	.10	75	54
L-dopa	10	66	29
clonidine	.10	0	0

Table 2

Effect on TD ratings (max. eff. and area above curve, AAC) of drugs active within the gaba-ergic system.

	Dose mg/kg	Effect %	
		max	AAC
saline		17	2
AOAA	1	0	0
–"–	2.5	50	38
baclophen	2.5	0	0
clonazepam	.001	0	0
–"–	.005	32	9
–"–	.010	73	32
–"–	.025	82	61
–"–	.050	100	84
diazepam	.200	50	49

Table 3

Effect on TD ratings (max. eff. and area above curve, AAC) of drugs active within the serotonergic system.

	Dose mg/kg	Effect %	
		max	AAC
saline		17	2
L-5HTP	20	67	68
methysergide	.10	25	9
–"–	.20	0	0
cyproheptadine	.20	TD increased	
–"–	.40	67	16

Table 4

Effect on TD ratings (max. eff. and area above curve, AAC) of drugs active within the cholinergic system.

	Dose mg/kg	Effect %	
		max	AAC
saline		17	2
oxotremorine	.03	89	34
deanol	10	25	14
– '' –	20	50	48
RS 86	.25	10	5
– '' –	.50	14	4
– '' –	1	70	24

CSF STUDIES

Figure 9 shows the response to an L-dopa infusion for 3 hours, with a drastic increase of the dopamine metabolite homovanillic acid (HVA), accompanied by a minor rise, followed by a depression of the serotonin metabolite 5HIAA. The noradrenaline metabolite MHPG remained mainly unchanged. There seemed to be only slight diurnal variations of the HVA and possibly of the 5HIAA level. The distinct circadian rhythm of HVA reported by Perlow *et al.* (7) in restrained monkeys was not seen in our experiments.

Figure 10 shows the HVA increase following 200 μg/kg of haloperidol in a drug-naive animal. Figure 11 illustrates the effect of two apomorphine infusions given at 2-day intervals. Each apomorphine infusion caused a slight depression of HVA, followed by a rise. The apomorphine dose (0.8 mg/kg/h delivered for 3 hours) was high enough to give rise to overt signs of scratching and motor unrest.

The general aim of the present studies is to either facilitate or inhibit one neurotransmitter system while monitoring the effects on some of the others. When dyskinetic animals will later be included in similar tests, we hope to be able to define at least some alterations in neurotransmitter balance, which might underlie neuroleptic-induced dyskinesias.

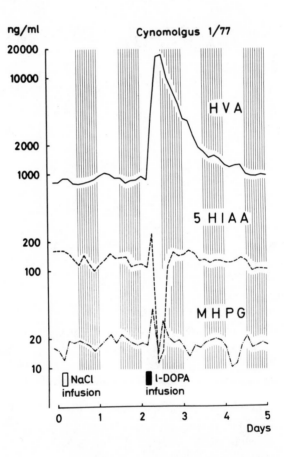

Figure 9.   Side ventricular CSF levels of HVA, 5HIAA, and MHPG during infusion of saline and L-dopa (20 mg/kg/h for 3 hours). Striped areas represent dark hours.

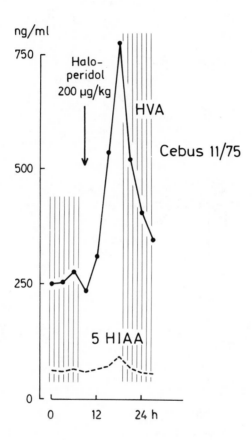

Figure 10.   Side ventricular CSF levels of HVA and 5HIAA. Effect of 0.2 mg/kg haloperidol
i.m. Striped areas represent dark hours.

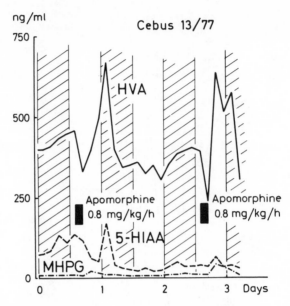

Figure 11.   Side ventricular CSF levels of HVA, 5HIAA and MHPG during 2 apomorphine infusions (0.8 mg/kg/h for 3 hours). Striped areas represent dark hours.

ACKNOWLEDGMENTS

This study has been supported by a Swedish Medical Research Council Grant B79–21X–04546–05C.

REFERENCES

1. Bedard, P., Larochelle, L., De Lean, J., Lafleur, J. Dyskinesias induced by long term administration of haloperidol in the monkey. *Physiologist, 15*:83, 1972.

2. Beard, P., Delean, J., Lafleur, J., Larochelle, L. Haloperidol-induced dyskinesias in the monkey. *Can. Sci. Neurol., 4*:197, 1977.

3. Gunne, L.M., Barany, S. Haloperidol-induced tardive dyskinesia in monkeys. *Psychopharmacology, 50*:237, 1975.

4. Marsden, C.D., Tarsy, D., Baldessarini, R.J. Spontaneous and drug-induced movement disorders in psychotic patients. In *Psychiatric Aspects of Neurological Disease*. Benson, D.F., Blumer, D. (eds). New York: Grune and Stratton, pp. 219–266, 1975.

5. Deneau, G., Yanagita, T., Seevers, M.H. Self-administration of psychoactive substances by the monkey. *Psychopharmacologia, 16*:30, 1969.

6. Gordon, E., Perlow, M., Oliver, J., Ebert, M., Kopin, J. Origins of catecholamine metabolites in monkey cerebrospinal fluid. *J. Neurochem., 25*:347, 1975.

7. Perlow, M., Festoff, B., Ebert, M., Gordon, E.K., Siegler, M.G., Lake, C.R., Hoffman, H., Johnson, D.K., Chase, T.N. The circadian variation of brain cyclic AMP and catecholamine metabolism in Rhesus primates. *Neurosci. Absts., 11*:499. 6th Annual Meeting of the Society for Neuroscience, Toronto, 1976.

2

Biochemical Studies After Chronic Administration of Neuroleptics to Monkeys

F.S. MESSIHA

The use of animal models often provides insight into human disease and into drug-induced side effects that cannot be acquired by other means. Treatment with phenothiazines involves risks for neurological complication which are frequently observed during chronic administration of neuroleptic drugs, i.e., chlorpromazine (CPZ), to psychiatric patients (1–6). Experimental dyskinesias have been produced in monkeys by administration of CPZ (7–10) over a long period of time, with large doses of L-dopa alone or combined with extracerebrally acting aromatic L-amino acid decarboxylase inhibitor (11), by means of stereotaxically produced lesions (12, 13) or with L-dopa subsequent lesions with 6-hydroxydopamine (14). However, a neuroleptic-induced dyskinesia is a better model of the abnormal movements seen in tardive dyskinesias than dyskinesias produced by other means. Reviewing structural and biochemical hypotheses of naturally occurring and drug-produced extrapyramidal disease, it soon became evident that there is a need for critical investigations in borderline areas among neurology, biochemical psychopharmacology, and pathophysiology, where a great variety of observations about movement disorders had accumulated. Furthermore, the implication of certain biogenic amines in the mechanism of action of the neuroleptic drugs, and the involvement of some of these monoamines in certain aspects of drug-produced abnormal repetitive movements and stereotyped behavior, suggest a relationship between the monamines and abnormal movement disorders seen in tardive dyskinesia. Accordingly, the present study was performed to investigate the effects of chronic administration of CPZ on the neurological status of the monkey, and to determine whether there is a relationship between alterations of biogenic amines and some of their metabolites to the dyskinetic manifestations.

METHODS

Behavioral Studies

The subjects were 3 female monkeys, aged 3–4 years. Monkeys were administered CPZ in a gradual dosage build-up from 100 mg to 120 mg/day over 4 months (short-term CPZ group). Four other animals received CPZ, from 10 to 180 mg/day, over 1 year (long-term CPZ group), and 5 monkeys remained drug-free during the study and served as controls. The highest dose of CPZ in the long-term group was maintained for 45 days. CPZ was administered by nasogastric tube. 2–4 hour baseline urine collections were obtained during the initial drug-free period for all 3 groups. 2–4 hour urine samples were then collected from each monkey at varied time intervals during CPZ administration, at which time the animals were symptom-free. Also, 24-hour urine samples were collected, 24 hours prior to sacrifice of the monkeys displaying oral dyskinesias (long-term group), as well as from monkeys on short-term CPZ administration, which failed to display dyskinesias, and the drug-free control.

The 24 hour urine specimens were collected over 10 ml of 2.0 N hydrochloric acid. The final urine volume was recorded and aliquots were kept frozen in dark-brown glass containers at −20°C for later analyses of the biogenic amines and their metabolites. Cerebrospinal fluid (CFS) samples were drawn immediately after sacrifice, mixed with 2 mg ascorbic acid per ml of CSF, and kept frozen at −20°C until assayed within 14 days.

Analytical Procedures

The fractionation technique utilized for the separation and purification of the catecholamines and their acid metabolites is summarized in Figure 1 and described in detail elsewhere (15–17). This method consists of chromatography on a Dowex 1x4 anion exchange resin and subsequent rechromatography on basic aluminum hydroxide at pH 4.5 for the separation of homovanillic acid (HVA) from vanillylmandelic acid (VMA), dihydroxyphenylmandelic acid (DOMA), and dihydroxyphenylacetic acid (DOPAC) by the differential elution of these acids. A second portion of the urine specimen was subjected to acid hydrolysis prior to isolation of the catecholamines dopamine (DA), norepinephrine (NE), and epinephrine (E) from their respective O-methylated metabolites. A third portion of the urine specimen was assayed for its content

Figure 1.   Fractionation of catecholamines & metabolites

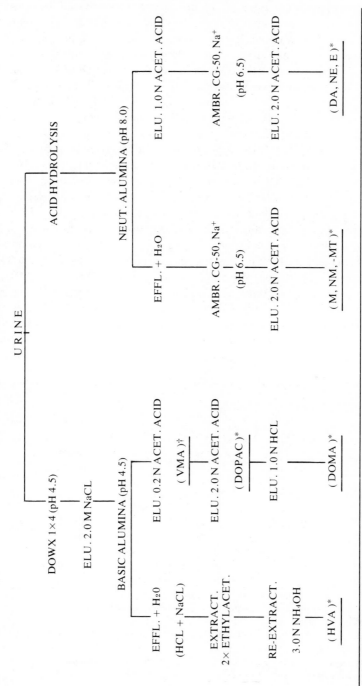

* SPECTROFLUOROMETRIC ASSAYS
⁑ SPECTROPHOTOMETRIC ASSAYS

of serotonin (5-HT) and its acid metabolite 5-hydroxyindole acetic acid (5-HIAA) by the procedures of Arterberry and Conley (18) and Ahlberg (19), respectively. Quantitative determinations of NE, E, and metanephrine (M) were made according to the procedures of Haggendal (20, 21). The ethylenediamine method was used for the estimation of DOPAC and DOMA (22). VMA and HVA were assayed by the methods of Pisano et al., (23) and Sato (24), respectively. Quantitative determinations of DA (25) and 3-methoxytyramine (26) followed a modification (27, 28) of the trihydroxyindole reaction (29) as outlined below.

In all experiments the Amberlite resin used was cycled by the procedure of Hirs *et al*. (30) and then washed with 8.0 N acetic acid. This was followed by washing with distilled water, reconverting to the Na^+ form, and cycling again as described by Hirs *et al*. (30). Prior to use, the resin was converted to the K^+ form by equilibration with potassium phosphate buffer 0.1 M pH 6.6.

Figure 2 (left panel) shows fluorescence blank as a function of resin treatment. The elution pattern of resin pretreated with acetic acid is compared to nontreated resin. The nature fluorescence of the eluate is measured at 330 nm with excitation at 285 nm. Washing with acetic acid stronger than that used for the cycling procedure eliminates fluorescent contaminants from the resin and reduces the fluorescence blank, leading to a greater sensitivity. This is analogous to the same beneficial effect observed for spectrophotometric assays (31).

Figure 2 (right panel) illustrates the fluorescence obtained as a function of

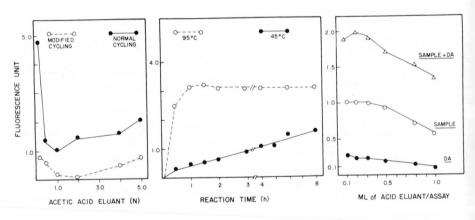

Figure 2. Experimental variables in trihydroxyindole reaction.
Left panel shows the effect of modified cycling procedure of the Amberlite resine on nature fluorescence intensity.
Middle panel shows the effect of temperature and reaction time on the development of stable fluorophore in the trihydroxyindole reaction.
Right panel shows the effect of the volume of acid eluant used on fluorescence intensity in the presence of and absence of authentic dopamine (DA).

the column eluate volume used for the fluoremetric assay. The fluorescence observed has been calculated to unit volume. This indicates that the aliquot of acid eluate used should not exceed 0.3 ml to avoid a marked decrease in fluorescence leading to a lower sensitivity (28).

The middle panel of Figure 2 shows fluorescence intensity as a function of reaction time and temperature. Development of the fluorophore formed in the hydroxyindole reaction in a boiling water bath resulted in approximately sixfold increase in fluorescence intensity as compared to that obtained at 45°C (32). The fluorescence reaches a maximum within 60 to 90 minutes and is stable for over 48 hours at room temperature. This modification of the trihydroxyindole reaction gives an increase in fluorescence intensity so that as little as 2.5 ng/ml of assay mixture can be determined.

The CSF samples obtained from the monkey experiments were assayed for DOPAC, HVA, and 5-HIAA, as described by Pullar *et al.* (33).

The results of the quantitative determination were corrected for percentage recovery of the authentic compounds used as internal standard, and given as total output for the monoamines, free + conjugates, and the free acid metabolites. Mean 24 hour urinary outputs of compounds measured were expressed in μg or mg/time unit indicated. The statistical significance of the results were analyzed by t-test for independent means.

RESULTS

Chronic administration of CPZ, in gradual dosage build-up, resulted in the appearance of involuntary dyskinetic symptoms in the buccal-lingual-oral area in monkeys. Their movements included abnormal mouth and lip movements, and frequent protrusion of the tongue. Conversely, monkeys administered CPZ for the short term failed to display such adverse reactions.

Figure 3 shows the effect of chronic administration of CPZ on the concentration of the biogenic amine acid metabolites DOPAC, HVA, and 5-HIAA in CSF of monkeys with demonstrable dyskinetic symptoms. There was a significant ($p < 0.05$) rise in 5-HIAA concentration in the CSF as a function of prolonged CPZ treatment compared to drug-free controls. Concomitantly, a nonsignificant (0.1 p 0.05) increase in the content of DOPAC and HVA were noted.

Table 1 lists the amounts of biogenic amine acid metabolites excreted in urine of the monkeys during an initial drug-free period, at variable time intervals during CPZ administration and at the time of onset of dyskinesias. The control animals remained drug-free throughout the experiment. Little changes occurred in the excretion of endogenous biogenic amine acid metabolites at the time intervals studied from their respective baseline values or from control animals.

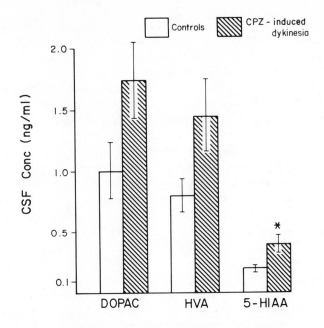

Figure 3.   The effect of chronic administration of chlorpromazine of CSF content of dihydroxyphenyl-acetic acid (DOPAC), homovanillic acid (HVA), and 5-hydroxyindole acetic acid (5-HIAA). Values are for means ± SD *p 0.05

Table 2 summarizes the effect of CPZ administration on mean 24 hour urinary excretion of the catecholamines DA, E, NE, their O-methylated metabolites 3-MT, and M, along with 5-HT. Compared to control values, long-term CPZ-treated monkeys with demonstrable dyskinesia excreted a significant increase in DA (p 0.05) and NE (p 0.05) by approximately 1.5 and 1.7 fold, respectively. There was a concomitant nonsignificant (0.1 p 0.05) increase in 3MT excretion, with little changes occurring in the 24 hour urinary output for E, M, VMA, and 5-HT.

DISCUSSION

CPZ was introduced in clinical psychiatry in 1952 (34, 35) and remains the most frequently used drug in the management of schizophrenia and related disorders. Apart from the antipsychotic effects of the neuroleptic drugs, i.e. CPZ, these agents produce different types of extrapyramidal syndrome, i.e., parkinsonian-like syndromes, akathisia, dystonic syndromes, or the late-appearing dyskinesia "tardive dyskinesia." Neuroleptic-produced tardive dyskinesia has attracted interest due to its frequent occurrences, 8%–22% in

Table 1
The Effect of Chlorpromazine (CPZ) on the Urinary
Excretion of Major Acidic Metabolites of the
Catecholamines and Serotonin in monkeys.

Phase of CPZ Treatment (Time of urine sampling)	DOPAC*	HVA (mg/24 h)	VMA	5-HIAA
Initial drug-free period (base-line)	0.38 ± 0.21	1.3 ± 0.7	0.15 ± 0.04	0.31 ± 0.23
Initial CPZ treatment (2–4 weeks of CPZ admin.)	0.41 ± 0.18	1.6 ± 0.9	0.17 ± 0.05	1.06 ± 0.78
Short-term CPZ treatment (4 months of CPZ admin.)	0.67 ± 0.29	2.5 ± 1.2	0.20 ± 0.05	0.55 ± 0.23
Long-term CPZ treatment (10–11 months of CPZ admin.)	0.31 ± 0.11	2.4 ± 0.7	0.29 ± 0.09	0.60 ± 0.11
Drug-free controls	0.42 ± 0.18	1.9 ± 1.4	0.23 ± 0.11	0.89 ± 0.37
Long-term CPZ treatment "During oral dyskinesia" (12–13 months of CPZ admin.)	0.43 ± 0.16	2.7 ± 0.80	0.23 ± 0.10	0.85 ± 0.26

*Means ± SD of 24 hour urinary output of dihydroxyphenylacetic acid (DOPAC), Homovanillic acid (HVA), vanillylmandelic acid (VMA), and 5-hydroxyindoleacetic acid (5-HIAA). Values are the means for at least 8 independent determinations obtained during the time indicated (n = 8–17). Data for drug-free controls derives from 24 hour urine samples obtained at the same days at which similar urine specimens were collected from the group of monkeys with CPZ-produced oral dyskinesia.

psychiatric patients treated chronically with CPZ (1, 2, 4–6, 36). Little is known about the pathophysiology and biochemical basis underlying CPZ-induced dyskinesia. However, with the increasing knowledge on catecholamine (CA) neurons and CA transmission mechanism, it has become possible to formulate certain hypotheses regarding the mode of action of the neuroleptics as well as of other psychotropic drugs (37–39). Accordingly, indirect evidence has advanced the hypothesis that CPZ-produced enhancement of DA metabolism is presumably a direct consequence of a feedback mechanism compensating for the blockade of the DA receptors by CPZ and/or is a result of a disturbance of the amine storage (40–49). Furthermore, CPZ-mediated increase in tyrosine hydroxylase activity, the rate limiting step in the biosynthesis of the CA, enhances not only the synthesis of the CA, but also of melanin, which is implicated in melanosis of the skin and eye, observed under chronic administration of CPZ (43). Since there is a relationship between cerebral DA and motor function (50–53), and since CPZ exerts an effect on cerebral DA metabolism (40–46), a relationship between the action of CPZ on these and subsequent developments of extrapyramidal movement disorders

Table 2

The Effect of Chlorpromazine (CPZ) on the Urinary Excretion of Dopamine, Some of Its Metabolites and Serotonin in Monkeys.

Phase of CPZ Treatment (Time of Urine Sampling)	DA†	3-MT	NE	E	M	5-HT
			(mg/24h)			
Initial drug-free period	201.2 ± 99.5	192.7 ± 26.0n	46.3 ± 5.0	2.1 ± 1.1	18.6 ± 3.7	80.3 ± 41.8
Initial CPZ treatment (2–4 weeks of CPZ admin.)	184.0 ± 106.1	226.0 ± 113.8	34.5 ± 4.8	3.2 ± 1.5	23.4 ± 13.0	112.0 ± 63.6
Short-term CPZ treatment (4 months of CPZ admin.)	276.0 ± 142.0	288.9 ± 122.5	69.0 ± 27.3	3.9 ± 0.9	39.7 ± 16.3	62.0 ± 33.6
Long-term CPZ treatment (10–11 months of CPZ admin.)	341.1 ± 60.4	368.8 ± 72.7	53.0 ± 6.0	5.7 ± 2.9	43.0 ± 7.4	69.2 ± 31.5
Drug-free controls	243.5 ± 101.7	210.6 ± 144.3	66.2 ± 22.2	6.0 ± 3.5	35.2 ± 14.7	115.0 ± 41.6
Long-term CPZ treatment "During oral dyskinesias" (12–13 months of CPZ admin.)	615.8 ± 120.2*	389.4 ± 77.2	115.4 ± 40.6*	6.2 ± 3.9	48.9 ± 15.5	83.5 ± 45.2

*Means ± SD of 24 hour urinary output of dopamine (DA), 3-methoxytyramine (3-MT), norepinephrine (NE), epinephrine (E), metanephrine (M), and serotonin (5-HT).

†Differs from drug-free controls at p 0.05.

seem likely. In the present study, long-term administration of CPZ to monkeys produced dyskinetic symptoms characterized by abnormal involuntary movements in the buccal-lingual-oral area, in addition to rotatory rhythmic movements of the jaw and frequent protrusion of the tongue similar to the symptoms seen in tardive dyskinesia. These drug-induced changes in the neurological states of the monkeys were associated with an increase in amounts of DOPAC, HVA, the major metabolites of DA, and 5HIAA, in the CSF as well as in urinary excretion of DA, 3MT, and NE. Conversely, subchronic administration of CPZ, which failed to produce dyskinetic symptoms in monkeys, did not produce alteration in the monoamines and their metabolites studied. These results suggest that increased turnover rates of 5HT and DA are associated with this type of dyskinetic manifestation produced by chronic treatment with CPZ.

Experimental evidence suggests that the content of HVA in the CSF is similar to that present in the caudate nucleus (54, 55), and that the concentration of 5HIAA in the CSF may originate from spinal cord (56). The concurrent rise in DA excretion and its acid metabolites DOPAC and HVA in CSF of monkeys with CPZ-produced dyskinesia suggests a relationship between cerebral and peripheral metabolism of DA. It seems likely that urinary DA, which does not originate in the CNS, might be indicative of similar changes occurring in CNS in this type of drug-induced dyskinesia. For example, decreased cerebral (50) and urinary DA (57) were determined in Parkinson's disease, as contrasted with increased HVA concentration in CSF in choreatic states (58) and increased urinary DA excretion from normal value in patients with choreatic movements, tremor, and segmental dystonia (59). In Gilles de la Tourette disease, another extrapyramidal motor hyperkinesia, a rise in DA excretion from normal was noted (60, 61).

It is of interest to correlate the clinical evidence suggesting a similar pathophysiological mechanism underlying tardive dyskinesia and involuntary tics (62) with the observed increase in urinary DA output from normal in drug-induced dyskinesia (63) and in Tourette's disease (60, 61), along with their favorable therapeutic responses to antidopaminergic agents, such as Li_2Co_3 (64). It seems likely that changes in DA excretion is associated with some of the manifested symptoms of extrapyramidal disorders and/or may reflect a "systemic" disease involving abnormalities in central and peripheral dopaminergic structures.

The present data suggest that although urinary DA is considered to be derived from peripheral sources, the deviation of its excretion from normal in certain neurological disorders of extrapyramidal disorders might be utilized as predictive measure for certain clinical and behavioral responses to pharmacotherapy. Moreover, modification of dopaminergic function by means of pharmacological interventions may be of value, not only in studying mechanisms underlying these symptoms but also in developing new approaches to their pharmacotherapy.

ACKNOWLEDGMENTS

This study was supported in part by U.S. Public Health Service Grant 1-R01 MH 20813.

REFERENCES

1. Sigwald, J., Bouttier, D., Raymondeaud, C. Quatre cas de dyskinesie facio-bucco-linguo-masticatirce a evolution prolongee secondaire a un traitement par les neuroleptiques, Rev. Neurol., 100:751–755, 1959.
2. Ayd, F.J. A survey of drug-induced extrapyramidal reactions. JAMA, 175:1054–1060, 1961.
3. Faurbye, A., Rasch, P., Pererson, P., .Bender, P., Brandberg, J., Pakkenberg, H. Neurological symptoms in pharmacotherapy of psychoses. Acta Psychiatry Scand., 40:10–27, 1964.
4. Degkwitz, R., Luxemburger, O. Das terminale Insuffizienz bzw. Defektsyndrom infolge chronischer Anwendung von Neuroleptika. Nervenarzt, 36:173–175, 1965.
5. Crane, G.E. Tardive dyskinesia in patients treated with major neuroleptics. A review of the literature. Am. J. Psychiatry, 124:40–48, 1968.
6. Crane, G.E. Dyskinesia and neuroleptics. Arch. Gen. Psychiatry, 19:700–703, 1968.
7. Deneau, G.A., Crane, G.E. Dyskinesia in Rhesus monkeys tested with high doses of chlorpromazine. In Crane, G.E., and Gardner, J.R. Jr. (eds.) Psychotropic Drugs and Dysfunctions of the Basal Ganglia, U.S. Public Health Service, Publ. No. 1938, Washington, D.C., pp. 12–14, 1969.
8. Deuel, R.K. Neurological examination of Rhesus monkeys treated with high doses of chlorpromazine. In Psychotropic Drugs and Dysfunctions of the Basal Ganglia, Crane, G.E., Gardner, J.R., Jr. (eds.). U.S. Public Health Service, Publ. No. 1938, Washington, D.C., pp. 15–18, 1969.
9. Paulson, G. Dyskinesias in rhesus monkeys. Trans. Am. Neurol. Assoc., 97:109–111, 1972.
10. Paulson, G. Dyskinesias in monkeys. Adv. Neurol., 1:647–650, 1973.
11. Mones, R.J. Experimental dyskinesias in normal rhesus monkey. Adv. Neurol., 1:665-669, 1973.
12. Ward, A., McCulloch, Magoun, H. Production of alternating tremor at rest in monkeys. J. Neurophysiol., 11:317–330, 1948.
13. Carpentar, M.B. Brain-stem and infratentorial neuraxis in experimental dyskinesia. Arch. Neurol., 5:504–524, 1961.
14. Ng, L.K.Y., Gelhard, R.E., Chase, T.N., Maclean, P.D. Drug-induced dyskinesia in monkeys: a pharmacologic model employing 6-hydroxydopamine. Adv. Neurol., 1:651–655, 1973.
15. Messiha, F.S., Hsu, T.H., Bianchine, J.R. Peripheral aromatic L-amino acids decarboxylase inhibitor in parkinsonism. I. Effect on 0-methylated metabolites of L-2-14 C-dopa. J. Clin. Invest., 51:452–455, 1972.
16. Messiha, F.S., Bakutis, E., Frankos, V. Simultaneous separation of acid metabolites of catecholamines: application to urine and tissue. Clin. Chim. Acta., 45:159–164, 1973.
17. Messiha, F.S. A study of biogenic amine metabolites in the cerebrospinal fluid and in urine of monkeys with chlorpromazine-induced dyskinesia. J. Neurol Sci., 21:39–46, 1974.
18. Arterbery, J.D., Conley, M.P. Urinary excretion of serotonin (5-hydroxytryptamine) and related indoles in normal subjects. Clin. Chim. Acta., 17:431–440, 1967.

19.   Ahlberg, C.D. Interference in the fluorometric quantitation of urinary 5-hydroxyindoleacetic acid by aspirin. *Biochem. Pharmacology, 20*:497–500, 1971.

20.   Haeggendal, J. Fluorometric determination of 3-0 methylated derivatives of adrenaline and noradrenaline in tissues and body fluids. *Acta Physiol. Scand., 56*:258–266, 1962.

21.   Haeggendal, J. An improved method for fluorometric determination of small amounts of adrenaline and noradrenaline in plasma and tissues. *Acta Physiol. Scand., 59*:242–254, 1963.

22.   Werdinius, B. Estimation of 3,4-dihydroxyphenylacetic acid from the blood. *Acta Pharmacol. Toxicol.* (Kbh.), *25*:9–17, 1967.

23.   Pisano, J., Croute, J., Abraham, D. Determination of 3-methoxy-4-hydroxy-mandelic acid in urine. *Clin. Chim. Acta., 7*:285–291, 1962.

24.   Sato, T. The quantitative determination of 3-methoxy-4-hydroxyphenylacetic acid in urine. *J. Lab. Clin. Med., 66*:517–525, 1965.

25.   Messiha, F.S., Agallianos, D., Clower, C. Dopamine excretion in affective states and following lithium carbonate therapy. *Nature, 225*:868–869, 1970.

26.   Messiha, F.S., Raval, R.P. Fluorometric determinations of 3-methoxytryamine and 3-methoxy-4-hydroxyphenyl-ethanol. *J. Pharm. Pharmacol., 25*:184–185, 1973.

27.   Laverty, R., Tylor, K.M. The fluorometric assay of catecholamines and related compounds. Improvements and extensions to the hydroxyindole technique. *Anal. Biochem., 22*:269–279, 1968.

28.   Messiha, F.S., Von Korff, R.W. An improved method for the determination of dopamine in urine. *Fed. Proc., 28*:543 (Abst.), 1969.

29.   Carlsson, A., Waldeck, B. A fluorometric method for the determination of dopamine (3-hydroxytyramine). *Acta Physiol. Scand., 44*:293–298, 1958.

30.   Hirs, C.H.W., Moore, S., Stein, W.H. A chromatographic investigation of pancreatic ribonuclease. *J. Biol. Chem., 200*:493–506, 1953.

31.   Gey, K.F., Messiha, F.S. Einfluss der Dopa-Transaminierung anf die Dopa-Decarboxylierung *in vitro. Experientia, 20*:498–499, 1964.

32.   Udenfriend, S. Fluorescence assay in biology and medicine, New York: Academic Press, pp. 130, 1962.

33.   Pullar, I.A., Weddell, I.A., Ahmed, R., Gillingham, J. Phenolic acid concentrations in the lumbar cerebrospinal fluid of Parkinsonian patients treated with L-dopa. *J. Neurol. Neurosurg. Psychiatry, 33*:851–857, 1970.

34.   Delay, J., Deniker, P., Harl, J.M. Utilisation en therapeutique psychiatrique d'une phenothiazine d'action Centrale elective. *Ann. Med. Psychol., 110*:112–131, 1952.

35.   Hamon, J., Paraire, J., Velluz, J. Remarques sur l'action du 4560 R.P. sur l'agitation manique. *Ann. Med. Psychol., 110*:331–335, 1952.

36.   Faurbye, A. The structural and biochemical basis of movement disorders in treatment with neuroleptic drugs and in extrapyramidal diseases. *Compr. Psychiatry, 11* (3): 205–225, 1970.

37.   Shore, P., Silver, S., Brodie, B.B. Interaction of reserpine, serotonin, and lysergic acid diethylamide in brain. *Science, 122*:284–285, 1955.

38.   Gey, K.F., Pletscher, A. Einfluss von chlorpromazine and chlorprothixen auf den monoamine Stoffwechsel des Rattenhirns. *Helv. Physiol. Pharmacol. Acta, 19*:22–24, 1961.

39.   Carlsson, A. Functional significance of drug-induced changes in brain monoamine levels. *Prog. Drug Res., 8*:14–24, 1964.

40.   Carlsson, A., Lindqvist, M. Effect of chlorpromazine or haloperidol on formation of 3-methoxytyramine and normetanephrine in mouse brain. *Acta Pharmacol., 20*:140–144, 1963.

41.   Gey, K.F., Pletscher, A. Influence of chlorpromazine and chlorprothixene on the cerebral

metabolism of 5-hydroxytryptamine, norepinephrine and dopamine. *J. Pharmacol. Exp. Ther.*, *133*:18–24, 1961.

42. Anden, N.E., Roos, B.E., Werdinius, B. Effects of chlorpromazine, haloperidol and reserpine on the levels of phenolic acids in rabbit corpus striatum. *Life Sci.*, *3*:149–158, 1964.

43. Pletscher, A. Pharmacological changes of the dopamine metabolism in the basal ganglia. In *Psychotropic Drugs and Dysfunctions of the Basal Ganglia*. Crane, G.E., and Gardner, R. Jr. (eds.). U.S. Publ. Health Serv. Public No. 1938, Washington, D.C., pp. 122–132, 1969.

44. Laverty, R., Sharman, D.F. Modification by drugs of the metabolism of 3,4-dihydroxyphenylethylamine, noradrenaline and 5-hydroxytryptamine in the brain. *Br. J. Pharmacol.*, *24*:759–772, 1965.

45. Neff, N., Costa, E. The effect of tricyclic antidepressants and chlorpromazine on brain catecholamine synthesis. In *Antidepressant Drugs*. Garattini, S., and Dukes, M. (eds.). Amsterdam: Excerpta Medica, pp. 28–34, 1967.

46. Nybaeck, H., Sedvall, G., Kopin, I.J. Accelerated synthesis of dopamine-C^{14} from tyrosine-C^{14} in rat brain after chlorpromazine. *Life Sci.*, *6*:2307–2312, 1967.

47. Gey, K.F., Pletscher, A. Acceleration of turnover of ^{14}C-catecholamines in rat brain by chlorpromazine. *Experientia*, *24*:335–336, 1968.

48. Bartholini, G., Pletscher, A. Enhancement of tyrosine hydroxylation within the brain by chlorpromazine. *Experientia*, *25*:919–920, 1969.

49. Gey, K.F., Burkard, W.P. Chlorpromazine-induced accumulation of pyridoxal-5-phosphate and activation of the decarboxylase of aromatic amino acids in rat brain. *Ann. N.Y. Acad. Sci.*, *166*:213, 1969.

50. Ehringer, H., Hornykiewicz, O. Verteilung von Noradrenalin und Dopamine (3-Hydroxytyramine) im Gehirn des Menschen und ihr Verhalten bei Erkrankungen des extrapyramidalen Systems. *Klin. Wochenschr.*, *38*:1236–1239, 1960.

51. Bernheimer, H., Birkmayer, W., Hornykiewicz O. Verteilung des 5-Hydroxytryptamines (Serotonin) im Gehirn des Menschen und sein Verhalten bei Patienten mit Parkinson-syndrome. *Klin. Wochenschr*, *39*:1056–1059, 1961.

52. Hornykiewicz, O. Die topische Lokalisation und das Verhalten von Noradrenaline und Dopamine in der substantia nigra des normalen und Parkinsokranksen Menschen. *Klin. Wochenschr.*, *73*:309–312, 1963.

53. Hornykiewicz, O. Dopamine and brain function. *Pharmacol. Rev.*, *18*:925–964, 1966.

54. Bartholini, G., Pletscher, A., Tissot, R. On the origin of homovanillic acid in the cerebrospinal fluid. *Experientia*, *22*:609–610, 1966.

55. Goldberg, H., Yates, C.M. Effects of chlorpromazine on the metabolism of catecholamines in dog brain. *Br. J. Pharmacol.*, *36*:535–548, 1969.

56. Bulat, M., Zivkovic, B. Origin of 5-hydroxyindoleacetic acid in the spinal fluid. *Science*, *173*:738–740, 1971.

57. Barbeau, A., Murphy, G.F., Sourkes, T.L. Excretion of dopamine in diseases of basal ganglia. *Science*, *133*:1706–1707, 1961.

58. Birkmeyer, W. Der alpha-methyl-p-tyrosin-Effect bei extra-pyramidalen Erkrankungen. *Clin. Wochenschr.*, *81*:10-12, 1969.

59. O'Reilly, S., Locin, M., Cooksey, B. Dopamine and basal ganglia disorders. *Neurology*, *15*:980–984, 1965.

60. Messiha, F.S., Knop, W., Vaneko, S., O'Brien, Corson, S.A. Haloperidol therapy in Tourette's syndrome: neurophysiological, biochemical, and behavioral correlates. *Life Sci.*, *10*:449–457, 1971.

61. Messiha, F.S., Knopp, W. A study of endogenous dopamine metabolism in Gilles de la Tourette's disease. *Dis. Nerv. Syst.*, *37*:470–473, 1976.

62.   Siomopoulos, V. Tardive dyskinesia: A clinical interpretation. *Dis. Nerv. Syst.*, *35*:138–143, 1974.
63.   Messiha, F.S., Larson, J.W. Biochemical changes associated with drug-produced alterations in motor function and the psyche. *Proc. West. Pharmacol. Soc.*, *20*:297–301, 1977.
64.   Messiha, F.S., Erickson, H.M., Goggin, J.E. Lithium carbonate in Gilles de la Tourette's disease. *Res. Commun. Chem. Pathol. Pharmacol.*, *15*:609–612, 1976.

3

"Tardive Dyskinesia" Resulting from Chronic Narcotic Treatment

KRISTIN R. CARLSON

In formulating the title of this chapter I felt it was only honest to put the term tardive dyskinesia in quotation marks. The syndrome I will describe bears a clear resemblance to the human condition in several critical respects, but in at least one aspect it does differ, and the underlying mechanism remains more speculative than is the case in neuroleptic-induced tardive dyskinesia. Nonetheless, I will present first the positive data linking chronic narcotic usage to symptoms which mimic those of tardive dyskinesia, and later consider the modifying evidence which may restrict the generality of this phenomenon.

The pathogenesis of tardive dyskinesia is usually ascribed to chronic blockade of striatal dopamine receptors by neuroleptics. It is thought that during blockade new receptors are synthesized (1), so that after the blockade is lifted by discontinuation of drug treatment, the striatal system is hypersensitive to stimulation by endogenous dopamine. As a consequence, the symptoms of tardive dyskinesia often appear when neuroleptic dosage is decreased or the drug is terminated (2, 3). Striatal hypersensitivity is implicated further by the fact that dopamine agonists can exacerbate present symptoms or precipitate them in symptom-free patients (4-6).

Oral dyskinesias, such as tongue protrusions and choreiform limb movements, are characteristic of tardive dyskinesia (7, 8). Emotional stress tends to exacerbate symptoms (9–11), whereas they can often be ameliorated by reinstituting dopaminergic blockade, i.e., resuming neuroleptic administration (5, 6, 12). Finally, the condition is often permanent (13, 14).

"TARDIVE DYSKINESIA" IN MONKEYS

We have found that the characteristics of tardive dyskinesia enumerated above can be produced by chronic narcotic treatment in Rhesus monkeys (15–17). Eight monkeys had access to low doses of methadone (0.5-2.6 mg/kg) mixed with Tang orange drink for 1 hour daily, for a total period of 10 to 22 months, and a control series of 11 monkeys had no experience with narcotics. The former methadone monkeys had been withdrawn from the narcotic 2–17 months prior to the beginning of this study. All subjects were challenged repeatedly with doses of methamphetamine, which in the normal monkey are well below threshold for eliciting oral dyskinesias (18). The control monkeys responded throughout with the expected stereotyped behaviors, such as body jerks, but in 7 of 8 former methadone monkeys methamphetamine immediately elicited pronounced and intense oral dyskinesias, the most common of which was tongue protrusions (see Fig. 1). In addition, 3 of these animals also exhibited choreiform limb movements. The oral dyskinesias were highly rhythmic and predictable, and could be elicited on every occasion by methamphetamine injection.

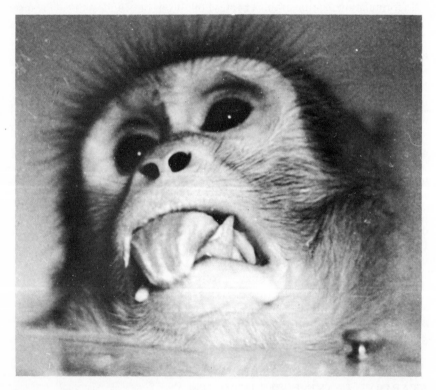

Figure 1.   Typical tongue protrusion elicited by 2.0 mg/kg methamphetamine in a former methadone monkey. This behavior occurred at a rate of approximately 30 protrusions/min. and persisted for 36 hours postinjection.

A much shorter course of parenteral methadone administration is also sufficient to sensitize monkeys. Two control subjects which had not exhibited oral dyskinesias in response to methamphetamine received increasing doses (1.0 to 10.0 mg/kg/day) of methadone s.c. for 45 days, and 10 days subsequently were challenged with 2.0 mg/kg methamphetamine. Both animals immediately exhibited tongue protrusions. Thus, following oral or parenteral methadone administration, low doses of a dopaminergic agonist elicit the oral dyskinesias which are so characteristic of tardive dyskinesia.

The former methadone monkeys were also susceptible to the effects of stress. When injected with a dose of methamphetamine, which by itself was subthreshold for the elicitation of dyskinesias, the addition of a stressful stimulus (a loud buzzer) immediately elicited tongue protrusions. This stressor had no effect on the other stereotyped behaviors exhibited by control monkeys, implying that the results were due not to a general augmentation of behavior, but to a specific stress-induced exaggeration of one type, oral dyskinesia.

In line with the amelioration of tardive dyskinesia symptoms by the resumption of neuroleptic therapy, we found that acute administration of dopaminergic blockers could prevent the appearance of dyskinesias when administered before methamphetamine, and could promptly abolish ongoing dyskinesias when administered after methamphetamine. Effective drugs were chlorpromazine, spiroperidol, and clozapine, whereas sedative doses of phenobarbital and diazepam had no effect.

Finally, there is some evidence that methadone treatment may induce a very long-lasting, if not permanent, alteration in brain function, producing hypersensitivity to dopaminergic agonists. One of the methadone monkeys described above had been drug free for 17 months, yet he responded with tongue protrusions to only 2.0 mg/kg methamphetamine. Another monkey which had terminated oral methadone treatment 26 months previously and had not received methamphetamine was challenged with a single s.c. dose of 0.5 mg/kg apomorphine, presumably a directly acting dopaminergic agonist (19, 20). This subject's elicited behaviors were exclusively oral, consisting primarily of very intense and prolonged bruxism, whereas a control monkey responded with milder limb movements of shorter duration. Further, the stress of being returned to the test cage 24 and 48 hours after apomophine challenge was sufficient to reinstate the methadone monkey's oral dyskinesia, but had no effect on the control monkey (21).

AN ANALOGOUS SYNDROME IN THE GUINEA PIG

Dopaminergic hypersensitivity can also be produced in rodents by neuroleptic treatment. Rats and guinea pigs are more sensitive to dopaminergic agonists—i.e., they emit more intense and prolonged stereotyped chewing and gnawing in response to amphetamines or apomorphine, for several weeks after such treatment (22, 23). Since this phenomenon in the guinea pig has been proposed as an animal model of tardive dyskinesia (23), we were interested in determining whether we could replicate with narcotics in this species the pattern resembling tardive dyskinesia which we had seen in monkeys.

Accordingly, guinea pigs were treated parenterally with methadone or chlorpromazine for 5 weeks. For 3 weeks thereafter, which was as long as they were tested, both groups responded with significantly more intense stereotyped behaviors in response to methamphetamine than did a saline control group. Stereotypies could be blocked by acute administration of methadone or chlorpromazine, and electric shock stress elicited stereotyped mouth movements in the methadone animals following treatment (24). In a subsequent experiment we found that a 3-week treatment period with increasing doses (20 to 40 mg/kg/day) of either methadone or morphine was sufficient to induce hypersensitivity to apomorphine. An interesting pattern of hypersensitivity emerged in this experiment, however, in that the morphine group was hypersensitive at 1 week but not at 5 weeks following chronic drug treatment, whereas the hypersensitivity of the methadone group actually increased from 1 to 5 weeks (25). In a recent unpublished work, we treated for 3 weeks with various dosage schedules of methadone or morphine, and challenged the subjects with apomorphine every week thereafter. In general, we not only replicated the study above (25), but found that methadone is a more efficient inducer of hypersensitivity than is morphine, and that the duration of hypersensitivity following treatment is a direct function of methadone dose. We do not yet know if a permanent condition of hypersensitivity can be induced in the guinea pig, but we have observed significant hypersensitivity for 8 weeks after methadone treatment.

DISCUSSION

This syndrome differs from the usual clinical picture of tardive dyskinesia in one important respect—the necessity of eliciting symptoms with a dopaminergic agonist. Spontaneous dyskinesias were never observed in either species following narcotic treatment. However, most animal models of neuroleptic-induced tardive dyskinesia have also been deficient in this regard, since agonist challenge has been necessary in order to demonstrate hypersensitivity in rats (22), guinea pigs (23), and macaque monkeys (26–28). Is it possible that there exists an important species difference in susceptibility to dyskinesias, since prolonged neuroleptic administration to Cebus monkeys (and, of course, humans) results in the emergence of oral dyskinesias upon drug withdrawal (28; and Gunne, this volume). Thus, a question of clinical relevance is whether methadone-maintenance patients are at risk to the development of oral dyskinesias when they terminate treatment. I am aware of only one report of extrapyramidal symptoms following narcotic use, a case involving abrupt Percodan withdrawal (29), but this patient's symptoms were atypical in that they did not respond to chlorpromazine, but were ameliorated by an anticholinergic agent, just the opposite of what would have been expected in the usual case of tardive dyskinesia. If methadone-maintenance patients are followed adequately after their participation in treatment programs, there may be an answer to this question within the next few years.

The mechanism underlying this phenomenon remains somewhat speculative, although the weight of evidence points to dopaminergic blockade in the striatum by narcotics, resulting in hypersensitivity after the blockade is lifted. Behaviorally, both neuroleptics and narcotics induce catalepsy (30–32), and both classes of drugs antagonize apomorphine-induced stereotypies (33). Biochemical studies have consistently revealed changes in the striatum indicative of dopaminergic blockade during narcotic administration, e.g., increased levels of homovanillic acid (30–32). On the other hand, narcotics do not antagonize the amphetamine-induced decrease in firing rates of substantia nigra neurons; with very rare exceptions, only neuroleptics with antipsychotic properties have this effect (34). It is known that chronic haloperidol treatment increases the number of receptor sites in the striatum without changing their affinity (1); an analogous binding study following chronic narcotic treatment would help determine the mechanism underlying narcotic-induced hypersensitivity.

ACKNOWLEDGMENTS

This research was supported by USPHS grants MH20121 and DA00883, and by grants from the Scottish Rite Schizophrenia Research Program, N.M.J., U.S.A. The collaboration of Dr. Robert D. Eibergen and the skilled technical assistance of John Almasi and Douglas Smith are gratefully acknowledged.

REFERENCES

1. Burt, D.R., Creese, I. Snyder, S.H. Antischizophrenic drugs: chronic treatment elevates dopamine receptor binding in brain. *Science, 196*:326–328, 1977.
2. Crane, G.E., Paulson, G. Involuntary movements in a sample of chronic mental patients and their relation to the treatment with neuroleptics. *Int. J. Neuropsychiat., 3*:286–291, 1967.
3. Curran, J.P., Tardive dyskinesia: side effect or not? *Am. J. Psychiatry, 130*:406–410, 1973.
4. Fann, W.E., Davis, J.M., Wilson, I.C. Methylphenidate in tardive dyskinesia. *Am. J. Psychiatry., 130*:922–924, 1973.

5. Gerlach, J., Reisby, N., Randrup, A. Dopaminergic hypersensitivity and cholinergic hypofunction in the pathophysiology of tardive dyskinesia. Psychopharmacologia, 34:21–35, 1974.

6. Kline, N.S. On the rarity of "irreversible" oral dyskinesias following phenothiazines. Am. J. Psychiatry, 124:48–54, Suppl., 1968.

7. Gerlach, J. Relationship between tardive dyskinesia, L-Dopa-induced hyperkinesia and parkinsonism. Psychopharmacology, 51:259–263, 1977.

8. Urhbrand, L., Faurbye, A. Reversible and irreversible dyskinesia after treatment with perphenazine, chlorpromazine, reserpine, and electroconvulsive therapy. Psychopharmacologia, 1:408–418, 1960.

9. Crane, G.E. Tardive dyskinesia in patients treated with major neuroleptics: A review of the literature. Am. J. Psychiatry, 124:40–48, Suppl., 1968.

10. Druckman, R., Seelinger, D., Thulin, B. Chronic involuntary movements induced by phenothiazines. J. Nerv. Ment. Dis., 135:69–76, 1962.

11. Jacobson, G., Baldessarini, R.J., Manschreck, T. Tardive and withdrawal dyskinesia associated with haloperidol. Am. J. Psychiatry, 131:910-913, 1974.

12. Simpson, G.M., Varga, E. Clozapine—a new antipsychotic agent. Curr. Ther. Res., 16:679–686, 1974.

13. Crane, G.E. Persistent dyskinesia. Br. J. Psychiatry, 122:395–405, 1973.

14. American College of Neuropsychopharmacology: Neurologic syndromes associated with antipsychotic drug use. N. Engl. J. Med., 289:20–23, 1973.

15. Eibergen, R.D., Carlson, K.R., Dyskinesias elicited by methamphetamine: susceptibility of former methadone-consuming monkeys. Science, 190:588–590, 1975.

16. Eibergen, R.D., Carlson, K.R. Dyskinesias in monkeys: interaction of methamphetamine with prior methadone treatment. Pharmacol. Biochem. Behav., 5:175–187, 1976.

17. Carlson, K.R. Eibergen, R.D. Susceptibility to amphetamine-elicited dyskinesias following chronic methadone treatment in monkeys. Ann. N.Y. Acad. Sci., 281:336–349, 1976.

18. Ellinwood, E.H. Effect of chronic methamphetamine intoxication in rhesus monkeys. Biol. Psychiatry, 3:25–32, 1971.

19. Ernst, A.M. Mode of action of apomorphine and dexamphetamine on gnawing compulsion in rats. Psychopharmacologia, 10:316–323, 1967.

20. Understedt, U., Butcher, L.L., Butcher, S.G. Direct chemical stimulation of dopaminergic mechanisms in the neostriatum of the rat. Brain Res., 14:461-471, 1969.

21. Carlson, K.R. Supersensitivity to apomorphine and stress two years after chronic methadone treatment. Neuropharmacology, 16:795–798, 1977.

22. Tarsy, D., Baldessarini, R.J. Behavioral supersensitivity to apomorphine following chronic treatment with drugs which interfere with the synaptic function of catecholamines. Neuropharmacology, 13:927–940, 1974.

23. Klawans, H.L., Rubovits, R. An experimental model of tardive dyskinesia, J. Neural Transm., 33:235–246, 1972.

24. Eibergen, R.D., Carlson, K.R. Behavioral evidence for dopaminergic supersensitivity following chronic treatment with methadone or chlorpromazine in the guinea pig. Psychopharmacology, 48:139–146, 1976.

25. Carlson, K.R., Almasi, J. Behavioral supersensitivity to apomorphine following chronic narcotic treatment in the guinea pig. Psychopharmacology, (In press.)

26. Paulson, G. Effects of chronic administration of neuroleptics: dyskinesias in monkeys. Pharm. Ther. [B]2:167–171, 1976.

27. Messiha, F.S. The relationship of dopamine excretion to chlorpromazine-induced dyskinesia in monkeys. Arch. Int. Pharmacodyn., Ther. 209:5–9, 1974.

28. Gunne, L-M, Barany, S. Haloperidol-induced tardive dyskinesia in monkeys. Psychopharmacology, 50:237–240, 1976.

29. Gardos, G. Dyskinesia after discontinuation of compound analgesic containing oxycodone. *Lancet, 8014*:759–760, 1977.
30. Sasame, H.A., Perez-Cruet, J., DiChiara, G. Evidence that methadone blocks dopamine receptors in the brain. *J. Neurochem., 19*:1953–1957, 1972.
31. Ahtee, L. Catalepsy and stereotyped behavior in rats treated chronically with methadone: relation to brain homovanillic acid content. *J. Pharm. Pharmacol., 25*:649–651, 1973.
32. Kuschinsky, K., Hornykiewicz, O. Morphine catalepsy in the rat: relation to striatal dopamine metabolism. *Eur. J. Pharmacol., 19*:119–122, 1972.
33. Puri, S.K., Reddy, C., Lal, H. Blockade of central dopaminergic receptors by morphine: effect of haloperidol, apomorphine or benztropine. *Res. Commun. Chem. Pathn. Pharmacol., 5*:389–401, 1973.
34. Bunney, B.S. Central dopaminergic systems: two *in vivo* electrophysiological models for predicting therapeutic efficacy and neurological side effects of putative antipsychotic drugs. In *Animal Models in Psychiatry and Neurology*, I., Hanin, and E., Usdin, New York: Pergamon Press, pp. 91–104, 1977.

4

On the Supersensitivity of DA-Receptors After Single and Repeated Administration of Neuroleptics

A.V. CHRISTENSEN
and I. MOLLER NIELSEN

It has always been a problem in experimental psychosis research that it is impossible to induce mental disorders in animals. When Delay *et al.* (1) in 1952 used chlorpromazine in the treatment of psychotic patients and found that the compound had a specific antipsychotic effect, no pharmacological tests were therefore available for testing such compounds.

The interest was later concentrated on the brain catecholamines. Based on the observation that abuse of amphetamine in man could induce schizophrenialike psychosis, and that the resemblance of the amphetamine-psychosis to schizophrenia was so close that misdiagnoses were made (2), the investigations of amphetamine-induced stereotyped behavior were initiated. Both amphetamine and methylphenidate release dopamine from presynaptic pools and induce in that way stereotypies in rates and mice (3–12). Antagonism against these stereotypies was then used as test for the postsynaptic dopamine–receptor blocking effect and correlated to the potency of the compounds against psychosis (8).

The above-mentioned pharmacological effect of neuroleptics was, however, an immediate effect, and in recognition of the fact that neuroleptic therapy in most cases entails long-term administration, and that the antipsychotic effect usually manifests itself only after prolonged treatment, many investigators have in recent years been concerned with the study of the pharmacological effects of neuroleptics after prolonged treatment. Several groups have found tolerance development to the amphetamine and methylphenidate antagonism of neuroleptics (13–17). In other experiments it was found that prolonged neuroleptic treatment led to increased sensitivity to dopamine agonists (18–24). In the experiments reported here it was intended to follow the effect of neuroleptics in prolonged studies after a single and repeated dosage.

As a model for dopamine, receptor-blockade antagonism against methylphenidate-induced compulsive gnawing in mice was used (7,10). Mice treated with a dose of methylphenidate (60 mg/kg) subcutaneously will, when placed on corrugated paper, bite holes in the paper. As mentioned above, this effect is antagonized by neuroleptics. Receptor supersensitivity was determined by assessment of apomorphine-induced gnawing. Apomorphine stimulates dopamine receptors directly (25) and induces stereotypies characterized by running, licking, and sniffing. However, when given apomorphine (10 mg/kg s.c.), normal mice do not show compulsive gnawing. Therefore, we considered induction of gnawing with apomorphine as a modified or increased sensitivity of dopamine receptors. In all tests performed, new groups of mice were used every day.

The time course of antagonism against methylphenidate-induced compulsive gnawing and of the occurrence of apomorphine-induced compulsive gnawing following a single dose of 12 different neuroleptics are shown in Figure 1. When given as a single dose, neuroleptics caused receptor blockade for varying periods of time, as judged by antagonism against methylphenidate-induced compulsive gnawing. During this time, apomorphine did not cause compulsive gnawing. As the degree of receptor blockade declined, an increasing degree of compulsive gnawing induced by apomorphine occurred. Since in our experimental set-up gnawing was not seen in nonpretreated mice, the occurrence of gnawing with apomorphine in mice pretreated with neuroleptics was taken as a sign of an altered response of dopamine receptors (supersensitivity) to the dopamine agonist apomorphine. Increased sensitivity of the receptor to dopamine agonists was also indicated by the finding that the dopamine turnover rate (decreased accumulation of ^{3}H-DA after ^{3}H-tyramine, and decreased HVA levels) was reduced at this stage (26–28). The results with various neuroleptics indicate it to be a universal phenomenon that receptor blockade is followed by a period of receptor supersensitivity, and that the degree and duration of the supersensitivity is related to the degree and duration of the preceding blockade. It is interesting to note that a short-lasting but clear-cut gnawing compulsion with apomorphine was observed after clozapine, although no preceding receptor blockade could be detected. However, this effect was seen on the day of drug administration; thus, it might be due to the anticholinergic effect of clozapine (29–30), since it has been shown that a combination of apomorphine and anticholinergics cause a marked gnawing compulsion in mice (31–33). In another experimental

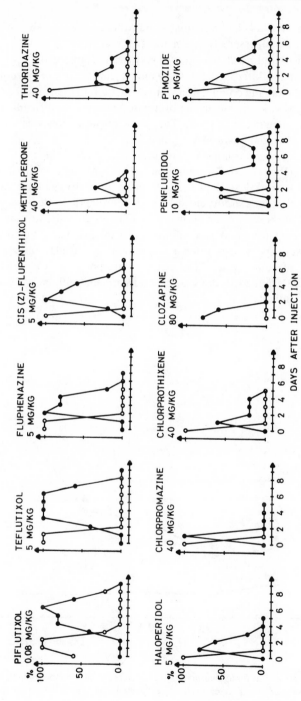

Figure 1. Influence of single doses of neuroleptics on methylphenidate- and apomorphine-induced stereotypies in mice. Ordinates indicate in case of methylphenidate percentage inhibition, and in case of apomorphine percentage occurrence of gnawing. All treatments performed i.p. on day zero. ○——○ Methylphenidate antagonism. ●——● Apomorphine gnawing.

model, Smith and Davis (24) and Gianutsos and Moore (34) have shown that clozapine also induces supersensitivity of the DA receptors.

Similarly, in the withdrawal phase (4 days) after a single dose of the neuroleptic compound teflutixol, the dose-response curves for apomorphine-induced stereotyped gnawing compulsion were estimated. In the control group almost no gnawing was seen, but in the pretreated group a significant (p < 0.05) induction of gnawing was seen. The same phenomenon was shown earlier with methylphenidate as a DA agonist (35).

The time course of apomorphine potentiation was studied after different doses of teflutixol (Fig. 3a) and flupenthixol (Fig. 3b). The induction of gnawing-compulsion was dose-dependent both in intensity and duration. Since tolerance to the antistereotypic effect of neuroleptics after repeated administration had previously been shown (13–17) and attributed to the development of supersensitivity to DA agonists (18–24), it was investigated whether the supersensitivity seen after a single dose might also reduce the antagonistic effect of neuroleptics. The antagonistic potency of a series of neuroleptics was determined 4 days after pretreatment with teflutixol, 5 mg/kg, or saline (Table 1).

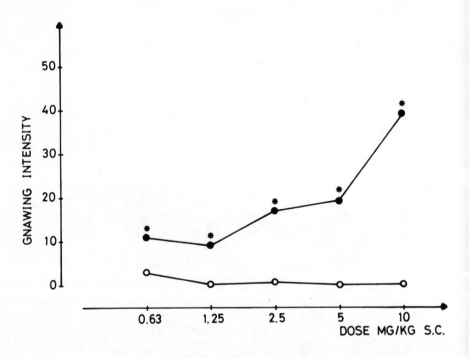

Figure 2.   Dose-response curves for apomorphine-induced stereotyped gnawing compulsion. O——O Treated with saline 4 days previously. ●——● Treated with teflutixol 4 days previously. * p < 0.05.

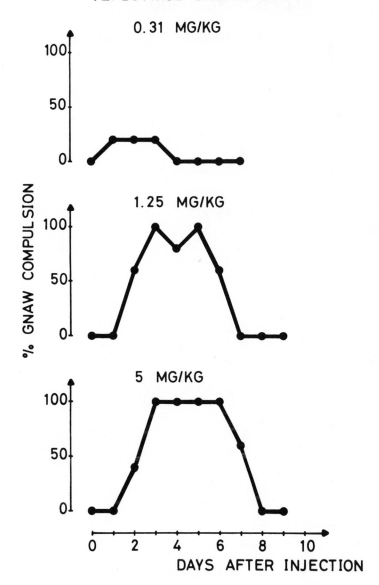

Figure 3.   Time course of teflutixol- (Fig. 3a) or flupenthixol- (Fig. 3b) induced potentiation of apomorphine. Teflutixol or flupenthixol was given i.p. on day zero: At various times after these treatments apomorphine, 10 mg/kg s.c., was given and % animals gnawing estimated.

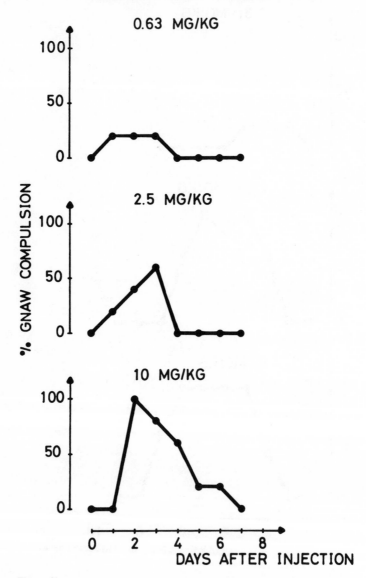

APOMORPHINE POTENTIATION,
FLUPENTHIXOL SINGLE DOSE

Figure 3b.

Table 1
The Methylphenidate Antagonistic Effect of Some
Compounds in Mice Treated 4 Days Previously with
Teflutixol, 5 mg/kg i.p., or Saline i.p.

Compound	Teflutixol-Pretreated Mice	Saline-Pretreated Mice
Teflutixol	1.2 (0.6–2.5)	0.13 (0.08–0.22)
Fluphenazine	0.34 (0.16–0.74)	0.04 (0.02–0.1)
Pimozide	1.4	0.05 (0.03–0.09)
Haloperidol	0.8 (0.5–1.4)	0.06 (0.04–0.09)
Cis (Z)-flupenthixol	0.6 (0.4–0.8)	0.07 (0.05–0.1)
Chlorprothixene	18 (12-29)	0.7 (0.4–1.8)
Chlorpromazine	61 (25–148)	4.0 (2.5–6.4)
Thioridazine	37 (22–62)	5.4 (7.6–38)
Clozapine	> 40	> 40
Azeperone	> 20	> 20
Acepromazine	> 10	> 10

In brackets 95% confidence limits
n = 5–20

The dose of neuroleptics required to antagonize methylphenidate by 50% was 5–15 times increased, as compared to saline-pretreated mice. Clozapine and the nonneuroleptic compounds azeperone and acepromazine had no effect at all, even in saline-pretreated animals.

As is the case in normosensitive animals (36), a balance between cholinergic and dopaminergic systems appears to exist in the supersensitive phase. Physostigmine causes cholinergic stimulation and decreases the gnawing intensity induced by methylphenidate in the supersensitivity phase. On the other hand, scopolamine, which possesses central anticholinergic properties, increases the effect of methylphenidate.

Similarly, one might expect that when given in the phase of receptor blockage, physostigmine could facilitate the receptor-blocking effect of neuroleptics (in this case teflutixol), and therefore intensify the later induction of supersensitivity. In contrast, scopolamine should then weaken the effect of teflutixol and then induce a lesser degree of supersensitivity. As it appears from Figure 5, no effect could be shown.

When a neuroleptic is given by repeated dosage, one would expect that the receptor blockade induced by each medication would be capable of overcoming the effect of any induced supersensitivity. This, however, is not the case.

When animals were given repeated daily doses of 1.25 mg/kg of teflutixol orally and tested with methylphenidate 2 hours after the daily dosage, full protection against methylphenidate compulsive gnawing was seen on days 0 and 1; after that inhibition declined (Fig. 6a). Animals tested with apomorphine 2 hours after the daily dose of teflutixol showed no compulsive gnawing

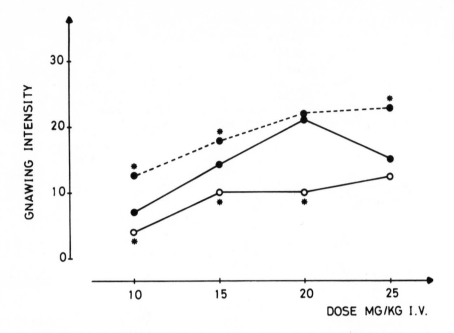

Figure 4.   Dose-response curves for methylphenidate-induced stereotyped gnawing compulsion. Teflutixol, 5 mg/kg i.p., was administered to all three groups 5 days before methylphenidate. Each point represents the mean of 10 × 2 mice. ●——● Teflutixol + water, ○——○ Teflutixol + physostigmine, 0.5 mg/kg i.p. ½ hour before methylphenidate, ●---● Teflutixol + scopolamine, 1 mg/kg i.p. ½ hour before methylphenidate. Ordinate: Gnawing intensity as percent of maximum. Abcisse: Dose of methylphenidate.

during the first 6 days, after which an increasing intensity of gnawing appeared (Fig. 6b). This trend was even more pronounced when animals were tested 24 hours after the daily dose of teflutixol (37).

When tested 24 hours after daily dosage, it could be shown that the induction of supersensitivity was dose-dependent (Fig. 7).

A daily dose of 0.8 mg/kg p.o. produced only marginal supersensitivity, while 1.25 mg/kg induced supersensitivity in all mice after 10 days of treatment, and 0.31 mg/kg produced intermediate supersensitivity.

Even when increasing dosages of teflutixol were administered, supersensitivity occurred (Fig. 8). The first dose was 1.25 and the last dose 10.25 mg/kg orally. When tested 24 hours after the preceding dose, the mice showed a very pronounced supersensitivity to apomorphine 3 days after the first injection. This supersensitivity persisted for the rest of the test period. In this experiment another observation was made. Normally, 10 mg/kg of teflutixol would induce sedation, but having been treated with increasing doses, mice did not show sedation with 10.25 mg/kg.

Finally, it was investigated whether a dose of teflutixol (0.08 mg/kg p.o.),

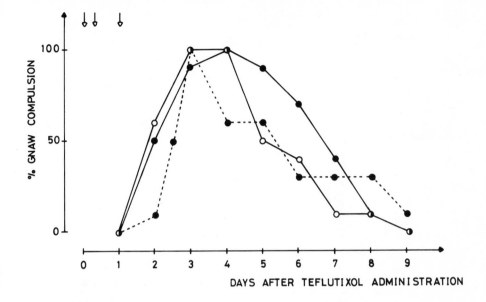

Figure 5.   Time course of teflutixol-induced potentiation of apomorphine after additional treatment with cholinergic compounds. Teflutixol was given i.p. on day zero in a dose of 5 mg/kg i.p. ●——● Teflutixol + saline, O——O Teflutixol + atropine, 2.5 mg/kg i.p. o, 6, and 24 hours after teflutixol administration, ● - - - ● Teflutixol + physostigmine, 0.63 mg/kg i.p. o, 6, and 24 hours after teflutixol administration. At various times after these treatments, apomorphine, 10 mg/kg s.c., was given and % animals gnawing estimated. Each point represents mean of 10 pairs of mice.

in itself too small to induce appreciable supersensitivity, would be able to maintain supersensitivity once induced by a higher dose — 1.25 mg/kg (Fig. 9). Under these circumstances, the supersensitivity was sustained more than 30 days. The level of apomorphine gnawing was significantly higher than that obtained with 0.08 mg/kg alone.

These results indicate that when given as single or repeated administrations, neuroleptics caused receptor blockade for varying periods of time as judged by antagonism against methylphenidate-induced compulsive gnawing. During this time, apomorphine did not cause compulsive gnawing. As the degree of receptor blockade declined, an increasing degree of compulsive gnawing induced by apomorphine occurred. Since in our experimental set-up gnawing was not seen in nonpretreated mice, the occurrence of gnawing with apomorphine was taken as a sign of an altered and intensified response of dopamine receptors (supersensitivity) to the dopamine agonist apomorphine (38, 39). An increased response of the dopamine receptors was also shown by shift to the left of the dose/response curves of methylphenidate-induced compulsive gnawing (19,35).

In the supersensitivity phase after teflutixol pretreatment, scopolamine

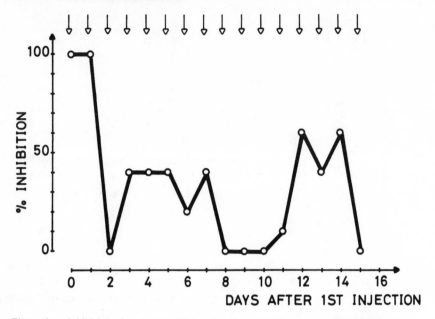

Figure 6a.   Inhibition of methylphenidate-induced gnawing in mice treated with teflutixol, 1.25 mg/kg p.o. (↓). Animals were tested with methylphenidate 2 hours after the preceding dose of teflutixol.

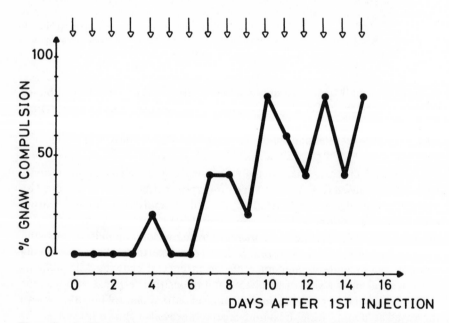

Figure 6b.   Incidence of apomorphine-induced gnawing compulsion in mice treated daily with teflutixol, 1.25 mg/kg p.o. (↓). Animals were tested with apomorphine 2 hours after the preceding dose of teflutixol.

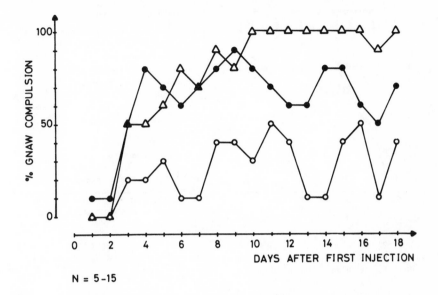

Figure 7.   Apomorphine potentiation after repeated dose of teflutixol. O——O 0.08 mg/kg
p.o., ●——● 0.31 mg/kg p.o.,   ——   1.25 mg/kg p.o. Each point represents mean of 5 to 15
pairs of mice.

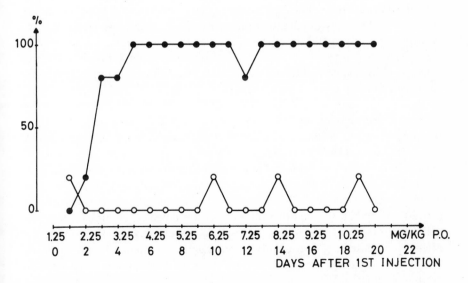

Figure 8.   Apomorphine potentiation ●——● and methylphenidate antagonism O——O in
mice daily dosed with teflutixol in increasing dose. Tested before the daily dose. Each point
represents mean of 5 to 10 pairs of mice.

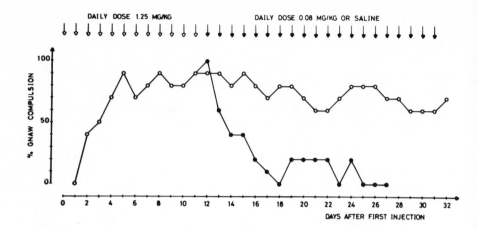

Figure 9.   Apomorphine gnawing after daily teflutixol treatment (1.25 mg/kg p.o.) for 12 days; thereafter 0.08 mg/kg p.o. O——O or saline ●——● for the rest of the period. Each point represents mean of 10 pairs of mice.

increased the gnawing intensity induced by methylphenidate, while physostigmine decreased it. This indicates that a dopaminergic-cholinergic balance is operative in the supersensitivity phase, as it is in normosensitive animals. In contrast, in the phase of receptor blockade, cholinergic/anticholinergic treatment had no influence on the subsequent development of supersensitivity.

In an attempt to overcome the supersensitivity, increasing doses of teflutixol were given. This way of administration only accelerated the supersensitivity. A dose of teflutixol 100 times the normal ED50 value could not counteract supersensitivity. The supersensitivity was reversible, but a dose in itself too small to induce appreciable supersensitivity was able to maintain supersensitivity once induced by a higher dose.

Thus the present and previous investigations (35,37–43) indicate that the effects of neuroleptics on DA-neuron systems is a dynamic process. First, receptor blockade is induced, which is accompanied by an increase in DA turnover (26–28,43). When the receptor blockade has declined, the receptor is not left in the same condition it was before the induction of receptor blockade. It has increased its sensitivity to DA agonists, which in turn results in a decreased DA turnover, or in other words, decreased dopaminergic firing (26–28,43). When the neuroleptic is given by repeated administration, the daily dose of neuroleptics becomes less and less effective in overcoming the effect of increased agonist sensitivity (tolerance development), and this leads to a return in the synthesis rate of DA from the initially increased level to normal level (22,42–47).

These observations are all made in mice. Using another experimental model in mice, Martres *et al.* (48) have shown a similar increase in sensitivity to apomorphine. Haloperidol pretreatment (single dose) induced a biphasic effect, starting with decreased climbing behavior (receptor blockade), followed by increased climbing behavior (supersensitivity). The effect of haloperidol on striatal HVA was also biphasic; in the receptor-blocking phase, HVA was increased, while it was decreased in the supersensitivity phase. This confirms the studies reported by Hyttel (26–28). In rats, indirect evidence of supersensitivity was obtained by the development of tolerance following neuroleptic treatment. Smith and Davis (24) have shown increased apomorphine-induced stereotypies in rats following chronic treatment with neuroleptics. In dogs, Svendsen (unpublished results) has demonstrated supersensitivity to apomorphine-induced stereotyped running, but not to apomorphine-induced vomiting.

If these phenomena are also operative in man, the question arises as to what clinical implications it might have. The first thing that comes into mind is tardive dyskinesia, since this side effect tends to develop especially upon discontinuation of neuroleptic treatment and is thought to be related to DA overactivity. This view is supported by the observations that levodopa and amphetamine increase the involuntary movements of tardive dyskinesia in affected patients (49–50), as well as by the finding that neuroleptic agents known to block DA receptors suppress the movements (51–52), and that anticholinergic compounds increase the frequency of tardive dyskinesia (53). Not in agreement with this hypothesis is the finding by Ettegi *et al.* (54) and Tamminga *et al.* (55) that no supersensitivity in the tuberoinfundibular DA tract (prolactin and growth hormone response to DA agonists) could be demonstrated in patients with tardive dyskinesia. Of course, supersensitivity in the nigro-striatal DA tract might not necessarily be paralleled by supersensitivity in the tuberoinfundibular DA system.

Although supersensitivity of dopamine receptors may be involved in tardive dyskinesia, supersensitivity as we see it in animals following neuroleptic treatment is a functional phenomenon which occurs and disappears within a rather short time after withdrawal. Since this is not the case with tardive dyskinesia, and since tardive dyskinesia does not develop in every patient treated with neuroleptics, we feel that functional supersensitivity, which probably follows in all cases of neuroleptic treatment, is not the cause of tardive dyskinesia, but that a more permanent damage must be involved. Elderly patients are more prone to develop tardive dyskinesia, indicating that these patients, perhaps due to preexisting disturbance in modulating neurone systems (ACh, GABA), are less able to compensate for the consequences of temporarily increased DA-receptor sensitivity. Once the functional balance has been disturbed, they have less ability, due to exhaustion of the modulating neurons, for reestablishing a normal balance; hence the symptoms tend to persist.

Another suggestion would be that the antipsychotic effect of neuroleptics is not necessarily, as previously implied, related to receptor blockade of DA receptors per se, but to the resulting supersensitivity, i.e., facilitation of DA transmission. Receptor blockade is the immediate effect, but it is declining during repeated administration, and thus does not correlate with the onset of antipsychotic effect. Both supersensitivity and antipsychotic effect are phenomena with delayed onset, and neither of them are subject to tolerance development. That schizophrenics could be in need of DA facilitation is indicated by the study of Rotrosen *et al.* (56), who found that schizophrenics responding to neuroleptic treatment had reduced response to apomorphine (growth-hormone increase) when tested in a drug-free period, while non-responders had increased response.

REFERENCES

1. Delay, J., Deniker, B., Harl, J.-H Traitement des états d'excitation et d'agitation par une méthode medicamenteuse dérivée de l'hibernothérapie. *Ann. Med. Psychol., 110*:267–273, 1952.
2. Randrup, A., Munkvad, I. Stereotyped activities produced by amphetamine in several animal species and man. *Psychopharmacologia* (Berl.), *11*:300-310, 1967.
3. Weissman, A., Koe, B., Tenen, S. Antiamphetamine effects following inhibition of tyrosine hydroxylase. *J. Pharmacol. Exp. Ther., 151*: 339-352, 1966.
4. Randrup, A., Munkvad, I. Role of catecholamines in the amphetamine excitatory response. *Nature* (Lond.), *211*:540, 1966.
5. Carlsson, A. Morphologic and dynamic aspects of dopamine in the central nervous system. In *Biochemistry and Pharmacology of the Basal Ganglia*. Costa, E., Coté, L., Yahr, M. (eds.). New York: Raven Press, pp. 107-114, 1966.
6. Rech, R.H., Carr, L.A., Moore, K.E. Behavioural effects of α-methyltyrosine after prior depletion of brain catecholamines. *J. Pharmacol. Exp. Ther., 160*:326-335, 1968.
7. Scheel-Krüger, J. Comparative studies of various amphetamine analogues demonstrating different interactions with the metabolism of the catecholamines in the brain. *Eur. J. Pharmacol., 14*:47–59, 1971.
8. Fog, R. On stereotypy and catalepsy: studies on the effect of amphetamines and neuroleptics in rats. Munksgård, Copenhagen 1972.
9. Pedersen, V., Christensen, A.V. Methylphenidate antagonism in mice as a rapid screening test for neuroleptic drugs. *Acta Pharmacol. Toxicol., 29*:suppl. 4, 44, 1971.
10. Pedersen, V., Christensen, A.V. Antagonism of methylphenidate-induced stereotyped gnawing in mice. *Acta Pharmacol. Toxicol., 31*:488-496, 1972.
11. Papeschi, R. Behavioural and biochemical interaction between AMT and (+)-amphetamine: relevance to the identification of the functional pool of brain catecholamines. *Psychopharmacologia* (Berl.), *45*:21-28, 1975.
12. Bræstrup, C. Biochemical differentiation of amphetamine vs methylphenidate and nomifensine in rats. *J. Pharm. Pharmacol., 29*:463–470, 1977.
13. Julou, L., Bardone, M.-C., Ducrot, R., Comparison des effets des neuroleptiques dans divers tests, en administration unique et en administrations répétées. Hypothèses sur la signification des tests utilisès et leur valeur prévisionelle. In *Neuro-Psycho-Pharmacology*. Brill, H. (ed.). Amsterdam: Excerpta Medica Foundation, pp. 293-303, 1967.

14. Schelkunov, E.L. Adrenergic effect of chronic administration of neuroleptics. *Nature* (Lond.), 214:1210-1212, 1967.
15. György, L., Pfeifer, K.A., Hajtman, B. Modification of certain central neurons effects of haloperidol during long-term treatment in the mouse and rat. *Psychopharmacologia* (Berl.), *16*:223–233, 1969.
16. Møller Nielsen, I., Fjalland, B., Pendersen, V., Pharmacology of neuroleptics upon repeated administration. *Psychopharmacologia* (Berl.) *34*:95–104, 1974.
17. Moore, K.E., Thornburg, J.E. Drug-induced dopaminergic supersensitivity. In *Advances in Neurology*. Calne, D.B., Chase, T.N., Barbeau, A. (eds.). New York: Raven Press, pp. 93-104, 1975.
18. Klawans, H.L., Rubovitz, R. An experimental model of tardive dyskinesia. *J. Neural Trans.*, *33*:235-246, 1972.
19. Fjalland, B., Møller Nielsen, I. Enhancement of methylphenidate-induced stereotypies by repeated administration of neuroleptics. *Psychopharmacologia* (Berl.),*34*:105-109, 1974.
20. Tarsy, D., Baldessarini, R.J. Pharmacologically induced behavioural supersensitivity to apomorphine. *Nature (New Biol.)*, *245*:Oct. 31, 1973.
21. Von Voigtlander, P.E., Losey, E.G., Triezenberg, H.J. Increased sensitivity to dopaminergic agents after chronic neuroleptic treatment. *J. Pharmacol. Exp. Ther.*, *193*:88-94, 1975.
22. Sayers, A.C., Bürki, H.R., Ruch, W., Neuroleptic-induced hypersensitivity of striatal dopamine receptors in the rat as a model of tardive dyskinesias. Effects of clozapine, haloperidol, loxapine and chlorpromazine. *Psychopharmacologia* (Berl.), *41*:97-104, 1975.
23. Smith, R.C., Davis, J.M. Behavioral supersensitivity to apomorphine and amphetamine after chronic high-dose haloperidol treatment. *Psychopharmacol. Commun.*, *1*:285-288, 1975.
24. Smith, R.C., Davis, J.M. Behavioural evidence for supersensitivity after chronic administration of haloperidol, clozapine and thioridazine. *Life Sci.*, *19*:725-732, 1976.
25. Andén, N.-E., Rubinson, A. Fuxe, K., Evidence for dopamine receptor stimulation by apomorphine. *J. Pharm. Pharmacol.*, *19*:627–629, 1967.
26. Hyttel, J. Long-term effects of teflutixol on the synthesis and endogenous levels of mouse brain catecholamines. *J. Neurochem.*, *25*:681–686, 1975.
27. Hyttel, J. Levels of HVA and DOPAC in mouse corpus striatum in the supersensitivity phase after neuroleptic treatment. *J. Neurochem.*, *28*: 227–228, 1977.
28. Hyttel, J. Changes in dopamine synthesis rate in the supersensitivity phase after treatment with a single dose of neuroleptics. *Psychopharmacology*, *51*:205-207, 1977.
29. Miller, R.J., Hiley, C.J. Antimuscarinic properties of neuroleptics and drug induced parkinsonism. *Nature* (Lond.), *248*:596-597, 1974.
30. Snyder, S., Greenberg, D., Yamamura, H.I. Antischizophrenic drugs and brain cholinergic receptors. *Arch. Gen. Psychiat.*, *31*:58-61, 1974.
31. Ther, L., Schramm, H. Apomorphin-synergismus (Zwangsnagen bei Mäusen) als Test zur Differenzierung psychotroper Substanzen.*Arch. Int. Pharmacodyn. Ther.*, *138*:302–310, 1962.
32. Pedersen, V. Potentiation of apomorphine effect (compulsive gnawing behaviour) in mice. *Acta Pharmacol. Toxicol.*, *25*:suppl. 4, 63, 1967.
33. Scheel-Krüger, J. Central effects of anticholinergic drugs measured by the apomorphine gnawing test in mice.*Acta Pharmacol. Toxicol.*, *28*:1–16, 1970.
34. Giantsos, G., Moore, K.E. Dopaminergic hypersensitivity in striatum and olfactory tubercle following chronic administration of haloperidol or clozapine. *Life Sci.*, *20*:1585-1592, 1977.
35. Christensen, A.V., Fjalland, B., Møller Nielsen, I. On the supersensitivity of dopamine receptors induced by neuroleptics. *Psychopharmacology*, *48*:1–6, 1976.

36. Fjalland, B., Møller Nielsen, I. Methylphenidate antagonism of haloperidol interaction with cholinergic and anticholinergic drugs. *Psychopharmacologia* (Berl.), *34*:111-118, 1974.
37. Møller Nielsen, I., Christensen, A.V. Long term effects of neuroleptic drugs. *J. Pharmacol.* (Paris), *6*:3, 277–282, 1975.
38. Christensen, A.V. Acute and delayed effect of a single dose of a neuroleptic drug. *Acta Physiol. Scand.*, *113*:suppl. 396, 78, 1973.
39. Christensen, A.V., Møller Nielsen, I. Influence of flupenthixol and flupenthixol-decanoate on methylphenidate and apomorphine induced compulsive gnawing in mice. *Psychopharmacologia* (Berl.), *34*:119–126, 1974.
40. Christensen, A.V., Moller Nielsen, I. The effect of repeated administration of neuroleptic drugs. *Acta Pharmacol. Toxicol.*, *35*:suppl. 1, 23, 1974.
41. Møller Nielsen, I., Christensen, A.V., Fjalland, B. Receptor blockade and receptor supersensitivity following neuroleptic treatment. In *Antipsychotic Drugs, Pharmacodynamics and Pharmacokinetics*. Sedvall, G., Uvnäs, B., Zotterman, Y., (eds.). New York: Pergamon Press, pp. 257–260, 1976.
42. Møller Nielsen, I., Christensen, A.V., Hyttel, J. Rezeptorblockade und Rezeptorhypersensibilität nach Behandlung mit Neuroleptika. *Arzneim. Forsch.*, *26*:6, 1090–1092, 1976.
43. Møller Nielsen, I., Christensen, A.V., Hyttel, J. Adaptational phenomena in neuroleptic treatment. Dopamine Symposia, Southampton, Aug. 8–Sept. 1, 1977. (In press).
44. Asper, H., Baggiolini, M., Bürki, H.R., Tolerance phenomena with neuroleptics. Catalepsy, apomorphine stereotypies and striatal dopamine metabolism in the rat after single and repeated administration of loxapine and haloperidol. *Eur. J. Pharmacol.*, *22*:287–294, 1973.
45. Scatton, B., Garret, C., Julou, L. Acute and subacute effects of neuroleptics on dopamine synthesis and release in the rat striatum. *Arch. Pharmacol.*, *289*:419, 1975.
46. Scatton, B., Glowinski, J., Julou, L. Neuroleptics: effects on dopamine synthesis in the nigroneostriatal, mesolimbic and mesocortical dopaminergic systems. In *Antipsychotic Drugs, Pharmacodynamics and Pharmacokinetics*. Sedvall, G., Uvnäs, B., Zotterman, Y., (eds.). New York: Pergamon Press, p. 243, 1976.
47. Scatton, B. Differential regional development of tolerance to increase in dopamine turnover upon repeated neuroleptic administration. *Eur. J. Pharmacol.*, *46*:363–369, 1977.
48. Martres, H.P. Costentin, J., Bandry, M., Long term changes in the sensitivity of pre- and postsynaptic dopamine receptors in mouse striatum evidenced by behavioural and biochemical studies. *Brain Res.*, *136*:319–373, 1977.
49. Gerlach, J., Reisby, N., Randrup, A. Dopaminergic hypersensitivity and cholinergic hypofunction in the pathophysiology of tardive dyskinesia. *Psychopharmacologia*, *34*:21–35, 1974.
50. Smith, R.C., Tamminga, C.A., Haraszti, J. Effects of dopamine agonists in tardive dyskinesia. *Am. J. Psychiatry*, *134*:763–768, 1977.
51. Klawans, H.L. The pharmacology of tardive dyskinesia. *Am. J. Psychiatry*, *130*:82–85, 1973.
52. Kobayashi, R.M. Drug therapy of tardive dyskinesia. *N. Engl. J. Med.*, *296*:257–260, 1977.
53. Gerlach, J. Tardive dyskinesier. Dan. Med. Bull. In press 1978.
54. Ettigi, P., Nair, N.P.U., Lal, S. Effect of apomorphine on growth hormone and prolactin secretion in schizophrenic patients, with or without oral dyskinesia, withdrawn from chronic neuroleptic therapy. *J. Neurol. Neurosurg. Psychiatry*, *39*:870–876, 1976.
55. Tamminga, C.A., Smith, R.C., Pandey, G., A neuroendocrine study of supersensitivity in tardive dyskinesia. *Arch. Gen. Psychiatry*, *34*: 1199–1203, 1977.
56. Rotrosen, J., Angrist, B.M., Gershon, S., Dopamine receptor alteration in schizophrenia: Neuroendocrine evidence. *Psychopharmacology*, *51*:1–7, 1976.

5

Alterations in Neuropharmacology of Apomorphine by Chronic Treatment with Haloperidol

HARBANS LAL
and GERALD GIANUTSOS

INTRODUCTION

Since the first report of its behavioral actions a century ago (1), apomorphine has been extensively employed as a tool to investigate the role of dopaminergic systems in medicine. This review has been prepared utilizing this approach. We briefly describe recent studies, using apomorphine in the investigation of the neurobiological mechanisms of extrapyramidal disorders which are frequently produced by the chronic use of potent neuroleptic (antipsychotic) drugs.

Apomorphine

Apomorphine can mimic certain behavioral effects of DOPA, which led Ernst and Smelik (2) to believe that apomorphine exerts its action through stimulation of central dopaminergic receptors. Ernst (3) further reported that interference with DA synthesis by inhibiting the enzymes tyrosine hydroxylase and dopamine decarboxylase, which produce dopamine, failed to block the action of apomorphine. These results suggest that apomorphine directly stimulates dopamine receptors.

More recently, more direct evidence has been presented to suggest that apomorphine indeed directly stimulates dopamine receptors. Using the binding of labeled dopamine to synaptic membranes of mammalian striatal tissue as a model of the dopamine receptor, Burt *et al.* (4) reported apomorphine to be

51

the most potent dopamine-receptor agonist. Similar experiments of Seeman *et al.* (5) also established the dopamine agonist properties of apomorphine. In addition to its affinity for the dopamine receptor, apomorphine also stimulates an adenylate cyclase in nerve tissue which is sensitive to dopamine. Low concentrations of apomorphine activate brain adenylate cyclase (6,7), an effect that is antagonized by dopamine antagonists.

Haloperidol

Haloperidol is a well-known prototype of specific dopamine-receptor antagonists that alleviate schizophrenia. The molecular structure of haloperidol can be conformed to that of dopamine in configuration studies (8). Haloperidol-like drugs show high binding affinity, with cellular constituents of dopaminergic neurons (4,5,9,10,11), and antagonize neurochemical and behavioral changes stimulated by dopamine (12). Biochemically, haloperidol increases turnover of brain dopamine (13). This is interpreted as a compensatory activation of dopamine neurons in response to receptor blockade by the drug. Haloperidol also inhibits dopamine-stimulated adenylate cyclase (7,14, 15,16). With respect to the behavioral effects of apomorphine and other dopamine-receptor stimulant drugs, all of them that are known are antagonized by haloperidol and other neuroleptics (12). They include motor stimulation, stereotypy, aggression, brain self-stimulation, and a number of other behaviors that are elicited experimentally. In addition, haloperidol-like drugs increase serum prolactin by antagonizing the tonic inhibitory control of the tuberinfundibular dopamine neurons of the hypothalamus (17).

When the dopamine receptors in the CNS are blocked for a prolonged period of time, as by chronic treatment with haloperidol, a number of compensatory mechanisms are thought to be triggered. As a result, an enhanced responsiveness of the behavioral and neurochemical effects of apomorphine is observed upon discontinuation of the dopamine-receptor antagonists. Because of a likely relationship of this enhanced responsiveness to iatrogenic diseases resulting from long-term use of neuroleptics, a review of the pharmacology of apomorphine in neuroleptic-induced 'supersensitive' subjects is undertaken in this chapter.

BEHAVIORAL ACTIONS OF APOMORPHINE

Apomorphine elicits several different types of behavior, which are thought to be largely dependent on the ability of the drug to stimulate dopamine receptors. An analysis of these behaviors follows.

Stereotypy

Apomorphine has been known to produce stereotyped behaviors for over a century. However, a detailed account of apomorphine-induced stereotyped behaviors was reported only in 1962 (18). Dependent upon doses employed, systemic injections of apomorphine induce intense and repetitive locomotion, sniffing, licking, gnawing, chewing, and increased reactivity to environmental stimuli. All these signs are usually included in stereotypy syndrome, although neuroanatomical sites of their origin may be different. Nigro-striatal and mesolimbic dopamine systems are considered to be the site of apomorphine action in producing stereotyped behaviors.

Some studies (19,20) consider the substantia nigra to be an important site of the apomorphine action. Other workers (21,22) differ with this view. Lesioning of caudate-putamen complex abolishes apomorphine stereotypy, according to some workers (23,24,25,26,27). Lesions of globus pallidus markedly reduce apomorphine stereotypy (27,28), as do the lesioning of neucleus amygdaloideus lateralis (20) and centralis (23,29). Ernst and Smelik (2) implanted crystalline Dopa or apomorphine in the dorsal part of the caudate nucleus and the globus pallidus of rats, which produced compulsive gnawing. Implantation in the ventral part of caudate, subthalamic structures, or substantia nigra were ineffective. Costall and Naylor (30), on the other hand, failed to observe stereotypy by intracaudate apomorphine injection. Whereas lesioning of tubercle olfactorium reduces apomorphine stereotypy (28), injection of apomorphine into tubercle olfactorium effectively induces stereotypy behavior (31). Lesions of nucleus accumbans septi have been found either to abolish apomorphine-induced sniffing (28) or to exert no effect at all (25). Lesions of nucleus interstitialis striatum terminalis do not affect apomorphine stereotypy (28).

Smelik and Ernst (2) also showed that application of the choline-esterase inhibitor physostigmine in the substantia nigra, but not in the caudate or pallidum, caused compulsive gnawing. This observation suggests that there may actually be cholinergic synaptic input on the nigral dopaminergic nerve cells involved in stereotypy behavior. These cells terminate in caudate where their terminals are located. This hypothesis is supported by the finding that accumulation of ACh in substantia nigra causes accumulation of dopamine at striatal nerve endings (2), and that electrical stimulation of substantia nigra causes a release of DA (32,33,34,35,36,37), as well as elicits unit cell activity (38,39,40) in the caudate nucleus.

That stereotypy behavior induced by apomorphine is mediated by dopamine stimulation is also suggested by the fact that dopamine-receptor antagonists are among the most effective agents that block apomorphine stereotypy (12).

Enhanced drug-induced stereotypy after chronic neuroleptics was first demonstrated by Schelkunov (41) using amphetamine and apomorphine as test drugs after chronic treatment with the neuroleptic perphenazine. Since then, numerous other reports have demonstrated an enhanced response to the stereotypy produced by apomorphine following chronic treatment with a large number of neuroleptics in rats, mice, and guinea pigs (42,43,44,45,46). Treatment with the nonneuroleptics promethazine, pentobarbital, and diazepam failed to alter the apomorphine effects (44). With chronic haloperidol, stereotypy induced by apomorphine is increased in intensity and duration (43), and this effect is similar to that seen by using amphetamine as stereotypic agent (47).

Since apomorphine-induced stereotypy is thought to be the result of stimulation of dopamine receptors in the brain, these results are evidence in favor of the development of dopaminergic supersensitivity with neuroleptics.

Aggression

Fighting in laboratory animals may be produced by a variety of pharmacological procedures which increase the stimulation of brain dopamine receptors (48). Apomorphine is the drug most often employed to elicit experimental aggression (31,48,49,50,51), but similar effects can also be produced by injection of other dopamine agonists when given in higher doses (52). Apomorphine-induced aggression is reduced by placing lesions in the amygdala of the substantia nigra. In contrast, lesions which destroy the septum or olfactory bulb enhance the degree of aggression (53,54).

Apomorphine-induced aggression is blocked either by cholinergic drugs (51) or by neuroleptics, such as haloperidol (48). Antagonism of apomorphine-induced aggression by neuroleptics is potentiated by cholinergic agonists and is reversed by anticholinergics (51). Apomorphine aggression is also antagonized by narcotic analgesics, but this antagonism is not reversed by anticholinergics (51).

When rats have been withdrawn from prolonged administration of haloperidol, the dose-response curve for apomorphine-induced aggression is shifted sharply to the left (43,52). While 20 mg/kg of apomorphine is usually required to produce substantial aggression in normal rats, the chronic haloperidol group responds to as little as 1.25 mg/kg of apomorphine. This effect is maximal 3–7 days after the haloperidol injections have been stopped. Once again, this is another sign of hypersensitivity to apomorphine and further evidence for the development of dopamine receptor supersensitivity after chronic haloperidol.

Locomotor Activity

Apomorphine has been reported to both increase (55,56,57) and decrease

(58,59,60) locomotor activity, the direction of the effect depending on the dose and the time interval after apomorphine injection (61). An interaction between dopaminergic and noradrenergic systems, as well as with an inhibitory serotonergic system (62,63), has been implicated in apomorphine-induced locomotion.

Following chronic treatment with haloperidol, the motor stimulation produced by apomorphine is increased in both rats and mice (45,47,64). Similarly, microinjections of dopamine into the nucleus accumbens results in enhanced stimulation in rats treated chronically with penfluridol (65). Following chronic clozapine, both an enhanced apomorphine stimulation (46,66) and no change in apomorphine effect (67) have been reported. This difference in results seems to be based upon clozapine doses employed for those studies.

There is also an increase in the locomotor stimulation produced by the noradrenergic drug clonidine after chronic haloperidol (68). These data are taken as a further support that receptor supersensitivity results from chronic treatment with neuroleptic drugs.

Circling Locomotion

Unilateral injections of apomorphine in the striatum elicit circling behavior (69). This effect is similar to that produced by intracaudate or intrapallidal injections of dopamine (30). These types of asymmetries can also be demonstrated in animals in which the dopaminergic nigro-striatal bundle has been unilaterally destroyed by a local injection of 6-hydroxy-dopamine. Administration of apomorphine causes these animals to circle away from the lesioned (presumed supersensitive) side (69,70). Circling behavior by apomorphine is readily blocked by haloperidol (71).

After repeated administration of haloperidol or chlorpromazine to unilaterally 6-hydroxy-dopamine lesioned rats, there is an increase in the turning response to apomorphine, suggesting an augmented supersensitivity (67). A somewhat less dramatic effect is noted after chronic treatment with thioridazine (72), which may produce a lower incidence of tardive dyskinesias than haloperidol.

NEUROCHEMICAL ACTIONS

Dopamine Turnover

Apomorphine reduces the neuronal activity of the presynaptic dopamine neurons (73) and the release and turnover of dopamine (32,50,74,75,76,77). These effects are thought to be secondary to neuronal feedback, brought about as a compensatory mechanism initiated by stimulation of dopamine receptors by apomorphine. These effects have traditionally been thought to be due to postsynaptic dopamine-receptor stimulation, but more recently it has been suggested that simulation of presynaptic receptors may play an important role in the biochemical effects of apomorphine (78,79,80). These various effects of apomorphine on dopamine neuronal activity and turnover are blocked by dopamine-receptor antagonists (13). Other actions of apomorphine, such as inhibition of tyrosine hydroxylase, monoamine oxidase, or the deamination of dopamine, are not fully understood and are often demonstrated only at very high drug concentrations.

Following chronic neuroleptics, it has been generally reported that brain dopamine concentrations remain unchanged (13,66,81), although there appears to be a transient reduction in the synthesis of brain dopamine during the withdrawal supersensitivity phase (81,82).

When rats are challenged with apomorphine after withdrawal of chronic haloperidol, there is an enhanced sensitivity to the ability of apomorphine to reduce the turnover of striatal dopamine, as measured by depletion of dopamine after synthesis inhibition (47). Similar effects are noted in both the striatum and olfactory tubercle of mice withdrawn from a chronic diet of either haloperidol or clozapine (66).

These results provide neurochemical support for the behavioral supersensitivity to apomorphine action seen after neuroleptic treatment.

Adenylate Cyclase

An adenylate cyclase system which is activated by dopamine has been proposed to be involved in the synaptic actions of dopamine (83). Low concentrations of apomorphine also activate this enzyme (6,7), an effect that is antagonized by neuroleptic drugs.

If this adenylate cyclase system, as proposed, represents the dopamine receptor (85), it would be expected that changes in adenylate cyclase should be exhibited in animals maintained on chronic neuroleptics. Earlier results have been largely negative. They were obtained with the administration of dopamine or apomorphine into various adenylcyclase assays conducted with tissue obtained from animals chronically treated with many different neuroleptic drugs (85,86,87). However, a recent report from Iwatsubo and Couet (88) described increased sensitivity of striatal adenylate cyclase to dopamine after chronic administration of haloperidol in the rat. These observations were recently replicated by Friedhoff et al. (89).

Receptor Binding

Another more recent approach has been to investigate the ability of radioactive dopamine and other ligands to stereospecifically bind to brain tissue as a measure of dopamine receptor concentration (4). Apomorphine and DA similarly bind to this receptor material (5).

Chronic treatment of rats with haloperidol, fluphenazine, or reserpine produced an increase in ^{3}H-haloperidol binding in the striatum, suggesting the synthesis of new receptor material (90,91). Enhanced ^{3}H-haloperidol as well as ^{3}H-apomorphine binding was noted in both the striatum and dopaminergic mesolimbic region of rats after long-term haloperidol (91). These results more closely correlate with the behavioral results and experiments with dopamine turnover, and support the hypothesis of dopamine receptor supersensitivity.

ENDOCRINE EFFECTS

Certain pituitary hormones (e.g., prolactin, growth hormone) are under dopaminergic control via the tuberoinfundibular tract in the medial basal hypothalamus (92,93,94). Dopaminergic stimulation inhibits prolactin release; thus, apomorphine reduces the plasma prolactin concentration in ovariectomized females treated with estrogen (95), as well as in intact male rats (96).

If dopamine supersensitivity occurs in the tuberoinfundibular dopamine receptors, it would be predicted that the ability of apomorphine to reduce prolactin would be enhanced after withdrawal of chronic neuroleptics. A number of investigators (17,97,98) failed to observe any increase in apomorphine-induced inhibition of prolactin release by chronic neuroleptic treatment. However, a careful study of dose-response relationship revealed that apomorphine effect reaches a plateau which is below the complete blockade of prolactin release. Therefore, beyond a small dose of apomorphine any increase in apomorphine dose does not result in any further increase in the prolactin inhibition. In view of this finding, recent experiments were repeated with very small doses of apomorphine (80). These doses were ineffective in normal animals. It was found that chronic treatment with haloperidol indeed increased apomorphine inhibition of prolactin release. This finding was recently replicated by A. Brown (personal communication).

CURRENT RESEARCH AND FUTURE PERSPECTIVES

Chronic treatment with antischizophrenic neuroleptic drugs produces a large variety of neurobiological changes. Many of these changes, such as those resulting in a relief from schizophrenia, are therapeutic and are desirable. Many other changes, such as appearance of several motor abnormalities, are undesirable. In order to develop new drugs in which therapeutic effects are enhanced and the side effects are eliminated, it is essential that the mechanisms underlying each category of effects be clearly identified. Responsiveness of biological systems to apomorphine is very frequently employed as a tool for mechanistic studies. Because of dopamine agonist's properties and the ease with which it penetrates into various brain structures, this drug makes an ideal tool to evaluate the functioning status of dopaminergic neurons in health and disease.

What has been known is reviewed in this chapter. These studies show that all of the neuroleptics that are potent antischizophrenics block apomorphine actions and render the neuronal system more sensitive to dopaminergic stimulation after prolonged administration. However, it is yet not established whether this supersensitivity is related to the therapeutic effectiveness of neuroleptics or their side effects. Most likely it will be proven to be an integral part of both categories of effects.

There are two areas of apomorphine action that have not been adequately studied. First, it is not known which of the pharmacological actions of apomorphine is related to its presynaptic effects and which to the postsynaptic actions. Release of dopamine is one clearly recognized presynaptic action of apomorphine (99). However, changes in its functioning after chronic neuroleptics is not known. Only an indirect evidence was recently reported (47). These actions of apomorphine in the chronically treated animals were compared to similar actions of amphetamine. While apomorphine is a direct agonist of dopamine receptors, amphetamine's predominant effect on dopamine receptors appear to be indirect (100), producing its central nervous system effects through release of dopamine (101) and blockade of reuptake (102). Following discontinuation of chronic haloperidol, rats exhibited enhanced spontaneous locomotor activity and an enhancement of stereotypy and locomotor stimulation, produced both by apomorphine and amphetamine. The effect on locomotor activity was not blocked by an inhibitor of dopamine synthesis, suggesting that changes in the release of dopamine were not the basis of this supersensitivity. In addition, whereas enhancement of apomorphine-induced aggression was reconfirmed, neither (+) nor (−) amphetamine was able to elicit aggression. In a similar experiment using chronic morphine, the ability of amphetamine to elicit aggression was clearly established (50,76,103). This experiment suggests that chronic haloperidol produces long-lasting presynaptic changes, so that a release of dopamine by amphetamine is differentially inhibited in brain areas related to aggressive behaviors. These animal data confirmed what has been reported clinically (104). Whereas a number of amphetamine actions are augmented in schizophrenic patients on neuroleptic drugs, other actions of amphetamine either are not affected or are actually reduced (105,106).

Another area of apomorphine that is critical but has not attracted attention is the interaction of apomorphine with other neurotransmitters. It is known that dopaminergic neurons are synaptically interconnected with neurons of many other neurotransmitters, such as acetylcholine, gamma-amino-butyric acid, glycine, serotonin, and endorphin. It is therefore very likely that changes in the functioning of dopaminergic systems by chronic neuroleptic treatment are reflected in the alteration of many other neurotransmitter systems. Some of these may be the basis of clinical changes that are reported. Tardive dyskinesia, for instance, is partially relieved by muscarinic drugs, which provide a sort of replacement therapy to correct cholinergic hyposensitivity that has been reported after chronic haloperidol treatment (48).

Whereas there has been a lot of work done with apomorphine pharmacology in the chronically treated subjects, there are glaring deficiencies, and some of them are pointed out as above to stimulate further work. Unless these areas are fully explored, mechanisms underlying long-term changes produced by neuroleptic drugs will not be understood.

REFERENCES

1. Harnack, E. Uber die Wirkuncor des Apomorphibes an Saugethier, und am Frosch. *Nauyn. Schmiedebergs. Arch. Pharmacol., 2*:254–306, 1974.
2. Ernst, A.M., Smelik, E. Site of action of dopamine and apomorphine on compulsive gnawing behavior in rats. *Experienta, 22*:837–839, 1966.
3. Ernst, A.M. Relation between the action of dopamine and apomorphine on gnawing compulsion in rats. *Psychopharmacologia, 10*:316–323, 1967.
4. Burt, D.R., Enna, S.J., Creese, I., Snyder, S.H. Dopamine receptor binding in the corpus striatum in mammalian brain. *Proc. Nat. Acad. Sci., 72*:4655–4699, 1975.
5. Seeman, P., Chau-Wong, M., Tedesco, J., Wong, K. Dopamine receptors in human and calf brains, using H^3 apomorphine and an antipsychotic drug. *Proc. Nat. Acad. Sci., 73*:4354–4358, 1976.
6. Bucher, M.G., Schorderet, M. Dopamine and apomorphine-sensitive adenylate cyclase in homogenates of rabbit retina. *Naunyn–Schmiedebergs. Arch. Pharmacol., 288*:103–107, 1975.
7. Kebabian, J.W., Petzold, G.L., Greengard, P. Dopamine-sensitive adenylate cyclase in caudate nucleus of rat brain and its similarity to the "dopamine receptor." *Proc. Nat. Acad. Sci., 69*:2145–2149, 1972.
8. Tollenaere, J.P., Moreels, H., Kock, M.H.J. On the conformation of neuroleptic drugs in the three aggregation states and their conformational resemblance to dopamine. *Eur. J. Med. Chem., 12*:199–211, 1977.
9. Seeman, P., Lae, T. Antipsychotic drugs: direct correlation between clinical potency and presynaptic action on dopamine neurons. *Science, 188*:1217–1219, 1975.
10. Creese, I., Iversen, S.D. The pharmacological and anatomical substrates of the amphetamine response in the rat. *Brain Res., 83*:419–436, 1975.
11. Leysen, J., Tollenaere, J.P., Koch, M.H.J., Laduron, P. Differentiation of opiate and neuroleptic receptor binding in rat. *Eur. J. Pharmacol., 43*:253–267, 1977.
12. Fielding, S., Lal, H. Behavioral actions of neuroleptics. In *Handbook of Psychopharmacology.* Iverson, L.L., Iverson, S.D., Snyder, S.H. (eds.). New York: Plenum, pp. 91–128, 1978.
13. Lal, H., Puri, S., Volicer, L. A comparison between narcotics and neuroleptics: effects on striatal dopamine turnover, cyclic AMP and adenylate cyclase. In *Tissue Responses to Addictive Drugs.* Ford, D., Clouet, D. (eds.). New York; Spectrum, pp. 187–207, 1976.

14.   Karobath, M., Leitich, H. Antipsychotic drugs and dopamine-stimulated adenylate cyclase prepared from corpus striatum of rat brain. *Proc. Nat. Acad. Sci., 71*:2915–2918, 1974.

15.   Miller, R.J., Horn, A.S., Iversen, L.I. The action of neuroleptic drugs on dopamine-stimulated adenosive cyclic 3′,5′-monophosphate production in rat neostriatum and limbic forebrain. *Mol. Pharmacol., 10*:759–766, 1974.

16.   Lauuron, P. Limiting factors in the antagonism of neuroleptics on dopamine sensitivity adenylate cyclase. *J. Pharm. Pharmacol., 28*:250–251, 1976.

17.   Meltzer, H.Y., Fan, V.S., Fessler, R., Simonovic, M., Stanisic, D. Neuroleptic-stimulated prolactin secretion in the rat as an animal model for biological psychiatry: comparison with anti-psychotic activity. In *Animal Models in Psychiatry and Neurology*. Hanin, I., Usdin, E. (eds.). New York: Pergamon Press, pp. 443–454, 1977.

18.   Janssen, P.A.J., Niemegeers, C.J.E., Verbruggeri, F. A propos d'une methode d'investigation de substances susceptibles de modifier le comprotement agressif in ne du rat blanc vis-a-vis de la souris blancke. *Psychopharmacologia, 3*:111–123, 1962.

19.   Baum, E., Etevenon, P., Piarrouse, M.C., Simon, P., Boissier, J.R. Behavioral modification and pharmacological sensitivity in rat following bilateral lesions of substantia nigra. *J. Pharm. Pharmacol., 2*:423–434, 1971.

20.   Costall, B., Naylor, R.J. Possible involvement of a noradrenergic area of the amygdala with stereotype behavior. *Life Sci., 11*:1135–1146, 1972.

21.   Amsler, C. Beitrage gur pharmakologie des gehirns. *Arch. Exp. Pathol. Pharmacol., 97*:1–14, 1923.

22.   Creese, I., Burt, D.R., Snyder, S.H. Dopamine receptor binding: differentiation of agonist and antagonist states with H³-dopamine and H³-haloperidol. *Life Sci., 17*:993–1002, 1975.

23.   Costall, B., Naylor, R.B. The role of elencephalic dopaminergic systems in the mediation of apomorphine-stereotyped behavior. *Eur. J. Pharmacol., 24*:8–24, 1973a.

24.   Divac, I. Drug-induced syndromes in rats with large chronic lesions in the corpus. *Psychopharmacologia, 27*:171–178, 1972.

25.   McKenzie, G.M. Role of the tuberculum olfactorium in stereotyped behavior induced by apomorphine in the rat. *Psychopharmacologia, 23*:212–219, 1972.

26.   Kelly, P.H., Seviour, P.W., Iversen, S.D. Amphetamine and apomorphine responses in the rat following 6-OHDA lesions of the nucleus accumbens septi and corpus striatum. *Brain Res., 94*:504–522, 1975.

27.   Wolforth, S. Reactions to apomorphine and spiroperidol of rats with striatal lesions—relevance of kind and size of lesion. *Pharmacol. Biochem. Behav., 2*:181–186, 1974.

28.   Costall, B., Naylor, R.J. On the mode of action of apomorphine. *Eur. J. Pharmacol., 21*:350–361, 1973b.

29.   Costall, B., Naylor, R.J. Specific asymmetric behavior induced by the direct chemical stimulation of neostriatal dopaminergic mechanisms. *Naunyn. Schmiedebergs. Arch. Pharmacol., 285*:83–98, 1974a.

30.   Costall, B., Naylor, R.J. The involvement of dopaminergic systems with the stereotyped behavior patterns induced by methylphenidate. *J. Pharm. Pharmacol., 26*:30–33, 1974b.

31.   McKenzie, G.M. Apomorphine-induced aggression in the rat. *Brain Res., 34*:323–330, 1972.

32.   Anden, N.E., Robenson, A., Fuxe, K., Hokfelt, T. Evidence for dopamine receptor stimulation by apomorphine. *J. Pharm. Pharmacol., 10*:627–629, 1964.

33.   Brodal, A. Some data and perspectives on the anatomy of the so-called extrapyramidal system. *Acta Neurol. Scand., 39*:17–38 (Suppl. 4), 1963.

34.   McLennan, A. The release of dopamine from the putamen. *Experientia, 21*:725, 1965.

35. Portig, P.J., Vogt, M. Activation of a dopaminergic nigrostriatal pathway. *J. Physiol.*, *197*:20–21, 1968.
36. Portig, P.J., Vogt, M. Release into the cerebral ventricles of substances with possible transmitter function in the caudate nucleus. *J. Physiol.*, *204*:687–715, 1969.
37. Vogt, M. Release from brain tissue of compounds with possible transmitter function: interaction of drugs with those substances. *Br. J. Pharmacol.*, *37*:325–337, 1969.
38. Connor, J.D. Caudate unit response to nigra stimulation: evidence for a possible nigro-neostriatal pathway. *Science*, *160*:899–900, 1968.
39. Connor, J.D. Caudate nucleus neurons: correlation of the effects of substantia nigra stimulation with iontophoretic dopamine. *J. Physiol.*, *208*:691–703, 1970.
40. Frigyesi, T.L., Purpura, D.F. Electrophysiological analyses of reciprocal caudo-nigral relations. *Brain Res.*, *6*:440–456, 1967.
41. Schelkunov, E.L. Adrenergic effects of chronic administration of neuroleptics. *Nature*, *214*:1210–1212, 1967.
42. Klawans, H.L., Rubovits, R., Patel, B.C., Weiner, W.J. Cholinergic and anticholinergic influences on amphetamine-induced stereotyped behavior. *J. Neurol. Sci.*, *17*:303–308, 1972.
43. Gianutsos, G., Drawbaugh, R.B., Hunes, M.D., Lal, H. Behavioral evidence for dopaminergic supersensitivity after chronic haloperidol. *Life Sci.*, *14*:887–898, 1974.
44. Tarsy, D., Baldessarini, R.J. Behavioral supersensitivity to apomorphine following chronic treatment with drugs which interfere with the synaptic function of catecholamines. *Neuropharmacology*, *13*:927–940, 1974.
45. Moore, K.E., Thornburg, J.E. Drug-induced dopaminergic supersensitivity. In *Advances in Neurology*, vol. 9. Calne, D.B., Chase, T.N., Barbeau, A. (eds.). New York: Raven Press, pp. 93-104, 1975.
46. Smith, R.C., Davis, T.M. Behavioral evidence for supersensitive after chronic administration of haloperidol, clozapine, and thioridazine. *Life Sci.*, *19*:725–732, 1976.
47. Gianutsos, G., Hynes, M.D., Drawbaugh, R., Lal, H. Similarities and contrasts between the effects of amphetamine and apomorphine in rats chronically treated with haloperidol. *Prog. Neuropsychopharmacol.*, *1*:1978. (In press).
48. Gianutsos, G., Lal, H. Alteration in the action of cholinergic and anticholinergic drugs after chronic haloperidol: indirect evidence for cholinergic hyposensitivity. *Life Sci.*, *18*:515–520, 1976a.
49. Senault, B. Comportement d'agressivite intraspecifique induit par l'apomorphine chez le rat. *Psychopharmacologia*, *18*:271–287, 1970.
50. Lal, H., Gianutsos, G., Puri, S.K. A comparison of narcotic analgesics with neuroleptics on behavioral measures of dopaminergic activity. *Life Sci.*, *17*:29–34, 1975.
51. Gianutsos, G., Lal, H. Blockade of apomorphine-induced aggression by morphine or neuroleptics: differential alteration by antimuscarinics and naloxone. *Pharmacol. Biochem. Behav.*, *4*:639–642, 1976b.
52. Lal, H., O'Brien, J., Pitteman, A., Gianutsos, G., Reddy, C. Aggression after amphetamines and dihydroxyphenylalanine. *Fed. Proc.*, *13*:529, 1972.
53. Senalut, B. Influence de la surrenalectomie, de l'hypophsyertomie, de la thyroidectomie, de la castration ainsi que de la testosterone sur le comportement d'agressivite intraspecifique induit par l'apomorphine chez le rat. *Psychopharmacologia*, *24*:476–484, 1972.
54. Senault, B. Amines cerebrales et comportement d'agressivite intraspecifique induit par l'apomorphine chez le rat. *Psychopharmacologia*, *34*:143–154, 1974.
55. Frommel, E., Ledebur, I.V, Seydoux, J., The cholinergic mechanism of psychomotor agitation in apomorphine-injected mice. *Arch. Int. Pharmacodyn.*, *154*:227–230, 1965.
56. Thomas, J. Hyperkinetic syndromes in the rat: the mode of action of amphetamine and apomorphine. *Fed. Proc.*, *29*:1488, 1970.

57. Maj, J., Grabowska, M., Gajda, L. Effect of apomorphine on motility in rats. *Eur. J. Pharmacol.*, *17*:208–214, 1972.

58. Puech, A.J., Simon, P., Chermat, R., Boissier, J.R. Profile neuropsychopharmacoligique de l'apomorphine. *J. Pharmacol.*, *5*:241–254, 1974.

59. Kulkarni, S.K., Dandiva, P.C. Influence of chemical stimulation of central dopaminergic system on the open field behavior of rats. *Pharakopsychiatrie*, *1:*45–50, 1975.

60. Strombom, V. On the functional role of pre and postsynaptic catecholamine receptors in brain. *Acta Physiol. Scan. Supply.*, *431*:1–43, 1975.

61. Sahakian, B.J., Robbins, T.W. Potentiation of locomotor activity and modification of stereotypy by starvation in apomorphine treated rats. *Neuropharmacology, 14*:251–257, 1975.

62. Grabowska, M. Influence of midbrain raphe lesion on some pharmacological and biochemical effects of apomorphine in rats. *Psychopharmacologia, 39*:315–322, 1974.

63. Grabowska, M., Mickaluk, J. On the role of serotonin in apomorphine-induced locomotor stimulation in rats. *Pharmacol. Biochem. Behav.*, *2*:263–266, 1974.

64. Dunstan, R., Jackson, P.M. The effect of apomorphine and clonidine on locomotor activity in mice after long-treatment with haloperidol. *Clin. Exp. Pharmacol. Physiol.*, *4*:131–141, 1977.

65. Jackson, D.M., Anden, N.E., Engel, J., Liljequiest, S. The effect of long-term penfluridol treatment on the sensitivity of the dopamine receptors in the nucleus accumbens and in the corpus striatum. *Psychopharmacologia, 45*:151–155, 1975.

66. Gianutsos, G., Moore, K.E. Dopaminergic supersensitivity in striatum and olfactory tubercle following chronic administration of haloperidol or clozapine. *Life Sci.*, *20*:1585–1592, 1977.

67. Sayers, A.C., Burki, H.R., Ruch, W., Asper, H. Neuroleptic-induced hypersensitivity of striatal dopamine receptors in the rat as a model of tardive dyskinesias. Effects of clozapine, haloperidol, loxapine on chlorpromazine. *Psychopharmacologia, 41*:97–104, 1975.

68. Dunstan, R., Jackson, D.M. The demonstration of a change in adrenergic receptor sensitivity in the central nervous system of mice after withdrawal from long-term treatment with haloperidol. *Psychopharmacology, 48*:105–114, 1976.

69. Ungerstedt, U. Postsynaptic supersensitivity after 6-hydroxydopamine induced degeneration of the nigro-striatal dopamine system. *Acta Physiol. Scand. 82, Suppl., 367*:69–93, 1969.

70. Von Voightlander, P.F., Moore, K.E. Involvement of nigrostriatal neurons in the in vivo release of dopamine by amphetamine, amantadine and tyramine. *J. Pharmacol. Exp. Ther., 184*:542–552, 1973.

71. Echols, S.D., Ursillo, R.C. Significance of species differences: rotational models. In *Animal Models in Psychiatry and Neurology.* Hanin I., Usdin, E. (eds.). New York: Pergamon Press, pp. 27–34, 1977.

72. Sayers, A.C., Burki, H.R., Ruch, W., Asper, H. Animal models for tardive dyskinesia. Effects of thioridazine. *Pharmocol. Psychia., 10*:291–295, 1977.

73. Bunny, B.S., Aghajanian, G.K., Roth, R.H. Comparison of effects of l-dopa, amphetamine and apomorphine on firing rate of rat dopaminergic neurons. *Nature, 245*:123–125, 1973.

74. Roose, B.E. Decrease in homovanillic acid as evidence for dopamine receptor stimulation by apomorphine in the neostriatum of the rat. *J. Pharm. Pharmacol., 21*:263–264, 1969.

75. Nyback, H., Schubert, J., Sedvall, G. Effect of apomorphine and pimozide on synthesis and turnover of labeled catecholamines in mouse brain. *J. Pharm. Pharmacol., 22*:622–624, 1970.

76. Puri, S.K., Lal, H. Effect of morphine, haloperidol, apomorphine and benztropine on

dopamine turnover in rat corpus striatum: evidence showing induced reduction in CNS dopaminergic activity. *Fed. Proc., 32*:758, 1973.

77. Scatton, B., Thiersy, A.M., Celowinski, J., Julou, L. Effects of thioperazine and apomorphine on dopamine synthesis in the mesocortical dopaminergic systems. *Brain Res., 88*:389–393, 1975.

78. Roth, R.H., Walters, J.R., Murrin, L.C., Morgenroth, V.H. Dopamine neurons: role of impulse flow and presynaptic receptors in the regulation of tyrosine hydroxylase. In *Pre- and Postsynaptic Receptors*. Usdin, E., Bunney, W.E. (eds.). New York: Dekker, pp. 5–48, 1975.

79. Carlsson, A. Dopaminergic auto-receptors. In *Chemical Tools in Catecholamine Research*. Almgren, O., Carlsson, A., Engel, J. (eds.). Amsterdam: North Holland Publishing, 1975.

80. Lal, H., Brown, W., Drawbaugh, R., Hynes, M., Brown, G. Enhanced prolactin inhibition following chronic treatment with haloperidol. *Life Sci., 20*:101–106, 1977.

81. Hyttel, J. Endogenous levels and turnovers of catecholamines in mouse brain after repeated administration of haloperidol. *Psychopharmacologia, 36*:237–241, 1974.

82. Hyttel, J., Moller-Nielsen, I. Changes in catecholamine concentrations and synthesis rate in mouse brain during the "supersensitivity" phase after treatment with neuroleptic drugs. *J. Neurochem., 27*:313–315, 1976.

83. Kebabian, J.W., Greengard, P. Dopamine-sensitive adenylate cyclase: role in synaptic transmission. *Science, 174*:1346–1348, 1971.

84. Clement-Cormier, YC., Kebabian, J.W., Petzold, G.L., Breengard, P. Dopamine-sensitive adenylate cyclase in mammalian brain: a possible site of action of antipsychotic drugs. *Proc. Nat. Acad. Sci., 71*:1113–1117, 1974.

84. Von Voigtlander, P.F., Losey, E.G., Triezenberg, M. Increased sensitivity to dopaminergic agents after chronic neuroleptic treatment. *J. Pharmacol. Exp. Ther., 193*:88–94, 1975.

86. Heal, D.J., Green, A.R., Boullin, D., Grahame-Smith, D.G. Single and repeated administration of neuroleptic drugs to rats: effects on striatal dopamine-sensitive adenylate cyclase and locomotor activity produced by tranyl-cypromin and l-tryptophan or l-dopa. *Psychopharmacology, 49*:287–300, 1976.

87. Rotrosen, J., Friedman, E., Gershon, S. Striatal adenylate cyclase activity following reserpine and chronic chlorpromazine administration in rats. *Life Sci., 17*:563–568, 1976.

88. Iwatsubo, K., Clouet, D.H. Dopamine-sensitive adenylate cyclase of the caudate nucleus of rats treated with morphine or haloperidol. *Biochem. Pharmacology, 24*:1499–1503, 1975.

89. Friedhoff, A.J., Bonnet, K., Rosengarten, J. Reversal of two manifestations of dopamine receptor supersensitivity by administration of l-dopa. *Res. Commun. Chem. Pathol. Pharmacol., 16*:411–416, 1977.

90. Burt, D.R., Creese, I., Snyder, S.H. Antischizophrenic drugs: chronic treatment elevates dopamine receptor binding in brain. *Science, 196*:326–328, 1977.

91. Muller, P., Seeman, D. Brain neurotransmitter receptors after long-term haloperidol, dopamine acetylcholine, serotonin, noradrenergic and naloxone receptors. *Life Sci., 21*:1751–1758, 1977.

92. Meites, J. Catecholamines and prolactin secretion. In *Advances in Biochemical Psychopharmacology*, vol. 16. Costa, E., Costa, G.L. (eds.). New York: Raven Press, pp. 139–146, 1977.

93. MacLeod, R.M., Lehneyer, T.E. Studies on the mechanism of the dopamine-mediated inhibition of prolactin secretion. *Endocrinology, 94*:1077–1085, 1974.

94. Hokfelt, T., Fuxe, K. On the morphology and the neuroendocrine role of the hypothalamic catecholamine neurons. In *Brain-Endocrine Interaction, Median Emi-*

nence: Structure and Function. Knigge, K.M., Scott, D.E., Weindle, A. (eds.). Basel: Karger, pp. 181–223, 1972.

95. Horowski, R., Neymann, F., Graf, R.J. Influence of apomorphine hydrochloride dibutyryl-apomorphine and lysenyl on plasma prolactin concentration in the rat. *J. Pharm. Pharmacol., 27*:532–534, 1975.

96. Brown, W.A., Drawbaugh, R., Gianutsos, G., Lal, H., Brown, G.M. Effect of apomorphine on serum prolactin level in the male rat. *Res. Commun. Chem. Pathol. Pharmacol., 4*:671–674, 1975.

97. Ravitz, A.J., Moore, K.E. Lack of effect of chronic haloperidol administration on the prolactin-lowering actions of piribedil. *J. Pharm. Pharmacol., 29*:384–386, 1977.

98. Ettigi, P., Nair, N.V.P., Lal, H., Cervantes, P., Guyda, H. Effect of apomorphine on growth hormone and prolactin secretion in schizophrenic patients, with or without oral dyskinesia, withdrawn from chronic neuroleptic therapy. *J. Neurol. Neurosurg. Psychiatry, 39*:870–876, 1976.

99. Ferris, R.M., Tang, F.L., Russell, A.V. Effects of apomorphine in vitro of the uptake and release of catecholamines in crude synaptosomal preparations of rat striatum and hypothalamus. *Biochem. Pharmacology, 24*:1523–1527, 1975.

100. Besson, M.J., Cheramy, A., Feltz, P., Glowinski, J. Release of newly synthesized dopamine from dopamine containing terminals in the striatum of the rat. *Proc. Nat. Acad. Sci., 62*:741–748, 1969.

101. Chiueh, C.C., Moore, K.K. Release of endogenously synthesized catechols from the caudate nucleus by stimulation of the nigrostriatal pathway and by the administration of d-amphetamine. *Brain Res., 50*:221–225, 1973.

102. Coyle, J.T., Snyder, S.K. Catecholamine uptake by synaptosomes in homogenates of rat brain: stereospecificity in different areas. *J. Pharmacol. Exp. Ther., 170*:221–231, 1969.

103. Lal, H., O'Brien, J., Puri, S.K. Morphine-withdrawal aggression: sensitization by amphetamines. *Psychopharmacologia, 22*:217–223, 1971.

104. Davis, J.M., Janowsky, D.S. Amphetamine and methylphenidate psychosis. In *Frontiers in Catecholamine Research.* Usdin, E., Snyder, S.H. (eds.). New York: Pergamon Press, pp. 977, 1973.

105. Modell, W., Hussar, A.E. Failure of dextroamphetamine sulfate to influence eating and sleeping patterns in obese schizophrenic patients. *JAMA, 19*:275–278, 1965.

106. Kornetsky, C. Hyporesponsitivity of chronic schizophrenic patients to dextro-amphetamine. *Arch. Gen. Psychiatry, 33*:1426, 1976.

6

Behavioral and Biochemical Effects of Chronic Neuroleptic Drugs: Interaction with Age

ROBERT C. SMITH
and D.E. LEELAVATHI

The hypothesis that one of the pathophysiological mechanisms underlying the syndrome of tardive dyskinesia in man involves a supersensitivity in the brain dopaminergic system (1) was derived partly from animal experiments. These studies, done in several laboratories, have provided behavioral and biochemical evidence for supersensitivity of presumed postsynaptic dopamine receptors in the brain after termination of treatment with chronic neuroleptic drugs in rats, mice and monkeys. This chapter will review some of the evidence that our own laboratory has collected about the effects of chronic neuroleptic drugs in rats, and will discuss the relevance of these animal models for the pathophysiology of tardive dyskinesia in man. In addition it will focus on recent work from our laboratory, which indicates that chronic treatment with neuroleptic drugs may also have important effects on biochemical processes in the presynaptic neuron, and on the interaction of age with the effects of chronic administration of neuroleptics.

EXPERIMENTAL RESULTS

Behavioral Evidence for Supersensitivity

We have shown that compared to saline controls, rats terminated from chronic administration of several neuroleptic drugs exhibit increased stereotyped behavior when they were given a direct-acting dopamine agonist, apomorphine, or indirect-acting dopamine agonist, amphetamine. This effect was found after 6–8 weeks of administration of several doses of haloperidol (ranging from 1 mg/kg to 5 mg/kg rat in different experiments), which is a potent blocker of dopamine receptors in the striatum (Fig. 1). However, it was also present in rats terminated from treatment with relatively high doses of thioridazine (20 mg/kg) and clozapine (25 mg/kg) (see Fig. 2). These drugs are considerably less potent blockers of dopamine receptors (2,3), and compared to haloperidol, these drugs have been reported to have a greater potency of affecting dopamine turnover in the limbic areas of the brain as compared to the striatum (4). In the Sprague-Dawley rats that we used in these initial experiments, the increased behavioral response to apomorphine usually peaked about 1 week after termination of neuroleptic administration and dissipated by 3 to 4 weeks after drug termination (Fig. 3).

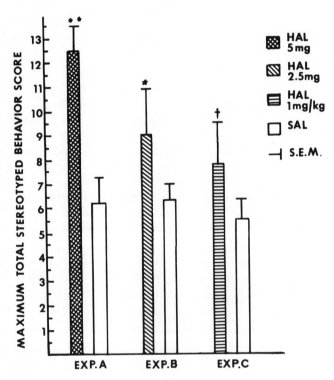

Figure 1.   The effects of apomorphine and amphetamine on stereotyped behavior in rats terminated from 6 to 8 weeks of chronic administration of one of several doses of haloperidol.
   a. The effects of apomorphine (1 mg/kg i.p.) on maximal stereotyped behavior during 60 minutes after drug administration in chronic haloperidol or saline control groups in 3 different experiments. Rats were administered apomorphine 6 or 7 days after termination of chronic administration of haloperidol or saline. Each bar graph represents the mean (± s.e.m.) of values based on 8 to 12 rats.

Concomitant treatment with other drugs may modify the behavioral super-sensitivity developed after chronic administration of neuroleptics. Rats administered benzotropine mesylate (1 mg/kg) together with haloperidol over a 2-month period showed a less marked supersensitivity to apomorphine (i.e., less severe stereotyped behavior) than rats administered haloperidol alone (Fig. 4). This apparent protective effect of benzotropine mesylate may be due to the biochemical effects of the drug on inhibiting dopamine uptake (5,6), and as a consequence, on increasing the functionally available dopamine in the synaptic cleft; this may partially antagonize the dopamine-receptor blockade produced by haloperidol. Since other studies (7) have shown that the concomitant administration of atropine together with chlorpromazine did not reduce the behavioral supersensitivity to apomorphine, it is less likely that this

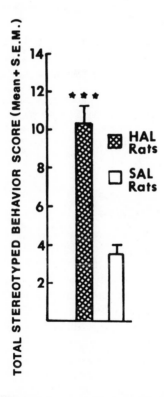

b. Effects of 1-amphetamine (5 mg/kg i.p.) on stereotyped behavior 5 days after termination of chronic haloperidol (5 mg/rat/day) or saline injections. Rats were scored for stereotyped behavior 15 to 60 minutes postamphetamine injection, and scores were *summed* for all time points. Each bar graph represents the mean (± s.e.m.) of 8 to 10 rats.

Statistical significance, compared to saline controls, analyzed by 2 sample t-test or LSD test after one-way analysis of variance are *** $p < .001$, ** $p < .05$ * $p < .01$, † $p < .10$.

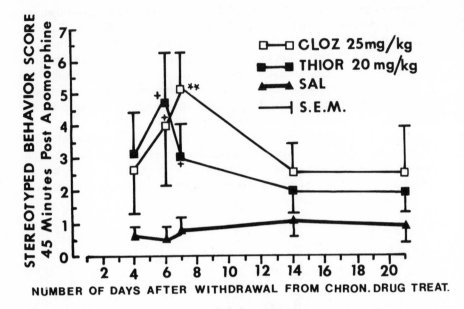

Figure 2.   The effect of apomorphine on stereotyped behavior at various times after termination of 7 weeks of chronic administration of clozapine (CLOZ 25 mg/kg/day), thioridazine (THIOR 20 mg/kg/day), or saline. Each point represents the mean ($\pm$ s.e.m.) of 8 to 12 rats. Symbols representing statistical significance of chronic drug versus saline control rats are indicated for each particular testing day. For interpretation of significance levels, see legend to Figure 1.

apparent protective effect of benzotropine mesylate is due to the anticholinergic properties that the drug also possesses. The behavioral supersensitivity induced by reserpine, a drug which depletes catecholamines, in mice is partially antagonized by the concomitant administration of L-dopa, which would also increase the functionally available dopamine (8).

In most of these experiments, both our own and those reported by other investigators (9,10), rats treated with chronic neuroleptic drugs did not exhibit *spontaneous* stereotyped behavior or other movement abnormalities either during administration or after the termination of chronic neuroleptic drugs, but only showed increased effects of dopamine agonists on evoking this behavior. At the very high dose of haloperidol (5 mg/rat/day) used in our initial experiment (11), some of the haloperidol rats did show spontaneous stereotyped behavior as well as apparent myoclonic seizures during the weeks they were receiving haloperidol, but they did not show spontaneous stereotyped behavior after the cessation of haloperidol. In recent series of experiments, however, in which we utilized Fisher 344 rats, we were able to observe another type of activity—mouthing and teeth-gnawing behavior—which occurred to a greater extent in rats receiving chronic neuroleptics than in saline controls; this

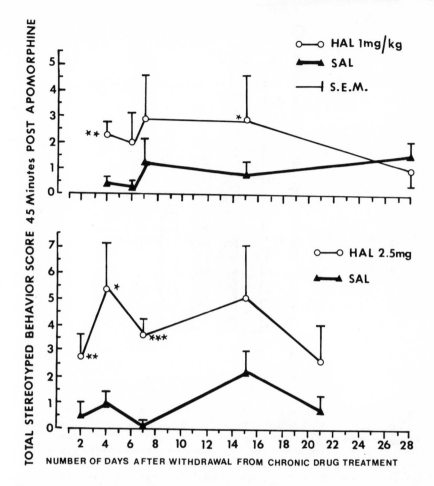

Figure 3. Persistence of behavioral supersensitivity to apomorphine for several weeks after termination of chronic (6–8 weeks) administration of 2 doses of haloperidol. Each point represents mean (± s.e.m.) based on 6 to 12 rats. For interpretation of statistical significance and other details see legends to Figures 1 and 2.

occurred during as well as after termination of chronic haloperidol or fluphenazine (see Fig. 5). On a phenomenological basis these mouthing movements may be similar to some of the oral-buccal symptoms in patients with tardive dyskinesia.

Biochemical Evidence for Dopaminergic Supersensitivity

In our biochemical studies we have used the effect of apomorphine on homovanillic acid (HVA) in rat caudate to investigate biochemical evidence

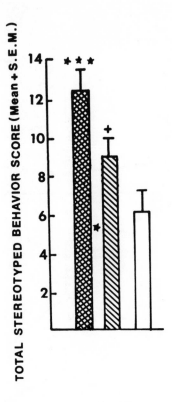

Figure 4.   The effects of chronic administration of benzotropine mesylate (BENZ 1 mg/kg/day), together with haloperidol (HAL 5 mg/rat/day), on attenuation behavioral super-sensitivity to apomorphine after termination of chronic administration of neuroleptics. Apomorphine (1 mg/kg) was administered 7 days after termination of each of the 3 chronic treatments. Each bar graph represents mean (± s.e.m.) based on 8 to 10 rats in the group.

   Symbols (*,†) above the bar indicate significant differences between the chronic drug group and the saline control group, and similar symbols between the 2 bar graphs indicate significant differences between the HAL and HAL + BENZ group. For interpretation of levels of statistical significance, see legends to Figures 1 and 2.

for postsynaptic supersensitivity of dopamine receptors after termination of chronic neuroleptic drugs. Apomorphine has been shown to cause a decrease in dopamine synthesis and turnover in rats; it decreases brain HVA, a metabolite of dopamine (12,13). This effect of apomorphine on striatal HVA is believed to be mediated primarily through indirect inhibition of dopamine synthesis in the presynaptic striatal dopaminergic neuron; this occurs via an interneuronal feedback loop from the postsynaptic neuron which is activated when apomorphine directly stimulates postsynaptic dopamine receptors. Recent research (14,15) has also indicated apomorphine may decrease dopamine synthesis by direct action on presynaptic dopamine neurons and receptors,

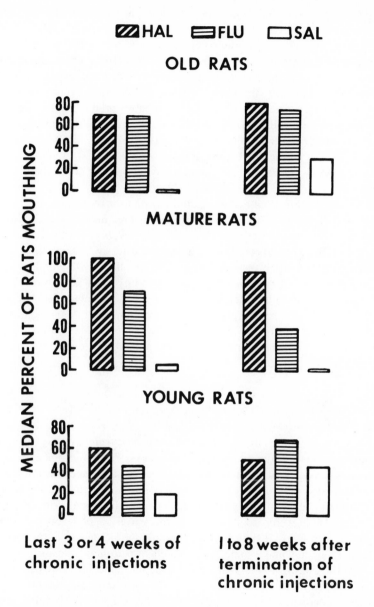

Figure 5. Percent of rats in each chronic administration group (n = 10–14 rats per group) who showed mouthing behavior during and/or after termination of chronic administration of haloperidol, fluphenazine, or saline. Each bar graph represents median percent averaged over several weeks of observation.

whose stimulation also inhibits tyrosine hydroxylase activity. The behavioral and biochemical effects of apomorphine which are attributable to its direct effects on presynaptic dopamine receptors may be the predominant effects of the drug at very low doses (i.e., .05—.10 mg/kg). However, at higher doses, such as 1 mg/kg apomorphine used in our biochemical experiments with chronic neuroleptic rats, the behavioral and biochemical effects of apomorphine on dopaminergic mechanisms are probably predominantly due to its direct stimulation of postsynaptic dopamine receptor. If the dopamine receptors of rats withdrawn from chronic neuroleptic treatment were supersensitive, then one would predict that apomorphine would have a greater effect on decreasing HVA in rats treated with chronic neuroleptic drugs than in saline controls.

Our results do show that one week after termination of the administration of chronic neuroleptics, rats who had been administered haloperidol (2.5 mg/rat) of clozapine (20 mg/kg) had considerably lower levels of HVA after apomorphine than saline controls (Fig. 6). The greater effectiveness of apomorphine in reducing HVA after termination of chronic haloperidol and clozapine provides biochemical evidence for supersensitivity of dopamine receptors in these rats. More direct evidence for supersensitivity comes from receptor-binding assays, which is presented in other chapters in this volume (see Chapters 10-13). Suprisingly, rats withdrawn from chronic administration of thioridazine did not show a greater effect of apomorphine on decreasing HVA than their saline controls.

Age and the Effects of Chronic Neuroleptic Drugs

Almost all the studies of the effects of chronic neuroleptic drugs in animals have utilized fairly young rats, mice, or monkeys. Epidemiological evidence, however, strongly indicates that the prevalence of tardive dyskinesia is definitely associated with old age, and that only in the older age group is there a fairly large incidence of tardive dyskinesia in patients treated with neuroleptic drugs (see Table 1 for an example of the variation of tardive dyskinesia symptoms with age). It may be that some of the processes associated with neuronal aging may make some of the effects of neuroleptic drugs more toxic, and, therefore, aging animals may provide better models for studying some of the pathophysiological processes associated with tardive dyskinesia.

We have begun to examine some of the effects of age on the biochemical and behavioral effects of chronic neuroleptic administration in rats. In these experiments we have utilized Fisher 344 rats (Charles River, NIA aging stock). At the beginning of our experiments, the three age groups of rats we used were about 2 months, 10 months, and 20 months of age, respectively. Initially, all three age groups of rats were tested for the stereotypy inducing effects of

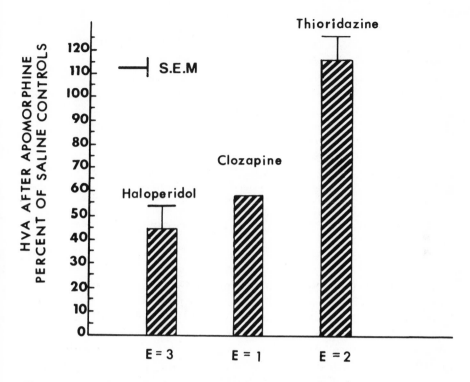

Figure 6.   Prior treatment with chronic neuroleptics increases the effect of apomorphine on decreasing striatal HVA.

Apomorphine (1 mg/kg) was administered to rats 6–7 days after termination of 6–8 week course of chronic neuroleptic or saline administration. Rats were sacrificed 45 minutes after apomorphine administration. Each bar graph represents mean percent (± s.e.m.) of striatal HVA levels in chronic neuroleptic rats compared to saline controls. E = number of separate *experiments*. In each experiment there were 1 or 2 groups of rats which previously received chronic neuroleptic drugs, as well as the saline control group. Each drug or saline group in each experiment had an N of 6 to 12 rats. HVA levels were analyzed separately in each striatum of each rat using GC-MS techniques.

apomorphine and d-amphetamine. After completion of these behavioral tests, the rats were begun on chronic injections of haloperidol and fluphenazine (starting at a dose of 1 mg/kg and increasing to 5 mg/kg) for a 2-month period. After termination of chronic neuroleptic administration, rats were retested with apomorphine at several time points over the following 8 weeks.

On the initial (preneuroleptic) testing, 20-month-old rats showed greater stereotypic and gnawing behavior after receiving the directly acting dopamine agonist apomorphine (1 mg/kg) and the indirectly acting dopamine agonist d-amphetamine (3.5 mg/kg) than the 2-month-old rats; the 10-month-old rats

Table 1
Relationship of Age to Prevalence of Tardive Dyskinesia

Percentage of Patients with Definite Oral-Buccal-Lingual Symptoms of Tardive Dyskinesia

Age	0–20	21–30	31–40	41–50	51–60	61+
Percent	0	3	5	19	24	34
(N)	(25)	(163)	(210)	(203)	(220)	(298)

N = total number of patients in age group. Statistics χ^2 = 107.49, df = 5, p< .001; χ^2 computed from actual number of patients in each cell and its companion, from which percentages shown in Table 1 were calculated. Data are from state survey in Illinois. Ratings were done using Smith Tardive Dyskinesia Scale.

usually fell between these two age groups (see Figs. 7 and 8). After termination of 2 months of treatment with haloperidol or fluphenazine, rats in all 3 age groups showed a greater stereotypic or gnawing response to 0.25 mg/kg apomorphine than age-matched saline controls (see Fig. 9). This increased response to apomorphine persisted over the full 2-month testing period. The greatest increase in gnawing behavior was seen in the youngest rats (who were 8–10 months of age during the time of postneuroleptic behavioral testing). The old-age group showed the smallest difference between drug and saline control rats because of the high baseline of stereotypic responsiveness to apomorphine in the old-age saline group. On the basis of absolute scores, however, the oldest (24–26 months) rats who had received chronic fluphenazine had slightly greater stereotypic scores during most weeks of testing than the youngest age group (see Fig. 10).

In another way fluphenazine appeared to be fairly toxic to the old-age rats. At the 5 mg/kg dose of fluphenazine, old-age rats began to lose a great deal of weight and appeared more toxic. This weight loss was substantially greater than the weight loss of the old-age rats receiving haloperidol, or of younger rats chronically treated with either of the neuroleptic drugs (see Table 2). Because of this apparent toxicity of fluphenazine, the dosage of fluphenazine had to be reduced from 5 mg/kg to 2 mg/kg in the old-age rats (and also correspondingly in the two younger age groups, so as to keep the design balanced). The apparently greater toxicity of fluphenazine in the older age group, as well as the higher absolute level of stereotypic behavior in old-age rats withdrawn from fluphenazine, may have relevance to the toxic side effects of tardive dyskinesia seen in man. Recent drug history studies (see Chapters 25–30 in this volume) suggest that fluphenazine may be particularly toxic in regard to inducing this movement disorder in man.

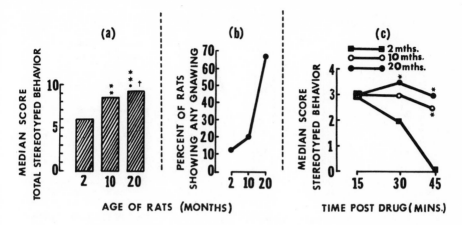

Figure 7.   Effects of apomorphine on gnawing or stereotyped behavior in young (2 months), mature (10 months), and old (20 months) rats. N = 24 rats in the two younger age groups, and 52 rats in the old-age group.

a.   Median stereotyped behavior score (sum of stereotyped behavior 15–45 minutes) after administration of apomorphine (1 mg/kg i.p.). There was a significant age effect on stereotyped behavior as shown by Kruskal-Wallis analysis of variance (Ho = 28.2, df = 2,p < .001).

b.   Percent of rats showing gnawing behavior at any time during 45 minutes after administration of apomorphine. Significant overall effect of age was shown by x^2 test (x^2 = 5.98, df = 2, p = .05). Difference between median scores of any two specific age groups were assessed in (a) and (c), the Dunn procedure. Statistical significance between 2-month-old and any other age group is as follows: * p < .05, ** p < .01, *** p < .001; between 20-month and 10-month-old rats: † p < .05, †† p< .01.

Biochemical Effects in the Presynaptic Neuron

Most research on the effects of chronic neuroleptic drugs has focused on changes related to the postsynaptic neurons or receptors in the striatum, and research on possible changes in the neurochemistry of presynaptic neurons, either during administration or after termination of chronic neuroleptics, has been relatively neglected. Preliminary results from our biochemical experiments with the Fisher rats indicate that chronic administration of neuroleptics may have an important effect on biochemical processes more readily localized in the presynaptic neurons. Following the behavioral experiments with the Fisher rats described above, these animals were reinjected with haloperidol (2 mg/kg) or fluphenazine (2 mg/kg) for a 4-week period. Seven days after termination of this second set of chronic neuroleptic injections, these rats were sacrificed for biochemical studies. (Some of the rats were given apomorphine, .25 mg/kg, 45 minutes before sacrifice, for the purpose of assessing the effects of dopamine agonists on HVA, although these results will not be reported here.)

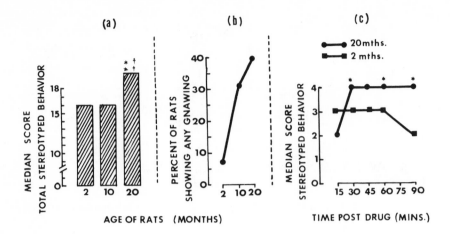

Figure 8.   Effects of d-amphetamine (3.5 mg/kg) on stereotyped behavior and gnawing in young, mature, and old rats.

   a. Median total stereotyped behavior 15–90 minutes after d-amphetamine administration. There was a significant overall effect (p < .001) by Kruskal-Wallis ANOV.

   b. Percent of rats showing any gnawing behavior during 90 minutes after administration of d-amphetamine. Overall age effects were significant by x^2 test (p < .02).

   c. Time course of stereotyped behavior after administration of d-amphetamine. For interpretation of symbols indicatins statistical significance between groups see legend to Figure 7.

In vitro studies of the uptake of ^{3}H-NE and ^{3}H-DA in rat cortex were performed according to standard procedures previously described in detail (16,17,18). There were clear effects of both age and prior chronic neuroleptic administration on the uptake of ^{3}H-NE and ^{3}H-DA in crude synaptosomal preparations from rat cortex. Rats who were 28 months old had substantially lower uptake of NE and DA than rats in the two younger age groups. Rats withdrawn from chronic haloperidol or fluphenazine generally had increased uptake of NE and DA in cortex synaptosomes compared to age-matched saline controls (except for DA uptake in 28-month-old rats; see Figs. 11 and 12).

Monoamine oxidase (MAO) activity was also effected by age and prior chronic neuroleptic administration. MAO activity was determined in mitochondrial fractions from rat cortex, with ^{14}C-PEA and ^{14}C-5-HT as substrates, following the methods of Wurtman and White (19,20). In agreement with reports of several other research groups (21,22), MAO activity for both substrates increased with age (see Fig. 13). Seven days after termination of treatment with neuroleptic drugs, rats previously treated with haloperidol or fluphenazine generally had lower MAO activities than their age-matched saline controls. Rats 11 and 18 months of age at time of sacrifice who had been withdrawn from chronic haloperidol or fluphenazine generally had 40%–60% lower MAO activity against the PEA substrate than age-matched saline con-

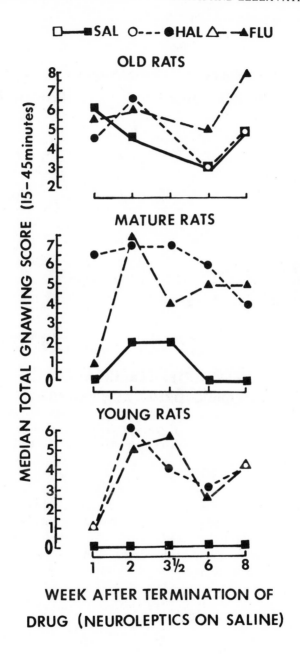

Figure 9. Gnawing behavior induced by apomorphine (0.25 mg/kg s.c.) in younger, middle-aged, and old-age rats terminated from 2 months of chronic administration of haloperidol, fluphenazine, or saline. Each point represents the median gnawing score at the indicated time after termination of chronic drug administration. (N = 10–13 rats in each group.)

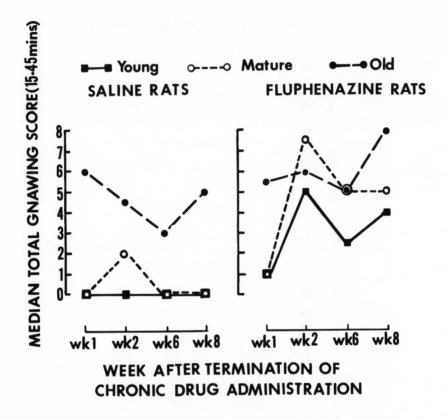

WEEK AFTER TERMINATION OF
CHRONIC DRUG ADMINISTRATION

Figure 10.   Older age rats show greater effects of apomorphine (.25 mg/kg) on stereotyped gnawing both in the chronic fluphenazine as well as the saline groups. For other details, see legend to Figure 9.

trols. The 28-month-old age group of rats, however, did not show any effect of chronic neuroleptic drugs on MAO activity using the PEA substrate, and overall, they had the highest MAO activity of the three age groups. There was a somewhat smaller 10%–30% decrease in MAO activity with the serotonin substrate in all three age groups of rats withdrawn from chronic neuroleptics (see Figs. 14 and 15).

DISCUSSION

The results of our studies clearly show that chronic administration of neuroleptics to rats produces behavioral and biochemical changes during the withdrawal period which indicate supersensitivity of postsynaptic dopamine

Table 2
Effects of Chronic Administration of Fluphenazine, Haloperidol, or Saline on Rat Weights

Drug Group	Week of Chronic Drug Administration			Week after Termination of Drug Administration	
	1	7	8	2	6
			Youngest Age Rats		
Fluphenazine	310 ± 6	267 ± 4 (−14%)	277 ± 5 (−11%)	300 ± 5 (−3%)	329 ± 6 (+6%)
Haloperidol	319 ± 8	297 ± 8 (−7%)	294 ± 8 (−8%)	311 ± 8 (−3%)	323 ± 8 (+1%)
Saline	308 ± 3	341 ± 4 (+11%)	347 ± 4 (+12%)	343 ± 4 (+11%)	350 ± 5 (+14%)
			Old Age Rats		
Fluphenazine	411 ± 10	261 ± 8 (−36%)	292 ± 7 (−29%)	344 ± 12 (−16%)	373 ± 10 (−9%)
Haloperidol	422 ± 11	347 ± 9 (−18%)	356 ± 9 (−16%)	378 ± 8 (−10%)	389 ± 9 (−8%)
Saline	415 ± 7	409 ± 7 (−10%)	423 ± 7 (+2%)	398 ± 9 (−4%)	387 ± 7 (−7%)

Each number represents mean ± s.e.m. of weights of 11 to 14 rats in a treatment group. Number in parentheses is percent increase (+) or decrease (−) in mean weights compared to the weight of the same group in week 1. Beginning in week 7, dose of fluphenazine was reduced from 5 mg/kg/day to 2 mg/kg/day. Dose of haloperidol was maintained at 5 mg/kg/ for the final 2 weeks of chronic drug administration.

receptors. What is the relevance of these and our other findings about the effect of chronic neuroleptics in the rat to the pathogenesis of the abnormal movements of tardive dyskinesia in man, a disorder which is increasingly being seen in patients who receive neuroleptic drugs for months or years? Several points relevant to these questions are discussed below.

Clinical Validity of the Supersensitivity Hypothesis for Tardive Dyskinesia in Man

On the basis of clinical evidence, is a dopamine supersensitivity model relevant to tardive dyskinesia in man? Some clinical experiments in patients with tardive dyskinesia provide support for the supersensitivity hypothesis. Administration of indirectly acting dopamine agonists, such as L-dopa (23) or amphetamine (24), which would stimulate supersensitive dopamine receptors, have been reported to increase dyskinetic symptoms in patients with tardive

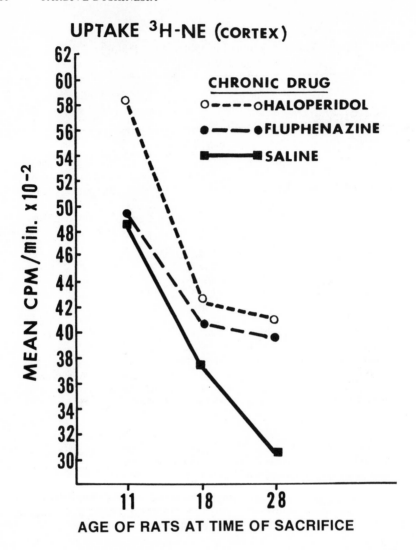

Figure 11.   Effects of age and prior administration of chronic neuroleptics on uptake of ^{3}H-NE in crude synaptosomal preparations from rat cortex. Rats were sacrificed 7 days after termination of chronic neuroleptic or saline administration.

UPTAKE ³H-DOPAMINE (CORTEX)

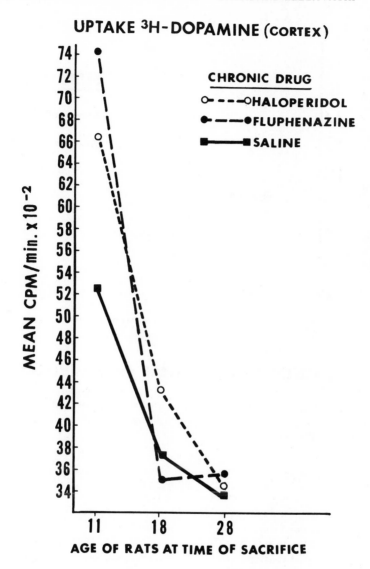

CHRONIC DRUG

O- - - -OHALOPERIDOL
●- - - -●FLUPHENAZINE
■————■SALINE

MEAN CPM/min. x10⁻²

AGE OF RATS AT TIME OF SACRIFICE

Figure 12.   Effects of age and prior chronic neuroleptic administration on ³H-DA uptake in crude synaptosomal preparations from rat cortex. See legend to Figure 11 for additional details.

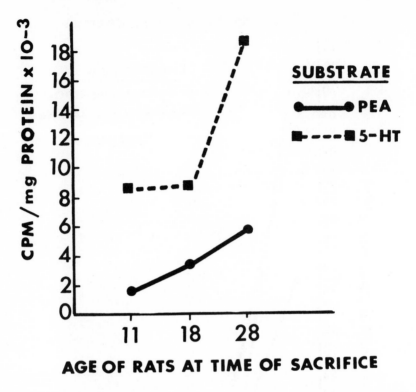

Figure 13.   Effects of age on MAO activity in mitochondrial preparation from rat cortex. Rats were sacrificed 7 days after termination of chronic saline administration. Only values of saline control rats are represented in this figure.

dyskinesia, whereas administration of neuroleptic drugs, which would reblock supersensitive dopamine receptors, often reduces or temporarily eliminates symptoms of tardive dyskinesia (25). Two recent reports (24,26), however, indicate that usual clinical doses of apomorphine may reduce rather than exacerbate symptoms of tardive dyskinesia. Gunne and Barney (see Chapter 1) have also reported that apomorphine reduced dyskinetic symptoms in their monkey model of tardive dyskinesia. Since apomorphine is the dopamine agonist drug which has been most frequently used in the experiments in rats and mice to assess the behavioral effects of chronic neuroleptics, the apparently dissimilar results in the human experiments suggest a lack of one-to-one analogy between the movement disorders produced by chronic neuroleptics in rat and man. However, since a relatively low dose of apomorphine was used in these human studies (.02–.12 mg/kg), compared to the doses used in the animal experiments (.25–1.0 mg/kg), it is possible that higher doses of apomorphine might have produced an increase of dyskinetic symptoms in

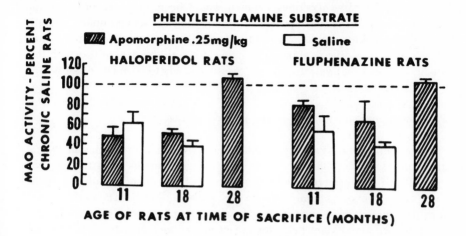

Figure 14.   Interaction of age and prior chronic treatment with neuroleptics on MAO activity to phenylthylamine (PEA) substrate. Each bar graph represents MAO activity in chronic haloperidol or chronic fluphenazine rats as mean percent (± s.e.m.) of the values in age-matched saline control rats. Rats were sacrificed 7–9 days after termination of chronic neuroleptic or chronic saline administration. Some rats received apomorphine (.25 mg/kg) 45 minutes before sacrifice and others received saline injection before sacrifice.

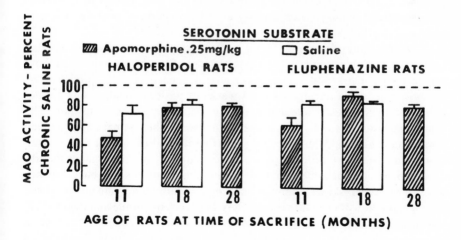

Figure 15.   Interaction of age and prior administration of chronic neuroleptics on MAO activity to serotonin substrate. For details, see legend to Figure 14.

patients with tardive dyskinesia which would be more in accord with the behavioral supersensitivity produced by this drug in rats and mice. Overall, there is some clinical evidence that the dopamine supersensitivity model may be relevant to tardive dyskinesia in man, although the degree to which this model applies to all varieties of the disorder needs to be further assessed.

Phenomenological Similarities and Choice of Species

Is the behavioral syndrome produced by chronic neuroleptics in the rat analogous in important respects to that seen in patients with tardive dyskinesia? Although stereotyped behavior in rats is not phenomenologically the same as the symptoms of tardive dyskinesia in man, they both consist of jerky, repetitive movements, and they may have similar pharmacological mediation. Increases in stereotyped behavior are primarily mediated by dopaminergic influences in the nigrostriatal system (27,28), and the movements of tardive dyskinesia probably represent pathophysiological mechanisms in the nigrostriatal system in man. Two important differences between the phenomena in the rat and tardive dyskinesia in man are that (a) in the rat model, the increases in the stereotyped behavior after termination of neuroleptics have usually not been reported to occur spontaneously, but are seen only after administration of dopamine agonists, such as apomorphine or amphetamine; and (b) the increase in stereotyped behavior that has usually been reported is fairly short-lived, peaking about 7 days after termination of chronic neuroleptics and often lasting less than 3 to 4 weeks in the Sprague-Dawley rats. The symptoms of tardive dyskinesia, on the other hand, occur without the provocation of dopamine agonist, often increase spontaneously after termination of neuroleptics, and can last indefinitely.

However, some of our more recent studies reported in this chapter show that some strains of rats may provide a better model of tardive dyskinesia in those respects. In Fisher 344 rats the behavioral supersensitivity produced by apomorphine lasted throughout the 8 weeks of postdrug testing, and did not appear to be markedly attenuated during the latter weeks of testing. The 2-month testing period in the lifespan of the rat may be comparable to a much longer time period in human aging. Furthermore, Fisher rats treated with chronic neuroleptics did develop a greater frequency of spontaneous mouthings, a behavior phenomenologically more similar to the oral-buccal symptoms of tardive dyskinesia in man, and these mouthing movements persisted after termination of chronic neuroleptics. The work of Gunne and Barany (29) has also shown that one species of monkeys, Cebus appella, develops a syndrome which more closely resembles, both phenomenologically and pharmacologically, that of tardive dyskinesia in man when these monkeys are administered haloperidol chronically, as compared to the syndrome developed in several other species of monkeys. These results point to the fact that strain or species differences may be one important factor in choosing the most appropriate animal for investigating the behavioral and biochemical pathophysiology of tardive dyskinesia.

Age Effects in Animal Models

Our results have shown that old-aged rats are more sensitive to the stereotypic inducing effects of dopamine agonists—i.e., they had a higher "baseline" response to the drugs even before chronic neuroleptic treatment. Subsequent chronic administration of neuroleptics brought the level of gnawing response to apomorphine in the youngest age group of neuroleptic-treated rats up to or above the level of saline control group of the old-age rats. The two older age groups of rats treated with fluphenazine, however, did tend to have higher absolute gnawing scores after apomorphine than the younger rats. The phenomenon in the rats may represent increases in the sensitivity of dopamine neurons or receptors which occur with age. If analogous increases in sensitivity also occur in man, then one could speculate that these behavioral results from our rat studies might provide the one clue to help explain the greater susceptibility of older age patients to tardive dyskinesia, using the rationale of a dopamine supersensitivity hypothesis of tardive dyskinesia. For example, a certain level of sensitivity to dopamine or dopamine agonists may be required to "trigger" the expression of tardive dyskinesia in man. If this were true, then older age patients might need less of an increase in sensitivity of their dopamine receptors (which is a consequence of chronic treatment with neuroleptics) to reach a critical level for the expression of these pathophysiological changes in dyskinetic movements. Even if, on the average, older patients showed only a slightly greater increase in sensitivity to dopamine or dopamine agonists after chronic treatment with neuroleptics as compared to young patients, this small difference might be enough to push more of the older patients over the threshold for dyskinetic response.

However, because the pharmacological mechanisms underlying these increased responses to dopamine agonists in old-age rats have not been determined, and because the analogous experimental pharmacological results in man have not been reported, our speculations about the implications of our behavioral results in old-age rats should be regarded as quite preliminary. These speculations are based on the idea that increased behavioral responses to dopamine agonists in old-age rats indicate a supersensitivity (i.e., an increase in number or affinity) of some postsynaptic dopamine receptors. However, biochemical evidence for an increase in number or affinity of brain dopamine receptors in old age has not been reported. On the contrary, some recent reports dealing with another receptor—the β-adrenergic receptor—indicate that the number of these receptors on peripheral cells in mouse and man, and also in mouse brain decrease rather than increase with age (30,31). Furthermore, it is also possible that the increased behavioral responses to apomorphine and amphetamine in our old-age rats are not mediated primarily by changes in receptor sensitivity, but may be due to decreased metabolism of these drugs in older animals. Several recent reviews of pharmacokinetics in the aged have indicated that older age is associated with slower metabolism or elimination of some drugs in both animals and man (32,33). One study (34) has reported no difference in brain levels of d-amphetamine in old-age gerbils, who also had shown a greater behavioral responsiveness to this drug, than in younger age gerbils, but preliminary results from other laboratories (35) reported increased brain levels of d-amphetamine in old age as compared to younger Wistar rats. There are no published studies of brain levels or metabolism of apomorphine in young rats as compared to very old rats or mice. If decreases in drug metabolism rather than increases in sensitivity were the main cause of the increased response to dopamine agonists seen in old-age rats, this would not support the pharmacological basis of our speculative hypothesis regarding old age and tardive dyskinesia.

Biochemical Changes in the Pre-Synaptic Neuron

Most biochemical research in animal models relevant to tardive dyskinesia has dealt with biochemical measures, such as changes in receptor binding or effects of apomorphine on HVA, adenyl cyclase, or dopamine turnover, which are more directly relevant to the supersensitivity of postsynaptic receptors. The results reported in this chapter show that chronic administration of neuroleptics may also produce biochemical changes in processes localized in the presynaptic neuron or receptor. The relevance of changes that we reported in MAO activity and reuptake of biogenic amines to the pathophysiology of tardive dyskinesia in man remains to be explored, but our results do indicate that more attention should be directed to changes in the functioning of presynaptic neurons or receptors after termination of chronic administration of neuroleptic drugs.

ACKNOWLEDGMENTS

Supported in part by NIA Grant 1 R23 AG00725-01 to Dr. Robert Smith.

REFERENCES

1. Rubovits, R., Klawans, H.L. Implications of amphetamine-induced stereotyped behavior as a model for tardive dyskinesia. *Arch. Gen. Psychiatry, 27*:502–507, 1972.
2. Burt, D.R., Cresse, I., Snyder, S. Dopamine receptor binding predicts clinical and pharmacological potencies of anti-schizophrenic drugs. *Science, 192*:481–485, 1970.

3.   Anden, H.E., Stock, G. Effect of clozapine in turnover of dopamine in corpus striatum and in limbic system. *J. Pharm. Pharmacol., 25*:346–348, 1973.

4.   Zivkovic, B., Guidotti, A., Rurvellta, A., Costa, E. Effects of thioridazine, clozapine, and other anti-psychotics on the kinetic state of tyrosine hydroxylase in striatum and nucleus accumbens. *J. Pharm. Exptl. Ther., 194*:37–46, 1976.

5.   Fuxe, K., Goldstein, M., Ljungdohol, ?., Antiparkinsonian drugs and central dopamine receptors. *Life Sci., 9*:811–824, 1970.

6.   Coyle, J.T., Snyder, S.H. Antiparkinsonian drugs: inhibition of dopamine uptake in corpus straitum as a possible mechanism of action. *Science, 166*:899–901, 1969.

7.   Tarsy, D., Baldessarini, R.J. Behavioral supersensitivity to apomorphine following chronic treatment with drugs which interfere with the synaptic function of catecholamines. *Neuropharmacology, 13*:927–940, 1974.

8.   Gudelsky, G.A., Thornburg, J.E., Moore, K.E. Blockade of 2-methyl paratyrosine induced supersensitivity to apomorphine by chronic administration of L-dopa. *Life Sci., 16*:1331–1339, 1975.

9.   Dianutsos, G., Drabargh, R., Hynes, M. Behavioral evidence of dopaminergic supersensitivity after chronic haloperidol. *Life Sci., 14*:887–898, 1974.

10. Sayers, A.C., Birki, H.R., Ruch, W., Asper, H. Animal models of dyskinesia: effects of thioridazine. *Pharmakopsychiatry, 10*:291–295.

11. Smith, R.C., Davis, J.M. Behavioral supersensitivity to apomorphine and amphetamine after chronic high-dose haloperidol treatment. *Psychopharma: Comm., 1*:285–293, 1975.

12. Roos, B.E. Decrease in homovanillic acid as evidence for dopamine receptor stimulation by apomorphine in the neostriatum of the rat. *J. Pharm. Pharmacol., 21*:263–264, 1969.

13. Kehr, W., Carlsson, A., Lindquist, M. Evidence for receptor mediated control of striatal tyrosine hydroxylase. *J. Pharm. Pharmacol., 24*:744–747, 1972.

14. Walters, J.R., Bunney, B.S., Roth, R.H. Piribedil and apomorphine. pre- and post-synaptic effects on dopamine synthesis and neurological activity. In *Advances in Neurology*, vol. 9. Calne, D.B., Chase, T.N., Barbeau, A. (eds.). New York: Raven Press, pp. 273–284, 1975.

15. Carlsson, A. Receptor mediated control of dopamine metabolism. In *Pre- and Postsynaptic Receptors.* Usdin, E., Bunney, W.E. (eds.). New York: Dekker, pp. 49–65, 1975.

16. Smith, R.C., Meltzer, H.V., Arora, R.C., Davis, J.M. Effects of phencyclidine on ^{3}H-catecholamine and ^{3}H-serotonin uptake in synaptosomal preparations from rat brain. *Biochem. harm., 26*:1435–1439, 1977.

17. Colburn, R.W., Goodwin, F.K., Murphy, D., Bunney, W.E., Davis, J.M. Quantitative studies of norepinephrine uptake by synatosomes. *Biochem. Pharm., 17*:957–964, 1968.

18. Janowsky, D.S., Davis, J.M., Fann, W.E., Freeman, J., Nixon, R., Michelabis, A.A. Angiotensin effect on uptake of norepinephrine by synaptosomes. *Life Sci., 11*:1–11, 1972.

19. Wurtman, R.J., Axelrod, J. A sensitive and specific assay for the estimation of monoamine oxidase. *Biochem. Pharm., 12*:1439–1441, 1963.

20. White, H., Wu, Joyce. Multiple binding sites of human brain monoamine oxidase as indicated by substrate competition. *J. Neurochem., 25*:21–26, 1975.

21. Neis, A. Robinson, D.S., Davis, J.M., Ravaris, C. Changes in monoamine oxidase with aging in Eisdorter and Fann, (eds.)*Adv. in Behavioral Biology, vol. 9, Psychopharmacology of Aging,* New York: Plenum Press, 1973.

22. Shinsen, D.S., Davis, J.M., Neis, A. Relation of sex and aging to monoamine oxidase activity in human brain, plasma, and platlets. *Arch. Gen. Psychiatry, 24*:536–539, 1971.

23. Gerlach, J., Reisby, N., Randrup, A. Dopaminergic hypersensitivity and cholin3rgic hypofunction in the pathophysiology of tardive dyskinesia. *Psychopharmacology, 34*:21–35, 1974.

24. Smith, R.C., Tamminga, C., Haraszti, J., Pandey, G., Davis, J.M. Effects of dopamine agonists in tardive dyskinesia. *Am. J. Psychiatry, 134*:769–774, 1977.

25. Kazamatsuri, H., Chien, C.-P., Cole, J.O. Long-term treatment of tardive dyskinesia with haloperidol and tetrabenazine. *Am. J. Psychiatry, 130*:470–482, 1973.

26. Carroll, B.J., Curtis, G.C., Kokmen, E. Paradoxical response to dopamine agonists in tardive dyskinesia. *Am. J. Psychiatry, 134*:785–788, 1977.

27. Cools, A.R., Van Rossum, J.M. Caudal dopamine and stereotyped behaviora in the cat. *Arch. nt. Pharmacodyn., 187*:163–173, 1977.

28. Fog, R. Stereotypy and catalepsy: studies of the effects of amphetamines and neuroleptics in rats. *Acta Neurol. Scand. Suppl., 50*:11–65.

29. Gunne, L.M., Barany, S. Haloperidol induced dyskenesia in monkeys. *Psychopharmacology, 50*:237–240, 1976.

30. Bylund, B., Tellez-Inon, M.T., Hollenberg, M.D. Age-related parallel decline in beta adrenergic receptors, adenylate cyclase, and phosphodiesterase activity in rat erythrocyte membranes. *Life Sci., 21*:403–410, 1977.

31. Schocken, D.D., Roth, G.S. Reduced B-adrenergic receptor concentrations in aging man. *Nature, 27*:856–858, 1977.

32. Triggs, E.J., Natia, R.L. Pharmacokinetics in the aged: a review. *J. Pharmacol. and Biopharmacol., 3*:387–418, 1977.

33. Crooks, J., O'Malley, K., Stevenson, I.H. Pharmacokinetics in the elderly. *Clin. Pharmacokinetics, 1*:280–296, 1976.

34. Tanner, R.H., Domino, E.F. Exaggerated response to (+) amphetamine in geriatric gerbils. *Gerontology, 23*:165–173, 1977.

7

Anatomical and Metabolic Changes after Long and Short-Term Treatment with Perphenazine in Rats

RASMUS FOG
and H. PAKKENBERG

Tardive dyskinesia is an increasing problem in neuroleptic treatment of psychiatric disorders. Symptoms seem to increase in severity with continued use of drugs (1,2). Tardive dyskinesia may be an irreversible syndrome, and it has therefore been attributed to a possible neurotoxic effect of neuroleptics.

An extensive literature exists on the effect of chlorpromazine on the animal brain following long-term administration (3). A series of changes in the brain have been described, including "degeneration" of nerve cells, satellitosis, neuronophagia, vascular changes, and minor haemorrhages (4, 5, 6, 7). On the other hand, only a few investigators have studied the long-term effect of promazine derivatives on the brain. Romasenko and Jacobson (8) administered trifluoperazine to rats in doses up to 250 mg/kg for up to 5 weeks. They found only small morphological changes, which were reversible. In the case of perphenazine, there are a few studies on cerebral changes. Grünthal and Walther-Büel (9) described pronounced cell changes in the inferior olive in a patient who had suffered from dyskinesia after the administration of perphenazine for 13 days. Nielsen and Lyon (10) found that this substance produced chromosome changes.

In an investigation (11), we tried to elucidate the long-term effect of perphenazine enanthate on the rat brain. The metabolism of nerve cells in the cortex and the basal ganglia was estimated by measuring the uptake of the nucleic acid precursor uridine and the amino acid lysine. Looking for anatomical changes, we counted the nerve cells in areas of the cortex and the basal ganglia. All investigations were made blind.

Perphenazine enanthate, 3, 4 mg/kg per injection, was administered sub-cutaneously to rats every second week over a period of a year, a total of 31 mg per animal being given. The animals were observed weekly, and only a few became cataleptic during brief periods. After treatment for one year, ^{3}H-uridine and ^{3}H-lysine were administered intravenously, and the labeling was studied by microautoradiography. Labeling of the cortical cells in the treated animals was found to be slightly greater than in the control animals. The converse was found in the basal ganglia in the case of uridine. None of these differences was significant.

In counting nerve cells in the cortex and the basal ganglia, a significantly lower number of nerve cells was found in the basal ganglia in the treated group. A cell loss of approximately 20% was found (Table 1). No changes were found in the substantia nigra (12).

As a consequence of this finding, we performed a study (13), to determine whether the administration of perphenazine over a shorter period was able to influence the number of nerve cells (and also the uridine uptake) in the rat brain.

A similar experiment was carried out on rats using the same dosage, 3.4 mg/kg, every second week, but for a period of 1 and 2 months, respectively. There were 10 animals in both the control and treated groups. Five animals

Table 1

Number of nerve cells per unit area in 12 treated and 8 control animals. Each figure is the average of counts in 2 sections. The difference found in the basal ganglia is significant (p $<$ 0.005). (Pakkenberg et al., 1973.)

Cortex		Basal Ganglia	
Treated Animals	Controls	Treated Animals	Controls
864	1075	825	1112
1019	1057	834	951
1022	828	804	724
955	869	834	866
1018	767	714	818
1111	933	693	997
954	838	626	1012
964		780	772
916		659	
1030		725	
833		773	
901		682	
965.6	903.8	745.8	906.5
difference = 61.8	s.e. = 42.3	difference = −160.7	s.e. = 45.9

s.e. = Standard error. No significant differences.

from each of the 4 groups were given 2 mCi ^{3}H-uridine intravenously 1 hour prior to being sacrificed to perform autoradiographic studies of the uridine uptake in the nerve cells of the cortex and basal ganglia and in the cells of the liver. No significant difference was found in the uptake in either the 1- or 2-month group. No loss of cells was found following cell counts in the cortex and basal ganglia after relatively short-term treatment. The weight of the brain was similar in both the control and treated groups. All the studies were carried out blind.

In a third study (14), we looked for the effect of higher dosages. In this investigation a treatment period of 6 months and a ten-fold higher dose of perphenazine enanthate (40 mg/kg s.c. every second week) was used. No significant differences from control animals were found by cell counting in the basal ganglia and the cortex, by electron microscopy investigation of the same structures, or by quantitative immunoelectrophoresis of proteins from the corpus striatum and the cortex. The uptake of ^{3}H-uridine measured by autoradiography in the cortex and in the liver was, however, 20%–50% higher in the experimental group (Table 2), but these differences were not significant.

Our findings show that prolonged neuroleptic treatment with perphenazine in a dosage 10 times higher than the usual clinical dose over a treatment period of approximately one sixth of a rat's life did not result in any morphologic alterations of the neurons of the basal ganglia. The only change was an increased uptake of uridine in the cortical nerve cells. This result is difficult to interpret, and kinetic studies are required to clarify if this is a consequence of increased metabolism, decreased catabolism, or any other change in the synthesis of RNA.

The results of the cell count contrast with our earlier findings of a cell loss in the basal ganglia of about 20%. The dose then was lower and "clinical," but the treatment period was longer. Thus, the time factor might be of greater

Table 2
Autoradiography Study of Rat Brains after
Long-Term Treatment with Perphenazine
Enanthate (Fog *et al.*, 1976.)

	Cortex, Fifth Layer					Liver			
	Nuclei	s.e.	Cytoplasm	Neuropil	s.e.	Nuclei	s.e.	Cytoplasm	s.e.
Controls	910		15	38		688		54	
		160			16		148		8
Treated Rats	1323		20	45		923		42	

Total grain counts from 25 cells from rats injected with uridine 1 hour before sacrifice. Each number is an average of counts from 10 animals.

s.e. = standard error.   No significant differences.

importance than the dose level. Furthermore, the animals were younger (8 months old) when they were sacrificed in this investigation than they were in the earlier one (14 months old). If our earlier results are correlated with the clinical syndrome of tardive dyskinesia, they seem to be in accordance with the clinical findings that the neurotoxic effects of neuroleptics are seen mostly in elderly patients after many years of constant neuroleptic treatment (15).

In another investigation from our group (10), the number of nerve cells in two different areas of the corpus striatum (i.e., ventrolateral and dorsomedial) has been estimated in rat brain following long-term (36 weeks) treatment with a neuroleptic drug (flupenthixol). Nine rats were given weekly injections of 4 mg/kg flupenthixol dissolved in Viscoleo i.m., and 7 rats received the Viscoleo alone. Fourteen to 18 weeks after the last drug injection, the animals were decapitated, with half of each brain being fixated with formalin for cell-count analysis, and the remaining half used for a biochemical analysis. Separate cell counts in the ventrolateral and dorsomedial corpus striatum yielded a significant cell loss of approximately 10%, but only in the ventrolateral striatum of treated animals. These results suggest at least one concrete anatomical basis for the behavioral and biochemical deficits found in the same animals, as reported earlier. The results further suggest that persistent irreversible anatomical changes can follow long-term neuroleptic treatment.

We are now revising our earlier studies, looking for anatomical changes by counting nerve cells in different areas of the basal ganglia; and we have started a new investigation of long-term neuroleptic treatment of older rats.

Effects on brain metabolism and anatomy of neuroleptic treatment may throw light upon mechanisms involved in various dyskinesias, and perhaps on those involved in psychoses as well.

REFERENCES

1. Klawans, H.L. *The Pharmacology of Extrapyramidal Movement Disorder*. Basel: Karger, 1973.
2. Gerlach, J. Relationship between tardive dyskinesia, l-dopa-induced hyperkinesia and parkinsonism. *Psychopharmacology, 51:*259–263, 1977.
3. Sommer, H., Quandt, J. Langzeitbehandlung mit Chlorpromazine im Tierexperiment. *Fortsch. Neurol. Psychiat. 38*:466–491, 1970.
4. Kemali, D., Scarlato, G., Pariante, F. Aspetti istologici ed istochemici del sistema nervoso dopo somministra zioni de chlorpromazina, reserpina e rauwolfina serpentina. *Acta Neurol.* (Napoli), *14*:414, 1958.
5. Gueyniseman, Y. Les modifications morphologiques du cerveau chez les animaux par l'action de l'aminazine et de l'amizine. Z Neuropath Psychiat *62*:190, 1962.
6. Mackiewicz, J., Gershon, S. An experimental study of the neuropathological and toxicological effects of chlorpromazine and reserpine. *J. Neuro-psychiat 5*:159, 1964.
7. Popova, E. On the effect of some neuropharmacological agents on the structure of neurons of various cyto-architectonic formations. *J. Hirn. Forsch. 9*:71, 1967.

8. Romasenko, V., Jacobson, J. Morpho-histochemical study of the action of trifluoperazine on the brain of white rats. *Acta Neuropathol.* (Berl.), *12*:23-32, 1969.

9. Grunthal, E., Walther-Buel, H. Uber Schadigung der Oliva inferior durch Chlorperphenazin (Trilafon). *Psychiat et Neurol* (Basal). *140*:249-257, 1960.

10. Nielson, E.B., Lyon, M. Evidence for cell loss in corpus striatum after long-term treatment with a neuroleptic drug (Flupenthixol) in rats. *Psychopharmacology,* 1978. (In press.)

11. Pakkenberg, H., Fog, R., Nilakantan, B. The long-term effect of perphenazine enanthate on the rat brain. Some metabolic and anatomical observations. *Psychopharmacologia* (Berl.), *29*:329–336, 1973.

12. Gerlach, J. Long-term effect of perphenazine on the substantia nigra in rats. *Psychopharmacologia* (Berl.), *45*:51–54, 1975.

13. Pakkenberg, H., Fog, R. Short-term effect of perphenazine enanthate on the rat brain. *Psychopharmacologia* (Berl.), *40*:165–169, 1974.

14. Fog, R., Pakkenberg, H., Juul, P., Bock, E., Jorgensen, O.S., Andersen, J. High-dose treatment of rats with perphenazine enanthate. *Psychopharmacology, 50*:305–307, 1976.

15. Faurbye, A., Rasch, P.J., Petersen, P.B., Brandborg, G., Pakkenberg, H. Neurological symptoms in pharmacotherapy of psychoses. *Acta Psychiat. Scand., 40*:10–27, 1964.

8

Modification of Dopamine-Acetylcholine Balance by Long-Term Neuroleptic Treatment

GERALD GIANUTSOS

INTRODUCTION

It is by now well established that prolonged use of antipsychotic drugs may lead to the development of transient or persistent dyskinetic disorders (1, 2). Clinical investigation of these disorders suggest that the underlying pathophysiological disturbance may be related to a hyperactive dopaminergic neuronal system in the CNS, possibly associated with a reduction in brain cholinergic function (3, 4). Interestingly, these changes are approximately opposite to the suspected neurochemical changes responsible for Parkinsonism.

Parallel results are evident in laboratory animals where repeated exposure to neuroleptic (antipsychotic) drugs is used. A hypersensitivity to dopaminergic drugs after chronic neuroleptics—presumably the result of a compensatory postsynaptic receptor supersensitivity—has been repeatedly demonstrated (5,6,7,8). More recently, evidence has been presented to support the hypothesis of a cholinergic hyposensitivity in chronic neuroleptic-treated animals (9,10).

DOPAMINE-ACETYLCHOLINE BRAIN INTERACTIONS

Numerous pharmacological studies have provided evidence for a reciprocal relationship between dopamine (DA) and acetylcholine (ACh) in the brain. In general, the behavioral effects of a dopaminergic drug such as apomorphine are antagonized by a cholinergic agonist and intensified by an anticholinergic. For example, the stereotyped behavior produced by apomorphine in mice is increased by pretreatment with anticholinergic drugs (11). Similarly, the aggression produced in rats by apomorphine is reduced by a cholinergic drug, pilocarpine, and enhanced by dexetimide, an anticholinergic (12). Furthermore, the behavioral effects of a DA-receptor antagonist (neuroleptic) may be reversed by an anticholinergic drug (13,14), and increased by cholinergic drugs (15).

Neurochemically, this relationship may be further explored. DA agonists appear to reduce the release of ACh, leading to increased ACh concentrations in the striatum (16,17). Neuroleptic drugs, on the other hand, increase the release of ACh, reduce its concentration in the striatum (18), and increase striatal ACh turnover (19). These results are interpreted as illustrated in Figure 1. DA is thought to inhibit the activity of cholinergic neurons in the striatum; blocking DA receptors with a neuroleptic disinhibits these cells and increases the firing rate of striatal cholinergic neurons. The degree of output from these cholinergic neurons may be an important component of some of the behavioral effects produced by drugs which act via DA.

CHRONIC NEUROLEPTICS

With chronic neuroleptic treatment, the relationship described above could be thought of as follows. Continuous DA-receptor blockade by a neuroleptic would lead to a persistent, unchecked release of ACh. The cholinergic receptor may be expected to compensate for this massive overstimulation by becoming less sensitive to the effects of ACh in an attempt to restore the normal balance and level of output in the striatum.

If this cholinergic hyposensitivity does in fact occur, it would be predicted that a cholinergic agonist would be less effective in stimulating the cholinergic receptor in animals treated chronically with a neuroleptic. In a broad sense,

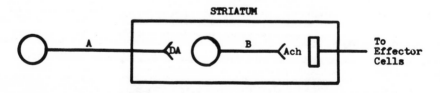

Figure 1.   Illustration of the dopamine-acetylcholine relationship in the striatum. Neuron A depicts a nigrostriatal dopamine-containing fiber. When stimulated, this fiber releases dopamine, which inhibits the activity of the cholinergic neuron, B, in the striatum. (Also see text.)

these animals would show a "tolerance" to the effects of a cholinergic drug. As an analogous example, it has been demonstrated that the behavioral effects of a cholinesterase inhibitor are reduced during chronic administration of the drug (20).

In experiments illustrated in Figure 2, the depressant effect of pilocarpine, a muscarinic-cholinergic-receptor stimulant, on motor activity was shown to be dramatically reduced in rats withdrawn from repeated injections of the neuroleptic haloperidol (9). Similar results have also been demonstrated by Dunstan and Jackson (10), who eliminated possible interference from the peripheral effects of the cholinesterase inhibitor physostigmine by blocking these peripheral actions with methylatropine. These results are consistent with the hypothesis stated above.

In addition, the motor stimulation produced by the anticholinergic drug dexetimide was increased in rats withdrawn from chronic haloperidol, as illustrated in Figure 3 (9). Although these results are more difficult to interpret, it may be suggested that anticholinergic drugs are more effective cholinergic-receptor blockers in the hyposensitive state. An alternative explanation may be that since many anticholinergics are also capable of blocking the reuptake of DA (21), it is the DA acting on supersensitive receptors that is responsible for the stimulation. In fact, depletion of DA partially antagonizes the stimulatory effects of anticholinergics (22), but the stimulation appears to be unrelated to DA uptake inhibition (10,22).

Unfortunately, these experiments have all been performed in animals treated chronically with haloperidol. It would be interesting to determine if chronic treatment with other neuroleptics such as thioridazine or clozapine—which, unlike haloperidol, possess intrinsic anticholinergic activity (23)—would produce similar alterations in cholinergic function.

Another interesting approach to this problem comes from experiments by Smith and Davis (24), who showed that coadministration of haloperidol with benztropine, a drug with mixed DA uptake blocking and anticholinergic activity, reduced the degree of apparent DA supersensitivity when compared with animals treated with haloperidol alone. It is possible that the presence of the anticholinergic prevents the development of hyposensitive cholinergic receptors, and that this is reflected by a reduced effect of DA agonists. However, other investigators have failed to show changes in DA supersensitivity in rats receiving a neuroleptic along with atropine (6,25).

Although these behavioral results are interesting, supportive neurochemical results have not yet been reported. Muller and Seeman (26) investigated the binding of various radioactive ligands in rats, following chronic haloperidol administration. There was an increase in apomorphine binding (consistent with supersensitive DA receptors), but they were unable to detect any changes in the binding of quinuclidinyl benzilate, a marker for cholinergic receptors.

One additional problem in the interpretation of these results is that the data

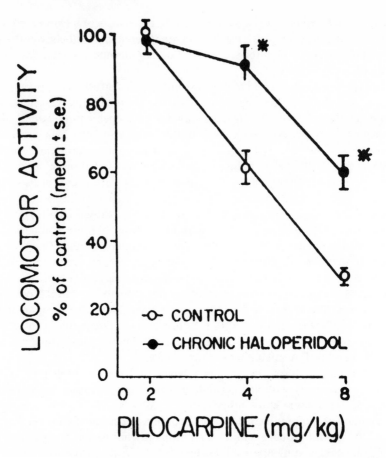

Figure 2.   Effect of pilocarpine on motor activity in normal rats and in rats withdrawn from chronic injections of haloperidol. Activity was measured for 1 hour, beginning 10 minutes after a subcutaneous injection of pilocarpine (at the indicated doses) or water (0 mg/kg). An asterisk indicates that the dose produced significantly less depression of motor activity in the groups maintained on chronic injections of haloperidol than in normal rats.

thus far collected involves only one behavioral measure, motor activity. Although the hypothesis stated earlier would be dependent upon an interaction between DA and ACh in the striatum, this site could be far less important for motor behavior than areas such as the nucleus accumbens (27,28). In the nucleus accumbens, evidence for a relationship as described in Figure 1 is much less convincing (29,30).

Although further experimentation is clearly necessary, the analysis of simultaneous changes in both cholinergic and dopaminergic activity with neuroleptics should be a fruitful approach to our understanding of both neuroleptics and tardive dyskinesias.

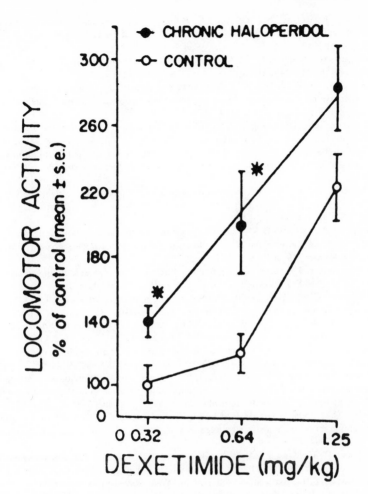

Figure 3.   Effect of dexetimide on motor activity in normal rats and in rats withdrawn from chronic injections of haloperidol. Activity was measured for 1 hour, beginning 30 minutes after a subcutaneous injection of dexetimide (at the indicated doses) or water (0 mg/kg). An asterisk indicates that the dose produced significantly greater stimulation of motor activity in the groups maintained on chronic injections of haloperidol than in normal rats.

REFERENCES

1.   Crane, G.E. High doses of trifluoperazine and tardive dyskinesia. *Arch. Neurol., 22*:176, 1970.
2.   Tarsy, D., Baldessarini, R.J. The pathophysiologic basis of tardive dyskinesia. *Biol. Psychiatry, 12*:431–450, 1977.
3.   Klawans, H.L. The pharmacology of tardive dyskinesias. *Am. J. Psychiatry, 130*:82–86, 1973.

4. Gerlach, J., Reisby, N., Randrup, A. Dopaminergic hypersensitivity and cholinergic hypofunction in the pathophysiology of tardive dyskinesias. *Psychopharmacologia, 34*:21–35, 1974.

5. Klawans, H.L., Rubovits, R. An experimental model of tardive dyskinesias. *J. Neural Transm., 33*:235–246, 1972.

6. Tarsy, D., Baldessarini, R.J. Behavioral supersensitivity to apomorphine following chronic treatment with drugs which interfere with the synaptic function of catecholamines. *Neuropharmacology, 13*:927–940, 1974.

7. Gianutsos, G., Drawbaugh, R.B., Hynes, M.D., Lal, H. Behavioral evidence for dopaminergic supersensitivity after chronic haloperidol. *Life Sci., 14*:887–898, 1974.

8. Von Voigtlander, P.F., Losey, E.G., Triezenberg, H.J. Increased sensitivity to dopaminergic agents after chronic neuroleptic treatment. *J. Pharm. Exp. Ther., 193*:88–94, 1975.

9. Gianutsos, G., Lal, H. Alteration in the action of cholinergic and anticholinergic drugs after chronic haloperidol: Indirect evidence for cholinergic hyposensitivity. *Life Sci., 18*:515–520, 1976a.

10. Dunstan, R., Jackson, D.M. The demonstration of a change in responsiveness of mice to physostigmine and atropine after withdrawal of long-term haloperidol pretreatment. *J. Neural Transm. 40*:181–189, 1977.

11. Scheel-Kruger, J. Central effects of anticholinergic drugs measured by the apomorphine test in mice. *Acta Pharmacol. Toxicol. (Kbh), 38*:1–16, 1970.

12. Gianutsos, G., Lal, H. Modification of apomorphine induced aggression by changing cholinergic activity in rats. *Neuropharmacology, 16*:7–10, 1976b.

13. Hanson, H.M. Stone, C.A. Witoslawski, J.J. Antagonism of the antiavoidance effects of various agents by anticholinergic drugs. *J. Pharmacol. Exp. Ther., 173*:117–127, 1970.

14. Costall, B., Naylor, R.J. On catalepsy and catatonia and the predictability of the catalepsy test for neuroleptic activity. *Psychopharmacologia, 34*:233–241, 1974.

15. Costall, B., Naylor, R.J., Olley, J.E. Catalepsy and circling behavior after intracerebral injections of neuroleptic, cholinergic and anticholinergic agents into the candate-putamen, globus pallidus and substantia nigra of rat brain. *Neuropharmacology, 11*:645–663, 1972.

16. Sethy, V.M., Van Woert, M.H. Modification of striatal acetylcholine concentration by dopamine receptor agonists and antagonists. *Res. Commun. Chem. Pathol. Pharmacol., 8*:13–28, 1974.

17. Guyenet, P.G., Javoy, F., Agid, Y., Beaujouan, J.C., Glowinski, J. Dopamine receptors and cholinergic neurons in the rat neostriatum. In *Advances in Neurology*, vol. 9, Calne, D., Chase, T.N., Barbeau, A. (eds.). New York. Raven Press, pp 43–51, 1975.

18. Stadler, H., Lloyd, K.G., Gadea-Ciria, M., Bartholini, G. Enhanced striatal acetylcholine release by chlorpromazine and its reversal by apomorphine. *Brain Res., 55*:476–480, 1973.

19. Trabucchi, M., Cheney, D., Racagni, G., Costa, E. Involvement of brain cholinergic mechanisms in the action of chlorpromazine. *Nature, 249*:664–667, 1974.

20. Russell, R.W. Overstreet, D.H., Cotman, C.W., Carson, V.G., Churchill, L., Dalglish, F.W., Vasquez, B.J. Experimental tests of hypotheses about neurochemical mechanisms underlying behavioral tolerance to the anticholinesterase, diisopropyl fluorophosphate. *J. Pharmacol. Exp. Ther., 192*:73–85, 1975.

21. Coyle, J.T., Snyder, S.H. Antiparkinson drugs: inhibition of dopamine uptake in the corpus striatum as a possible mechanism of action. *Science, 166*:899–901, 1969.

22. Thornburg, J.E., Moore, K.E. Inhibition of anticholinergic drug-induced locomotor stimulation in mice by α-methyltyrosine. *Neuropharmacology, 12*:1179–1185, 1973.

23. Snyder, S.H., Greenberg, D., Yamamura, H. Antischizophrenic drugs and brain cholinergic receptors; affinity for muscarinic sites predicts extrapyramidal effects. *Arch. Gen. Psychiatry, 31*:58–61, 1974.

24. Smith, R.C., Davis, J.M. Behavioral supersensitivity to apomorphine and amphetamine after chronic high dose haloperidol treatment. *Psychopharmcol. Commun.*, *1*:285–293, 1975.

25. Burki, H.R., Eichenberger, E., Sayers, A.C., White, T.G. Clozapine and the dopamine hypothesis of schizophrenia, a critical appraisal. *Pharmakopsychiat. Neuropsychopharmakol.*, *8*:115–121, 1975.

26. Muller, P., Seeman, P. Brain neurotransmitter receptors after long-term haloperidol: dopamine, acetylcholine, serotonin α-noradrenergic and naloxone receptors. *Life Sci.* (In press).

27. Pijnenberg, A.J.J., Van Rossum, J.M. Stimulation of locomotor activity following injection of dopamine into the nucleus accumbens. *J. Pharm. Pharmacol.*, *25*:1004–1005, 1973.

28. Kelly, P.H., Sevoiour, P.W., Iversen, S.D. Amphetamine and apomorphine responses in the rat following 6-OHDA lesions of the nucleus accumbens septi and corpus striatum. *Brain Res.*, *94*:507–522, 1975.

29. Consolo, S., Ladinsky, H., Bianchi, S., Ghezzi, D. Apparent lack of a dopaminergic-cholinergic link in the rat nucleus accumbens septituberculum olfactorium. *Brain Res.*, *135*:255–263, 1977.

30. Bartholini, G., Stadler, H., Gadea-Ciria, M., Lloyd, K.G. Interaction of dopaminergic and cholinergic neurons in the extrapyramidal and limbic systems. In *Advances in Biochemical Psychopharmacology*, pp. 391–395, Costa, E., Gessa, G.L. (eds.). New York: Raven Press, pp. 391–395, 1977.

9

Striatal Dopaminergic Activity During Withdrawal from Chronic Neuroleptic Treatment in Rats

EMANUEL MELLER
and EITAN FRIEDMAN

INTRODUCTION

In the 15 years that have elapsed since the pioneering work of Carlsson and his associates (1) demonstrated an effect of antipsychotic drug treatment on dopaminergic neuronal activity in the corpus striatum, a great deal of effort has been directed toward elucidating a possible relationship between central dopaminergic function and schizophrenia (2). The major portion of these experimental studies has been conducted with acutely treated animals, and only in the last few years has extensive interest been focused on the effects of repeated neuroleptic administration vis-à-vis dopaminergic activity.

The well-documented demonstration of behavioral supersensitivity to dopaminergic agonists, such as apomorphine and amphetamine, following withdrawal from chronic neuroleptic treatment (3–7) or chemical sympathectomy (7–9) has lent credence to the suggestion (2,5,10) that this altered state may be related to the development of tardive dyskinesia (11,12), which is seen in some 10% to 20% (13) of all patients withdrawn from chronic neuroleptic treatment. This hypothesis postulates that the clinical dyskinetic manifestations result from a hypersensitivity of dopamine (DA) receptors in the basal ganglia after dose reduction or termination of antipsychotic drug treatment (10).

From a biochemical standpoint, it is of interest to determine if the behavioral supersensitivity phenomenon can be correlated to changes in the striatal dopaminergic system in vitro. Specifically, one might expect (a) an increased response of striatal adenylate cyclase, which has been postulated to be the dopaminergic receptor (14); (b) an increase in binding of agonists and/or antagonists to striatal dopamine receptors (15,16); and (c) a concomitant compensatory decrease in presynaptic DA synthesis and turnover, secondary to overstimulation of the postulated nigrostriatal neuronal feedback mechanism (17).

The present report describes results of experiments designed to furnish information on the last of the above expectations. Rats were treated for several weeks with low to moderate doses of antipsychotics. On withdrawal from drug treatment, changes in postsynaptic dopaminergic activity (behavioral super-sensitivity to apomorphine) and two parameters of presynaptic activity —synaptosomal tyrosine hydroxylase (TH) activity and 3, 4-dihydroxyphenylacetic acid (DOPAC) levels (17)—were measured.

MATERIALS AND METHODS

Apomorphine stereotypy

Powdered rat chow (Wayne lab-blox) was thoroughly dry-mixed with haloperidol HCl to yield a concentration of 12.5 mg drug/kg chow. Male Sprague-Dawley rats, 250–300 g. were fed drug-treated or control chow for 25 days, and daily food intake was recorded. Drug-treated animals ingested an estimated average of 0.8 mg/kg haloperidol/day. After 25 days, untreated chow was substituted for 5 to 6 days, and then groups of 6 animals were administered various doses of apomorphine subcutaneously. Stereotypy was scored as previously described (18).

Tyrosine hydroxylase

Male Sprague-Dawley rats (250 g) were administered haloperiodol (0.5 mg/kg) i.p. for 4 weeks. Control animals received saline throughout, while acutely treated rats received saline followed by haloperidol as the last injec-tion. Animals were sacrificed one and 24 hours and 6 to 7 days after the last injection. Striatal tissue from the right side of the brain was homogenized in 0.32M sucrose. (The left striata from the same animals were frozen for later DOPAC determinations; see below.) Tyrosine hydroxylase activity was measured in aliquots of the 1000 x g supernatant (synaposomal P_2 fraction) by the method of Nagatsu et al. (19), utilizing the conversion of 3, 5-di-^{3}H-tyrosine to ^{3}H-H_2O as an index of tyrosine hydroxylation.

DOPAC

DOPAC was measured by a modification of the enzymatic radioisotopic method of Kebabian *et al.* (20). Duplicate incubations were carried out essentially as described (20), except for the following modifications: (a) Partially purified catechol-O-methyltransferase (COMT) was prepared without addition of dithiothreitol, as this compound increased the blank; and (b) identically treated cerebellar tissue (rather than perchloric acid) was used for estimation of the blank and recovery of added DOPAC. A different and less laborious procedure was devised for extraction of the product, as follows: incubations were terminated by addition of 0.2 ml of 1.5 N HCl containing 25 mg of homovanillic acid (HVA) and extracted with 6 ml of toluene-isoamyl alcohol (95:5, v/v). Five ml of the extract were back-extracted into 1 ml of 5% NaHCO₃ containing 160 mg of solid NaHCO₃, and the aqueous suspension was treated with 0.1 ml of acetic anhydride. After 45 minutes the tubes were extracted twice with 5 ml of ethyl acetate (discarded), acidified with 0.4 ml of 12 N HCl, and again extracted with 6 ml of the organic solvent. Five ml of the final extract was counted. The assay was linear up to at least 50 pmol of added DOPAC, and although the blank (v2000 cpm) was somewhat higher than that reported (20), the sensitivity limit was essentially identical (about 1 pmol).

RESULTS

Five to 6 days after withdrawal from oral haloperidol treatment, there was an obvious and highly significant shift in the dose response to apomorphine-induced stereotypy (Fig. 1). These results are qualitatively in agreement with those reported by others (3–5) and indicate that the postulated striatal supersensitivity of DA receptors is readily apparent with the indicated treatment duration, drug dosage level, and drug washout period.

Tyrosine hydroxylase activity was not significantly altered 6 to 7 days after withdrawal from repeated haloperidol injection (Fig. 2). One hour after the last injection, on the other hand, complete tolerance to the ability of the neuroleptic to increase striatal TH activity was seen in these animals (Fig. 2). At 24 hours after the last injection, TH activity in both acute and chronically treated animals was reduced, but this effect did not attain statistical significance.

Similarly, attenuation of the increased DOPAC levels seen after acute haloperidol treatment was observed in the chronic animals one hour after the final injection (Fig. 3). However, DOPAC levels during withdrawal (6–7 days) were unchanged. One day after termination of treatment, there was a 20% decrease in DOPAC levels relative to controls, but again (cf. TH activity) this drop did not reach statistical significance. A similar nonsignifi-

cant decline in DOPAC at this time period has been reported (21). HVA
levels, however, were significantly depressed (21).

DISCUSSION

Since the duration of treatment, the drug dosage level, and the drug withdrawal period were similar in the behavioral and biochemical experiments
described herein, a direct comparison of the results appears reasonable and
valid. Synaptosomal TH activity and tissue levels of DOPAC (17) appear to
be reliable indexes of the level of neuronal activity in the nigrostriatal
dopaminergic pathway. As shown in Figures 2 and 3, TH activity and
DOPAC levels were unchanged one week after withdrawal of drug treatment
when behavioral supersensitivity was readily apparent (Fig. 1). Gianutsos *et
al*. (22) likewise found no change in striatal DA turnover after treatment with
much larger doses of haloperidol, though there was an increased sensitivity to

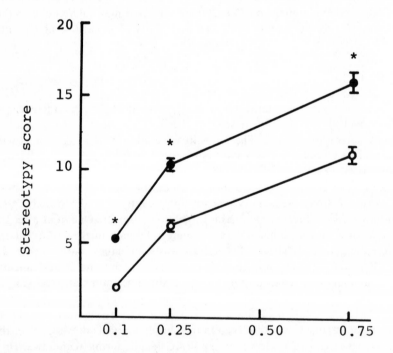

Figure 1.   Dose-response curves for apomorphine in control (o) and haloperidol (o) (0.8
mg/kg/p.o./day) treated rats. Stereotypy was scored as previously described (18). Shown are
mean scores ± SEM, 6 animals per group.

*p < .001 vs. corresponding control, Student's t test.

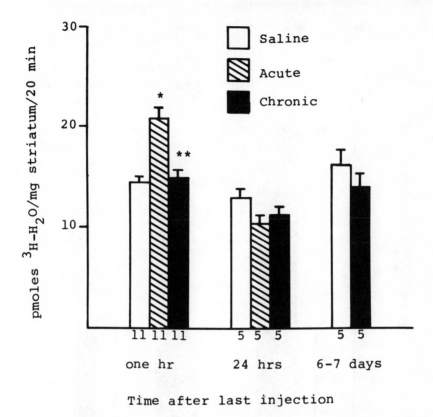

Figure 2.   Synaptosomal tyrosine hydroxylase activity at various times after withdrawal from
acute or chronic haloperidol (0.5 mg/kg 1.p.) treatment. Mean ± SEM; number of animals in
each group is shown under the bars. Statistics. One-way analysis of variance, followed by
Neuman-Kuels test.

*p < .01 vs. saline group.
**p < .01 vs. acute group.

apomorphine in effecting a reduction of DA turnover. The latter effect is an
expected biochemical correlate of DA-receptor supersensitivity. Similarly,
Hyttel (23) found no change in DA synthesis in the mouse brain after withdrawal from chronic haloperidol.

Other data, although not strictly comparable because of differences in drug
dosage, duration of treatment, drug washout period, species, and methodological criteria, have yielded somewhat different results. Hyttel and Møller
Nielson (24) have reported a decrease of DA synthesis (in the mouse) following withdrawal from chronic haloperidol; however, the ability of a challenge
dose of the drug to increase DA synthesis was not diminished. Hyttel (25) has

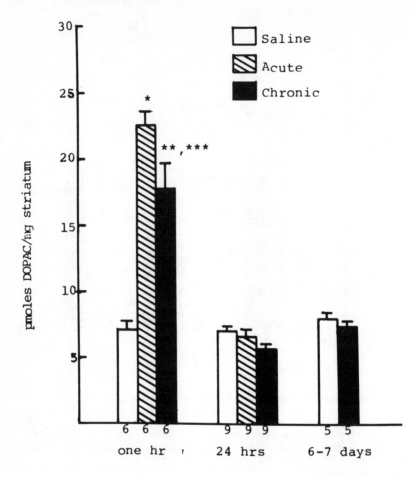

Figure 3.   Striatal DOPAC levels after haloperidol treatment. See legend to Figure 2 for explanation.

*p < .01 vs. saline group.

**p < .05 vs. acute group.

***p < .01 vs. saline group.

also measured DOPAC and HVA in mouse brain after a single injection of tefluxitol, which produces an apparent receptor supersensitivity within 2 days (26). An initial increase in both metabolites was followed by a decline to below normal levels within several days before returning to baseline. Scatton et al. (27) found a similar biphasic response in DA synthesis (and turnover) after injection of a depot form of a neuroleptic (pipotiazine palmitic ester). Comparison of this data with results of treatment on a daily schedule is difficult, however, since in the former instance there is no clear period of drug withdrawal.

Measurements of changes in postsynaptic receptor activity following chronic neuroleptic treatment or lesioning of the nigrostriatal pathway have been reported by several laboratories. Initial reports of alterations in striatal dopamine-sensitive adenylate cyclase have led to some confusion, since some groups (6,28–30) reported no change in this parameter after such treatments, whereas other data (31–33) are at variance with these conclusions. The disparity in results may be due to differences in methodology. As has been elegantly demonstrated by Kreuger et al. (34), electrothermal or 6-hydroxydopamine lesions of the nigrostriatal pathway result in an observable increased sensitivity of adenylate cyclase to DA in striatal slices, but not in the usual homogenate preparation. Furthermore, Friedhoff et al. (33) have found an increased adenylate cyclase response to dopamine in striatal slices after withdrawal from chronic neuroleptics. Gnegy et al. (35) have also obtained positive results using a particulate membrane fraction of rat striatum.

In contrast to the somewhat confusing results obtained regarding changes in adenylate cyclase activity, several groups have now reported increased DA-receptor binding of tritiated dopaminergic agonists and/or antagonists after chronic neuroleptic treatment. Thus Friedhoff et al. (33), Burt et al. (36), and Muller and Seeman (37) have all reported such increases. The small increase in apparent receptor density, however, is poorly correlated with the large increase observed in behavioral sensitivity to apomorphine (36).

The results reported here (Figs. 2 and 3) are somewhat surprising in view of the reasonable expectation that during the supersensitivity phase, neuronal feedback regulation should effect a reduction in presynaptic activity (10). However, as others do find transient compensatory decreases in presynaptic synthesis and turnover (24,25,27), measurement of these parameters at more closely spaced intervals (cf. one hour and 24 hour results in Figs. 2 and 3) may yield more detailed information regarding the dynamic alterations in presynaptic activity on withdrawal of chronic neuroleptics. Such experiments are presently in progress. On the other hand, if such alterations are only transient, then these data may have some bearing on the development of tardive dyskinesia, since the net dopaminergic activity would be increased on drug withdrawal.

During the behavioral supersensitive phase after withdrawal from chronic antipsychotic drug treatment, tolerance to the protective effect of the neuroleptic vis-à-vis amphetamine- and apomorphine-induced stereotypies is observed (38,39). This tolerance appears within several days after drug withdrawal, is long-lasting, and displays cross-tolerance with other antipsychotic drugs (39). Biochemically, tolerance development appears to be dependent on several factors, including treatment duration and drug dosage (27,38,40–44). Thus, tolerance to the increase in DA synthesis and DOPAC and HVA levels occurs earliest and at the lowest doses in striatum. Higher doses and/or longer treatment periods are required to produce tolerance in the mesolimbic areas (40; unpublished observations). In the mesocortical dopaminergic neurons, no tolerance has been observed (40; unpublished observations), at least with the treatment schedules and dosage levels thus far employed.

Almost all the biochemical estimations of tolerance development (DA synthesis and/or turnover [22–24,27,39]; DOPAC and/or HVA levels [25,38,40–44]) have been performed shortly after the last of a chronic series of treatments (cf. Figs. 2 and 3), whereas pharmacological tolerance has been measured during the supersensitivity phase (38,39). Clearly missing are experiments designed to demonstrate tolerance to the neurochemical effects *during* this period of receptor hypersensitivity. Interestingly, in the only such experiment reported (24), to our knowledge there was no attenuation of the neuroleptic effect in increasing striatal DA synthesis during this phase. Experiments addressing this question are currently in progress.

The development of dopaminergic supersensitivity, and tolerance to neuroleptic drugs at this time, may have important relevance to the therapeutic effect of neuroleptics in schizophrenia as well as to the appearance of tardive dyskinesia. Recently, a new treatment paradigm for tardive dyskinetic patients has been formulated by Friedhoff (10), based on current concepts of dopaminergic receptor dynamics, whereby the postulated supersensitive receptor in this pathological state is "tuned" down by increasing the agonist supply (dopamine) via-L-dopa administration. Recent preliminary clinical (45) and experimental evidence (33) lend support to the potential therapeutic value of this approach.

Clinical manifestations of extrapyramidal side effects decrease after prolonged antipsychotic drug treatment (46,47); these diminished effects may therefore result from tolerance to the drug's effect in the striatum where, as mentioned earlier, behavioral and biochemical tolerance occurs earliest. On the other hand, no tolerance has been noted to the therapeutic effects of neuroleptics, which may therefore be mediated *via* an action of these drugs on dopaminergic systems in mesocortical areas (27,40; unpublished observations).

It should be noted that dopamine-receptor supersensitivity and pharmacologic neuroleptic tolerance may be inseparable phenomena. This suggestion is supported by the observation that neither tolerance (48) nor receptor supersensitivity (49) appears to occur in the tubero-infundibular dopaminergic system. If the supposition that tolerance and supersensitivity phenomena are closely linked is true, it might be expected, based on the observation that tolerance develops in the mesolimbic system (40,41; unpublished observations), that DA-receptor supersensitivity should also develop in this area after prolonged and/or higher dosage treatment with neuroleptics. Pharmacological observation of such supersensitivity might be accomplished in a behavioral circling paradigm with the use of a new ergolene derivative reported to activate mainly limbic DA receptors (48).

A final cautionary note regarding the anatomical locus of the postulated receptor supersensitivity in tardive dyskinesia appears in order. As mentioned earlier, neuroleptic tolerance (and/or supersensitivity) appears to occur most easily, and most rapidly, in the striatum. The time course of the appearance of tardive dyskinetic symtomatology, which apparently develops only after drug withdrawal or dosage reduction following prolonged but not short-term treatment (13), thus correlates poorly with the time course for development of striatal supersensitivity. The possibility of a nonstriatal etiology for this syndrome should therefore be borne in mind.

ACKNOWLEDGMENTS

Expert technical assistance of Ms. Marilyn Hallock is greatly appreciated. Supported by PHS grants MH 28350 and MH 08618.

REFERENCES

1. Carlsson, A. Lindqvist, M. Effect of chlorpromazine on formation of 3-methoxytyramine and normetanephrine in mouse brain. *Acta Pharmacol. Toxicol.* (Kbh),*20*:140–144, 1963.
2. Snyder, S.H., Banerjee, S.P., Yamamura, H.I., Greenberg, D. Drugs, neurotransmitters and schizophrenia. *Science, 184*:1243–1253, 1974.
3. Tarsy, D., Baldessarini, R.J. Behavioral supersensitivity to apomorphine following chronic treatment with drugs which interfere with the synaptic function of catecholamines. *Neuropharmacology, 13*:927–940. 1974.
4. Gianutsos, G., Drawbaugh, R.B., Hynes, M.D., Lal, H. Behavioral evidence for dopaminergic supersensitivity after chronic haloperidol. *Life Sci., 14*:887–898, 1974.
5. Sayers, A.C., Burki, H.R., Ruch, W., Asper, H. Neuroleptic-induced hypersensitivity of striatal dopamine receptors in the rat as a model of tardive dyskinesias. Effects of clozapine, haloperidol, loxapine and chlorpromazine. *Psychopharmacologia, 41*:97–104, 1975.
6. Von Voigtlander, P.F., Losey, E.G., Triezenberg, H.J. Increased sensitivity to dopaminergic agents after chronic neuroleptic treatment. *J. Pharmacol. Exp. Ther., 193*:88–94, 1975.
7. Moore, K.E., Thornburg, J.E. Drug-induced dopaminergic supersensitivity. In *Advances in Neurology*, vol. 9, Calne, D., Chase, T.N., Barbeau, A. (eds.). New York, Raven Press, pp. 93–104, 1975.
8. Ungerstedt, U. Postsynaptic supersensitivity after 6-hydroxydopamine induced degeneration of the nigrostriatal dopamine system., *Acta Physiol. Scand., 367*:69–93, 1971.
9. Iversen, S.D., Creese, I. Behavioral correlates of dopaminergic supersensitivity. In *Advances in Neurology*, vol. 9., Calne, D., Chase, T.N., Barbeau, A. (eds.). New York: Raven Press, pp. 81–92, 1975.
10. Friedhoff, A.J. Receptor sensitivity modification—a new paradigm for the potential

treatment of some hormonal and transmitter disturbances. In *Psychopathology and Brain Dysfunction*. Shagass, C., Gershon, S., Friedhoff, A.J. (eds.). New York: Raven Press, pp. 139-148, 1977.

11. Paulson, G.W. Tardive dyskinesia. *Annu. Rev. Med., 26*:75-81, 1975.

12. Klawans, H.L. The pharmacology of tardive dyskinesia. *Am. J. Psychiatry, 130*:82-86, 1973.

13. Hippius, H. On the relations between antipsychotic and extrapyramidal effects of psychoactive drugs. In *Antipsychotic Drugs, Pharmacodynamics and Pharmacokinetics*. Sedvall, G., Uvnas, B., Zotterman, Y. (eds.). Oxford: Pergamon Press, pp. 437-448, 1976.

14. Kebabian, J.W. Petzold, G.L., Greengard, P. Dopamine-sensitive adenylate cyclase in the caudate nucleus of rat brain and its similarity to the dopamine receptor. *Proc. Natl. Acad. Sci. USA, 69*:2145-2149, 1972.

15. Seeman, P., Chau-Wong, M., Tedesco, J., Wong, K. Brain receptors for antipsychotic drugs and dopamine: direct binding assays. *Proc. Natl. Acad. Sci. USA, 72*:4376-4380, 1975.

16. Burt, D.R., Enna, S.J., Creese, I., Snyder, S.H. Dopamine receptor binding in the corpus striatum of mammalian brain. *Proc. Natl. Acad. Sci. USA, 72*:4655-4659, 1975.

17. Roth, R.H., Murrin, L.C., Walters, J.R. Central dopaminergic neurons: effects of alterations in impulse flow on the accumulation of dihydroxyphenylacetic acid. *Eur. J. Pharmacol., 36*:163-171, 1976.

18. Friedman, E., Rotrosen, J., Gurland, M., Lambert, G.A., Gershon, S. Enhancement of reserpine-elicited dopaminergic supersensitivity by repeated treatment with apomorphine and alpha-methyl-p-tyrosine. *Life Sci., 17*:867-874, 1975.

19. Nagatsu, T., Levitt, M., Udenfriend, S. A rapid and simple radioassay for tyrosine hydroxylase activity. *Anal. Biochem., 9*:122-126, 1964.

20. Kebabian, J.W., Saavedra, J.M., Axelrod, J. A sensitive enzymatic radioisotopic assay for 3, 4-dihydroxypheny-lacetic acid. *J. Neurochem., 28*:795-801, 1977.

21. Lerner, P., Nose, P., Gordon, E.K., Lovenberg, W. Haloperidol: effect of long-term treatment on rat striatal dopamine synthesis and turnover. *Science, 197*:181-183, 1977.

22. Gianutsos, G., Hynes, M.D., Lal, H. Enhancement of apomorphine-induced inhibition of striatal dopamine turnover following chronic haloperidol. *Biochem. Pharmacol., 24*:581-582, 1975.

23. Hyttel, J. Endogenous levels and turnover of catecholamines in mouse brain after repeated administration of haloperidol. *Psychopharmacologia, 36*:237-241, 1974.

24. Hyttel, J., Møller Nielsen, I. Changes in catecholamine concentrations and synthesis rate in mouse brain during the supersensitivity phase after treatment with neuroleptic drugs. *J. Neurochem., 27*:313-315, 1976.

25. Hyttel, J. Levels of HVA and DOPAC in mouse corpus striatum in the supersensitivity phase after neuroleptic treatment. *J. Neurochem., 28*:227-228, 1977.

26. Christensen, A.V., Fjalland, B., Møller Nielsen, I. On the supersensitivity of dopamine receptors induced by neuroleptics. *Psychopharmacology, 48*:1-6, 1976.

27. Scatton, B., Boireau, A., Garret, C., Glowinski, J., Julou,. Action of the palmitic ester on pipotiazine on dopamine metabolism in the nigro-striatal, meso-limbic and meso-cortical systems. *Naunyn. Schmiedebergs. Arch. Phalmacol., 296*:169-175, 1977.

28. Rotrosen, J., Friedman, E., Gershon, S. Striatal adenylate cyclase activity following reserpine and chronic chlorpromazine administration in rats. *Life Sci., 17*:563-568, 1975.

29. Palmer, G.C., Wagner, H.R. Supersensitivity of striatal and cortical adenylate cyclase following reserpine: lack of effect of chronic haloperidol. *Res. Commun. Psychol. Psychiatr. Behav., 1*:567-570, 1976.

30. Roufogalis, B.D., Thornton, M., Wade, D.N. Specificity of the dopamine sensitive adenylate cyclase for antipsychotic antagonists. *Life Sci., 19*:927-934, 1976.

31. Mishra, R.K., Gardner, E.L., Katzman, R., Makman, M.H. Enhancement of dopamine-stimulated adenylate cyclase activity in rat caudate after lesions in substantia nigra: evidence for denervation supersensitivity. *Proc. Natl. Acad. Sci. USA, 71*:3883–3887, 1974.

32. Iwatsubo, K., Clouet, D.H. Dopamine-sensitive adenylate cyclase of the caudate nucleus of rats treated with morphine or haloperidol. *Biochem. Pharmacol., 24*:1499–1503, 1975.

33. Friedhoff, A.J., Bonnet, K., Rosengarten, H. Reversal of two manifestations of dopamine receptor supersensitivity after administration of L-dopa. *Res. Commun. Chem. Pathol. Pharmacol., 16*:411–423, 1977.

34. Kreuger, B.K., Forn, J., Walters, J.R., Roth, R.H., Greengard, P. Stimulation by dopamine of adenosine cyclic 3', 5'-monophosphate formation in rat caudate nucleus: effect of lesions of the nigro-neostriatal pathway. *Mol. Pharmacol., 12*:639–648, 1976.

35. Gnegy, M., Uzunov, P., Costa, E. Participation of an endogenous calcium binding protein activator in the development of drug-induced supersensitivity of striatal dopamine receptors. *J. Pharmacol. Exp. Ther., 202*:558–564, 1977.

36. Burt, D.R., Creese, I., Snyder, S.H. Antischizophrenic drugs: chronic treatment elevates dopamine receptor binding in brain. *Science, 196*:326–328, 1977.

37. Muller, P., Seeman, P. Brain neurotransmitter receptors after long-term haloperidol: dopamine, aceytlcholine, serotonin, a-noradrenergic and naloxone receptors. *Life Sci., 21*:1751–1758, 1977.

38. Asper, H., Baggiolini, M., Burki, H.R., Lauener, H., Ruch, W., Stille, G. Tolerance phenomena with neuroleptics. Catalepsy, apomorphine stereotypes and striatal dopamine metabolism in the rat after single and repeated administration of loxapine and haloperidol. *Eur. J. Pharmacol., 22*:287–294, 1973.

39. Møller, Nielsen, I., Fjalland, B., Petersen, V., Nymark, M. Pharmacology of neuroleptics upon repeated administration. *Psychopharmacologia, 34*:95–104, 1974.

40. Scatton, B. Differential regional development of tolerance to increase in dopamine turnover upon repeated neuroleptic administration. *Eur. J. Pharmacol., 46*:363–369, 1977.

41. Bowers, Jr., M.B., Rozitis, A. Brain homovanillic acid: regional changes over time with antipsychotic drugs. *Eur. J. Pharmacol., 39*:109–115, 1976.

42. Scatton, B., Bischoff, S., Dedek, J., Korf, J. Regional effects of neuroleptics on dopamine metabolism and dopamine-sensitive adenylate cyclase activity. *Eur. J. Pharmacol., 44*:287–292, 1977.

43. Waldmeier, P.C., Maitre, L. Clozapine: reduction of the initial dopamine turnover increase by repeated treatment. *Eur. J. Pharmacol., 38*:197–203, 1976.

44. Burki, H.R., Ruch, W., Asper, H., Baggiolini, M., Stille, G. Effect of single and repeated administration of clozapine on the metabolism of dopamine and noradrenaline in the brain of the rat. *Eur. J. Pharmacol., 27*:180–190, 1974.

45. Friedhoff, A.J., Alpert, M. Receptor sensitivity modification as a potential treatment. In *Psychopharmacology: A Generation of Progress*. Lipton, M.A., DiMascio, A., Killam, K.F. (eds.). New York: Raven Press, pp. 797–801, 1978.

46. Ayd, F.J. Do antiparkinson drugs interfere with the therapeutic effects of neuroleptics? *Int. Drug Ther. Newsletter, 9*:29–31, 1974.

47. Orlov, P., Kasparian, G., DiMascio, A., Cole, J.O. Withdrawal of antiparkinson drugs. *Arch. Gen. Psychiatry., 25*:410–413, 1971.

48. Fuxe, K., Agnati, L., Tsuchiya, K., Hokfelt, T., Johansson, O., Jonsson, G., Lidbrink, P., Lofstrom, A., Ungerstedt, U. Effect of antipsychotic drugs on central catecholamine neurons of rat brain. In *Antipsychotic Drugs, Pharmacodynamics and Pharmacokinetics*. Sedvall, G., Uvnas, B., Zotterman, Y. (eds.). Oxford: Pergamon Press, pp. 117–132, 1976.

49. Ravitz, A.J., Moore, K.E. Lack of effect of chronic haloperidol administration on the prolactin-lowering actions of piribedil. *J. Pharm. Pharmaol., 29*:384–386, 1977.

10

Effect of Long-Term Neuroleptic Treatment on Neurotransmitter Receptors: Relation to Tardive Dyskinesia

PAVEL MULLER
and PHILLIP SEEMAN

INTRODUCTION

This chapter will deal with the effects of long-term administration of neuroleptics on brain receptors for neurotransmitters. A central question is whether the observed alterations in receptors can be meaningfully related to the clinical problem of neuroleptic-induced tardive dyskinesia.

It is now clear that a single injection of most, if not all, neuroleptic drugs will elicit a short-term dopaminergic supersensitivity within 1 day (see Fig. 1) after the direct neuroleptic actions start to wear off. The clinical phenomenon of tardive dyskinesia, on the other hand, takes many months or years to develop in patients who are taking neuroleptics. One of the objectives in this chapter, therefore, is to examine whether it is possible to resolve this apparent discrepancy in these time courses by reviewing and analysing the animal data on long-term neuroleptic treatment.

DOPAMINERGIC SUPERSENSITIVITY—TIME COURSE

Dopaminergic supersensitivity can be experimentally demonstrated after a single injection of neuroleptics (1,2) and it appears to increase over a period of a week (Fig. 1). It is possible that the supersensitivity continues to develop, but at a substantially slower rate, as is evident after lesions (3).

This very rapid development of dopaminergic supersensitivity under experimental conditions is much faster than the rate of development of tardive dyskinesia in patients. This discrepancy in the time course is one of the reasons why Tarsy and Baldessarini (4) suggest that neuroleptic-induced dopaminergic supersensitivity may not be an appropriate model for tardive dyskinesia. Thus, according to Crane (5), the tardive dyskinesia develops usually in the patients treated with the neuroleptics for a year or more and very rarely in less than 6 months. It is important to note that while the behavioral experimental models induce supersensitivity by administration after neuroleptic withdrawal of dopaminergic agonists (e.g., Tarsy and Baldessarini [15], tardive dyskinesia is demonstrated in the absence of stimulation and most often in the presence of the neuroleptic that would mask any demonstration of dopaminergic supersensitivity. Interestingly, removal or reduction of neuroleptic dosage precipitates signs of tardive dyskinesia in apparently nondyskinetic patients (5). We propose that in experimental animals on long-term neuroleptics, as well as in patients taking neuroleptics, the dopaminergic supersensitivity is masked by the neuroleptics and possibly by the compensatory changes in the function of other neurotransmitters (Fig. 2) (6,7).

In order to assess the role of dopaminergic supersensitivity in tardive dyskinesia, it is worthwhile to see if chronically neuroleptic-treated patients without the signs of dyskinesia are more sensitive to the dopaminergic agonists or cholinergic agonists than are the patients not treated with these drugs (8).

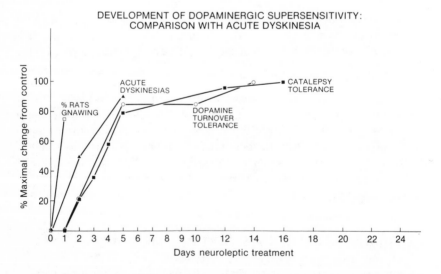

Figure 1.   Time course of dopaminergic supersensitivity. Maximal observed change from the control was taken as 100%. Rat gnawing—from Christensen *et al.*, 1976; acute dyskinesias—from Marsden *et al.*, 1975; turnover tolerance—Lerner and Nosé, 1977; catalepsy tolerance—Ezrin-Waters and Seeman, 1977.

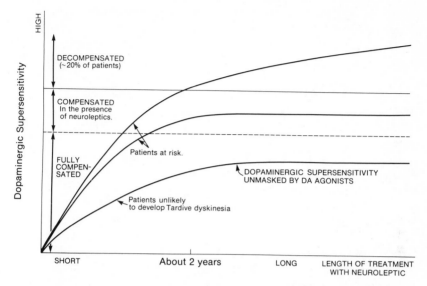

Figure 2.   The compensation of dopaminergic supersensitivity in tardive dyskinesia—a
model. Decompensated dopaminergic supersensitivity leads to spontaneous appearance of dyskinetic symptoms. Dopaminergic supersensitivity compensated in the presence of the neuroleptics will be clinically dormant until the neuroleptics are discontinued or the dose is lowered.
Fully compensated dopaminergic supersensitivity could be precipitated by dopamine agonists
or anticholinergic drugs.

DOPAMINERGIC SUPERSENSITIVITY—RATE OF LOSS

Although tardive dyskinesia is generally considered irreversible or poorly
reversible, several authors report a reversal or diminution of the dyskinetic
symptoms, particularly in patients under fifty (9,10,11). Another important
factor, according to Quitkin et al. (9), is the length of time for which the
dyskinesia is manifested before the neuroleptics are discontinued. The
patient's prognosis improves if the neuroleptics are withdrawn soon after the
treatment is discontinued. Similarly, a review of the literature suggests that the
length of persistence of dopaminergic supersensitivity is directly proportional
to the length of treatment (Fig. 3).

DOPAMINERGIC SUPERSENSITIVITY—EFFECT OF DOSE

The increase in the dopaminergic sensitivity appears to be dose-independent
over the dose range tested (Fig. 3, inset). This might indicate that the doses
used for pretreatment in the binding experiments might be supramaximal.
According to Crane (5), there is also no clear dose-dependence in the incidence of tardive dyskinesia.

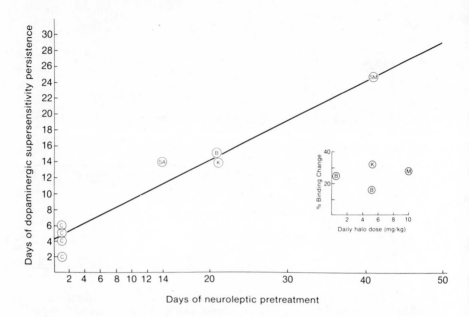

Figure 3.   Correlation of the persistence of dopaminergic supersensitivity with the length of neuroleptic pretreatment. C—Christensen *et al.*, 1976, stereotypy; S.A.—Sayers *et al.*, 1975, turning; B—Burt *et al.*, 1977, neuroleptic binding; K—Kobayashi *et al.*, 1978, neuroleptic binding; S.M—Smith *et al.*, 1976, stereotypy. Inset: correlation of the daily dose with the maximal neuroleptic binding increase over controls—Muller and Seeman, 1977.

To study the specificity of chronic neuroleptic treatment, we have studied the effect of chronic neuroleptic treatment on several neurotransmitter receptor bindings in several brain areas (12).

RESULTS

The long-term haloperidol pretreatment resulted in a 34% increase in ^{3}H-haloperidol binding and a 77% increase in ^{3}H-apomorphine binding in the rat striatum (Fig. 4). These increases were significant at the 0.05 and 0.02 levels, respectively, using the Wilcoxon's rank test.

In the mesolimbic brain areas, ^{3}H-haloperidol binding increased by 45% and apomorphine binding by 55%. These increments were significant at the P < 0.02 level.

Striatal ^{3}H-serotonin binding increased by 20% (P < .05), although the hippocampal and cortical binding of ^{3}H-serotonin was not significantly affected by the chronic haloperidol treatment.

There was no significant change in ^{3}H-naloxone or ^{3}H-QNB binding in any of the areas tested.

The chronic haloperidol administration induced a small, but significant, increase of ^{3}H-WB 4101 binding in the cortex, but not in the striatum. To test whether the increase in the striatal serotonin binding after chronic haloperidol was or was not due to a true increase in ^{3}H-serotonin binding sites, we also measured specific ^{3}H-serotonin binding in the presence of excess (500 nM) apomorphine. This ought to have eliminated any binding of ^{3}H-serotonin to dopamine binding sites. Under these conditions, the ^{3}H-serotonin binding was possibly somewhat reduced, but the increase in specific ^{3}H-serotonin binding was no less prominent than in the assays without the apomorphine present (Fig. 5). The assays were done using only two haloperidol-treated striatal preparations with their matched controls. The assays were done in duplicates. The same design was used for the cortex (Fig. 5).

DISCUSSION

These results indicate that long-term haloperidol treatment selectively increased the amount of specific bonding of ^{3}H-haloperidol and ^{3}H-apomorphine in both the striatum and mesolimbic tissues without much change in other receptors. This increase may reflect a higher affinity of the receptor for these ligands, or there may have been an increase in the number of receptors (13).

These results are compatible with past behavioral observations made on animals undergoing long-term neuroleptic treatment. Such animals are apparently supersensitive to dopaminergic agonists (14,15,16,17), as measured by stereotypy, for example. Some evidence has previously been presented indicating an increase in dopamine/neuroleptic receptors following chronic neuroleptic treatment in the striatum (12,13,18,19,20,21). Stereotypy, however, is not exclusively mediated by the striatal dopaminergic system. It is known that the mesolimbic system is also involved in eliciting stereotypy (22,23). It is known, furthermore, that locomotor activity also increases following chronic neuroleptic pretreatment (24–27). In locomotor behavior, however, the striatal dopaminergic system seems to play a minor role, while the mesolimbic dopaminergic system is dominantly involved (23,27–30).

It has been observed that rats display more locomotor behavior (upon intra-accumbens injection of dopamine) following chronic penfluridol pretreatment than do control rats. Our results, showing increased haloperidol and apomorphine binding in the mesolimbic system, are consistent with dopaminergic supersensitivity in the mesolimbic system.

The dopaminergic receptor binding increase appears to be at least somewhat specific to the neuroleptic, since repeated ethanol treatment results in

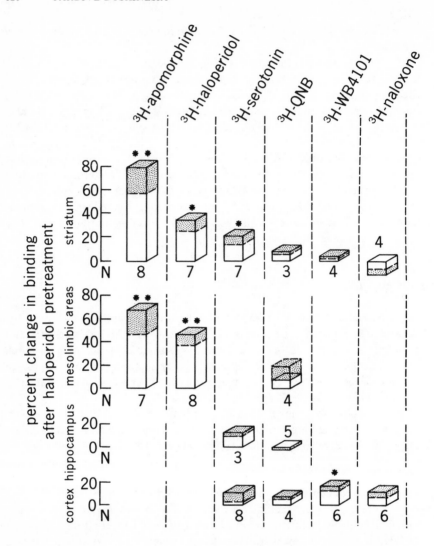

Figure 4. Percentage changes in neurotransmitter receptors (rat brain regions) following long-term haloperidol treatment (10 mg/kg/day for at least 3 weeks). The height of the bars indicates the mean percentage change. The shaded portion indicates the standard error of the mean. The number of completely independently assayed membrane preparations (from 2 to 15 rats per preparation) used in each experiment (N) is indicated below each bar (* = P< .05; ** = P < .02, using Wilcoxon's rank test). The long-term haloperidol treatment selectively increased the dopamine/neuroleptic binding without significant effects on acetylcholine receptors (^{3}H-QNB), alpha-adrenergic receptors (^{3}H-WB-4101), or opiate receptors (^{3}H-naloxone).

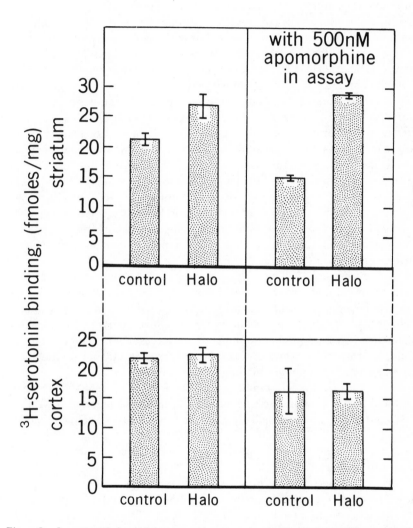

Figure 5.   Long-term haloperidol treatment increases the specific binding of ^{3}H-serotonin in the striatum. Left: Tissues from control rats and haloperidol-treated rats showing an increase in the striatum, but no change in the cortex. Right: Same membrane preparations, but the assays were done in the presence of an excess (500 nM) apomorphine to preclude any ^{3}H-serotonin from binding to dopamine sites.

dopaminergic subsensitivity in the limbic system and no change in the striatal dopaminergic binding (31). Similarly, chronic agonists do not increase the dopaminergic binding (13,20,32). We have seen no change in striatal or mesolimbic dopaminergic binding after chronic kindling (31).

Considerable supersensitivity (after chronic haloperidol) of both the mesolimbic system and the nigrostriatal system may arise from only rather small percentage changes in numbers of receptors. For example, Kelly and Moore (33) reported that the limbic dopaminergic system might be functioning as a modulator of the striatal dopaminergic system. Thus, if both systems are supersensitive as a result of chronic neuroleptic pretreatment, it is possible that the effect of these two regional supersensitivities is multiplied.

Behavioral supersensitivity might not necessarily be due to changes exclusively in the two dopaminergic systems. Other neurotransmitters and receptors might be involved. Serotonin is an example of one such possible influence of other neurotransmitters on dopaminergic behavior (34). It appears that serotonin exercises a negative influence on dopaminergic activity; thus 5-hydroxytryptophan inhibits apomorphine-induced stereotyped behavior (35), while lesions of the raphe nuclei augment apomorphine-induced locomotor behavior (36). In addition, serotoninergic antagonists potentiate dopaminergic action (35,37).

In the present experiments, we observed an increase in the specific ^{3}H-serotonin binding following chronic haloperidol pretreatment. This increase was not seen in the cortex or the hippocampus. The increase was not due to ^{3}H-serotonin binding to dopamine receptors, since excess of apomorphine in the incubation media did not eliminate the increase. Serotonin increase in binding appears to be rather nonspecific, as repeated ethanol pretreatment induces increase of serotonin binding as well (31).

We have also measured the binding to the alpha-noradrenergic binding in the striatum. Alpha-noradrenergic binding in the striatum was reported previously (33), even though the functional significance is not clear, since there is little noradrenaline found in the striatum (39). We would not, therefore, have expected any increase in the binding in the striatum following chronic haloperidol pretreatment.

We were unable to observe any significant change in opiate receptors following chronic neuroleptic pretreatment. Opiates are interesting drugs to study in relation to the striatal dopaminergic system. They share many properties with the neuroleptics. They increase the turnover of dopamine, induce catalepsy (40), and block apomorphine-induced stereotyped behavior (41). Furthermore, cross-tolerance to some opiate-neuroleptic actions has been observed (42,43). Because of this close relation between the opiates and the neuroleptics, one might have expected a change in the striatal ^{3}H-naloxone binding (44). Both cortex and striatum, however, showed no significant change in ^{3}H-naloxone binding.

ACKNOWLEDGMENTS

We thank Mrs. Joan Dumas for excellent technical assistance, and Dr. L. Endrenyi for statistical analysis. Supported by the Ontario Mental Health Foundation and the Medical Research Council of Canada (MT–2951). We are grateful to Dr. W. Forgiel, McNeil Laboratories, for kindly donating haloperidol.

REFERENCES

1. Christensen, A.V., Fjalland, B., Møller Nielsen, I. On the supersensitivity of dopamine receptors induced by neuroleptics. *Psychopharmacology*, *48*:1–6, 1976.
2. Martes, M.P., Constentin, J., Baudry, M., Marcais, H., Protais, P., Schwartz, J.C. Long-term changes in the sensitivity of pre- and postsynaptic dopamine receptors in mouse striatum evidenced by behavioural and biochemical studies. *Brain Res.*, *136*:319–337, 1977.
3. Ungerstedt, U. Postsynaptic supersensitivity after 6-hydroxydopamine induced degeneration of the nigro-striatal dopamine system. *Acta Physiol. Scand. Suppl.*, *367*:69–93, 1971.
4. Tarsy, D., Baldessarini, R.J. The pathophysiologic basis of tardive dyskinesia. *Biol. Psychiatry*, *12*:431–450, 1977.
5. Crane, G.E. Persistent dyskinesia, *Br. J. Psychiatry*, *122*:395–405, 1973.
6. Mao, C.C., Cheney, D.L., Marco, E., Revuelta, A., Costa, E. Turnover of gamma-aminobutyric acid and acetylcholine in nucleus caudatus, nucleus accumbens, globus pallidus and substantia nigra: effects of repeated administration of haloperidol. *Brain Res.*, *132*:375–379, 1977.
7. Lloyd, K.G., Shibuya, M., Davidson, L., Hornykiewicz, O. Chronic neuroleptic therapy: tolerance and GABA systems. In *Advances in Biochemical Pharmacology*, vol. 16. New York: Raven Press, pp. 409–415, 1977.
8. Granacher, R.P., Baldessarini, R.J., Cole, J.O. The pharmacologic evaluation of tardive dyskinesia. *N. Engl. J. Med.*, *292*:326, 1975.
9. Quitkin, F., Rifkin, A., Gochfeld, L., Klein, D.F. Tardive dyskinesia: are first signs reversible? *Am. J. Psychiatry*, *134*:84–87, 1977.
10. Uhrbrand, L., Faurbye, A. Reversible and irreversible dyskinesia after treatment with perphenazine, chlorpromazine, reserpine and electroconvulsive therapy. *Psychopharmacologia*, *1*:408–418, 1960.
11. Rosenbaum, A.H., Niven, R.G., Hanson, N.P., Swanson, D.W. Tardive dyskinesia: relationship with primary affective disorder. *Dis. Nerv. Syst.*, *38*:423–427.
12. Muller, P., Seeman, P. Brain neurotransmitter receptors after long-term haloperidol: dopamine, acetylcholine, serotonin, α-noradrenergic and naloxone receptors. *Life Sci.*, *21*:1751–1758, 1977.
13. Burt, D.R., Creese, I., Snyder, S.H. Antischizophrenic drugs: chronic treatment elevates dopamine receptor binding in brain. *Science*, *196*:326–328, 1977.
14. Tarsy, D., Baldessarini, R.J. Pharmacologically induced supersensitivity to apomorphine. *Nature (New Biol.)*, *245*:262–263, 1973.
15. Tarsy, D., Baldessarini, R.J. Behavioral supersensitivity to apomorphine following chronic treatment with drugs which interfere with synaptic function of catecholamines. *Neuropharmacology*, *13*:927–940, 1974.
16. Gianutsos, G., Moore, K.E. Dopaminergic supersensitivity in striatum and olfactory

tubercle following chronic administration of haloperidol or clozapine. *Life Sci.,* 20:1585–1592, 1977.

17. Møller Nielsen, I., Fjalland, B., Pedersen, V., Nymark, M. Pharmacology of neuroleptics upon repeated administration. *Psychopharmacologia, 34*:95–104, 1974.

18. Burt, D.R., Creese, I., Pardo, J., Coyle, J.T., Snyder, S.H. Dopamine receptor binding: influence of age, chronic drugs and specific lesions. *Soc. Neurosci., Abstracts II,* 775, #1103, 1976.

19. Muller, P., Seeman, P. Increased specific neuroleptic binding after chronic haloperidol in rats. *Soc. Neurosci., Abstract II,* 874, No. 1266, 1976.

20. Friedhoff, A.J., Bonnet, K., Rosengarten, H. Reversal of two manifestations of dopamine receptor supersensitivity by administration of L-DOPA. *Res. Commun. Chem. Pathol. Pharmacol., 16*:411–423, 1977.

21. Kobayashi, R.M., Fields, J.Z., Hruska, R.E., Beaumont, K., Yamamura, H.I. Brain neurotransmitter receptors and chronic antipsychotic drug treatment: a model for tardive dyskinesia. In *Animal Models in Psychiatry.* Usdin, E. (ed.). Oxford: Pergamon Press, 1978.

22. Costall, B., Naylor, R.J. Extrapyramidal and mesolimbic involvement with the stereotypic activity of d- and l-amphetamine. *Eur. J. Pharmacol., 25*:121–129, 1974.

23. Pijnenburg, A.J.J., Honing, W.M.M., Van Der Heyden, J.A.M., Van Rossum, J.M. Effects of chemical stimulation of the mesolimbic dopamine system upon locomotor activity. *Eur. J. Pharmacol., 35*:45–58, 1976.

24. Stolk, J.M., Rech, R.H. Enhanced stimulant effects of d-amphetamine in rats treated chronically with reserpine. *J. Pharmacol. Exp. Ther., 163*:75–83, 1968.

25. Smith, R.C., Davis, J.M. Behavioural evidence for supersensitivity after chronic administration of haloperidol, clozapine and thioridazine. *Life Sci., 19*:725–732, 1976.

26. Dustan, R., Jackson, D.M. The demonstration of a change in adrenergic receptor sensitivity in the central nervous system of mice after withdrawal from long-term treatment with haloperidol. *Psychopharmacol., 48*:105–114, 1976.

27. Jackson, D.M., Andén, N.-E., Dahlstrom, A. A functional effect of dopamine in the nucleus accumbens and in some other dopamine-rich parts of the rat brain. *Psychopharmacologia, 45*:139–149, 1975b.

28. Jackson, D.M., Andén, N.-E., Engel, J., Liljequist, S. The effect of long-term penfluridol treatment on the sensitivity of the dopamine receptors in the nucleus accumbens and the corpus striatum. *Psychopharmacologia, 45*:151–155, 1975a.

29. Costall, B., Naylor, R.J. The behavioural effects of dopamine applied intracerebrally to areas of mesolimbic system. *Eur. J. Pharmacol., 32*:87–92, 1975.

30. Creese, I., Iversen, S.D. The role of forebrain dopamine systems in amphetamine-induced stereotype behavior in the rat. *Psychopharmacologia, 39*:345–357, 1974.

31. Muller, P., Seeman, P. Presynaptic subsensitivity as a possible basis for sensitization by long-term dopamine-mimetics. (Submitted for publication, 1978.)

32. Muller, P., Britton, B., Seeman, P. Brain neurotransmitter binding after long-term ethanol. (In preparation, 1978.)

33. Kelly, P.H., Moore, K.E. Mesolimbic dopaminergic neurons in the rotational model of nigrostriatal function. *Nature, 263*:695–696, 1976.

34. Barbeau, A. The pathogenesis of parkinson's disease: a new hypothesis. *Can. Med. Assoc. J., 87*:802–807, 1962.

35. Goetz, C., Klawans, H.L. Studies on the interaction of reserpine, d-amphetamine, apomorphine and 5-hydroxytryptophan. *Acta Pharmacol., Toxicol., 34*:119–130, 1974.

36. Grabowska, M. Influence of midbrain raphe lesion on some pharmacological and biochemical effects of apomorphine in rats. *Psychopharmacologia, 39*:315–322, 1974.

37. Scheel-Krüger, J., Hasselager, E. Studies of various amphetamines, apomorphine and clonidine on body temperature and brain 5-hydroxytryptamine metabolism in rats. *Psychopharmacologia, 36*:189–202, 1974.

38. Coyle, J.T., Henry, D. Catecholamines in fetal and newborn rat brain. *J. Neurochem.*, *21*:61–67, 1973.
39. Ahtee, L., Kaariainen, I. The effect of narcotic analgesics on the homovanillic acid content of rat nucleus caudatus. *Eur. J. Pharmacol.*, *22*:206–208, 1973.
40. Sasame, H.A., Perez-Cruet, J. Evidence that methadone blocks dopamine receptors in the brain. *J. Neurochem.*, *19*:1953–1957, 1972.
41. Puri, S.K., Lal, H. Tolerance to the behavioural and neurochemical effects of haloperidol and morphine in rats chronically treated with morphine or haloperidol. *Naunyn. Schmiedebergs. Arch. Pharmacol.*, *282*:155–170, 1974.
42. Kuhar, M.J., Pert, C.B., Snyder, S.H. Regional distribution of opiate receptor binding in monkey and human brain. *Nature, 245*:447–450, 1973.
43. Ezrin-Waters, C., Seeman, P. Haloperidol-induced tolerance to morphine catalepsy. *Life Sci., 21*:419-422, 1977.
44. U'Prichard, D.C., Greenberg, D.A., Snyder, S.H. Binding characteristics of radiolabeled agonist and antagonist at central nervous system alpha noradrenergic receptors. *Mol. Pharmacol., 13*:454-473, 1977.

*Ezrin-Waters, C., Seeman, P. Tolerance to haloperidol catalepsy. *Eur. J. Pharmacol., 41*:321–327, 1977.
**Lerner, P., Nosé, P. Haloperidol: effect of long-term treatment on rat striatal dopamine synthesis and turnover. *Science, 197*:181–183, 1977.
***Marsden, C.D., Tarsy, D., Baldessarini, R.J. Spontaneous and drug-induced movement disorders in psychotic patients. In *Psychiatric Aspects of Neurologic Disease*. Benson, D.F., Blumer, D. (eds.). Grune and Stratton, pp. 219–265, 1975.
****Sayers, A.C., Bürki, H.R., Ruch, W., Asper, H. Neuroleptic-induced hypersensitivity of striatal dopamine receptors in the rat as a model of tardive dyskinesias. Effects of clozapine, haloperidol, loxapine and chlorpromazine. *Psychopharmacologia, 41*:97–104, 1975.

11

Chronic Neuroleptic Treatment and Dopamine Receptor Binding: Relevance to Tardive Dyskinesia

SOLOMON H. SNYDER
and IAN CREESE

Several items of clinical evidence suggest that the motor symptoms of tardive dyskinesia may reflect a supersensitivity of dopamine receptors. Whereas neuroleptic drugs actually cause a decrease in motor activity, tardive dyskinesia symptoms resemble the opposite, namely an increase in motor activity. Though the symptoms are caused by chronic treatment with neuroleptics, stopping drug administration frequently exacerbates symptoms, whereas increase in the dose of neuroleptics may often decrease symptoms. This suggests that after prolonged blockade by neuroleptic drugs, the dopamine receptors in the corpus striatum of patients with tardive dyskinesia "fight back" and "hypertrophy" to become hypersensitive to dopamine. Hypersensitivity of dopamine receptors in tardive dyskinesia is also suggested by the fact that these symptoms resemble, to a certain extent, those produced by L-dopa in parkinsonian patients, whose striatal dopamine receptors are thought to be supersensitive.

The clinical syndrome of tardive dyskinesia points toward an important and little studied aspect of synaptic function in the brain, namely the influence of altered neurotransmitter availability on the sensitivity of postsynaptic receptors to neurotransmitters in the central nervous system. During the past several years, we have developed techniques for labeling biochemically the binding sites for numerous neurotransmitter receptors in the brain. The present essay reviews the influence of chronic neuroleptic treatment upon dopamine receptors, which may have relevance for the pathogenesis of tardive dyskinesia.

PRINCIPLES OF NEUROTRANSMITTER BINDING ASSAYS

In principle, the techniques utilized in labeling neurotransmitter receptors are quite simple. One merely measures the binding of a radioactive drug to brain membranes. However, developing procedures that permit selective labeling of transmitter receptors can be quite difficult, because nonspecific binding sites on brain membranes greatly exceed the number of specific receptors. It is quite easy to be deceived into believing that binding involves the receptor site in question, since even if binding characteristics satisfy a limited number of criteria for specificity, one may still be not dealing with the specific receptor in question, or indeed with any neurotransmitter receptor. For instance, stereospecificity is frequently cited as an important criterion of receptor selectivity. In the case of the opiate receptor, ($-$)-isomers possess all the pharmacological activity, and a necessary but *not sufficient* criterion for identification of opiate receptor binding is that binding should be displaced much more by ($-$)-than by ($+$)-isomers of opiates. However, stereospecific binding alone does not ensure that one is dealing with the opiate receptor. Thus, numerous acidic lipids from a wide variety of tissues bind radioactive opiates stereospecifically, but have no relationship to the pharmacologically relevant opiate receptor. Indeed, even synthetic filters can bind ^{3}H-opiates in a saturable fashion with stereospecificity in which the ($-$)-isomer is more potent than the ($+$)-isomer (1).

Even if the ^{3}H-drug employed binds to relatively selective sites, these may not involve only a single neurotransmitter. Thus, ^{3}H-ergots label dopamine, -noradrenergic and serotonin receptors at the same time in certain brain regions (2). Stereospecificity for isomers of the neuroleptic drugs flupenthixol and butaclamol at the dopamine receptors have been thought to represent a screening device to ensure that one is dealing with dopamine receptors. Flupenthixol, but not its β-isomer, and ($+$)-butaclamol, but not its ($-$)-isomer, exhibit potent neuroleptic and antidopamine activity in vivo. However, these drugs also display stereospecificity at α-noradrenergic and serotonin receptors (3). Clearly, before conducting valid studies of the receptor binding of a radiolabeled drug or neurotransmitter, one must fulfill a number of stringent criteria of specificity. The ligand must bind saturably with high and appropriate affinity. The relative potencies of a reasonably extensive series of agents including antagonist and agonist drugs and transmitter analogues, should parallel closely their relative biological activities, thought to be mediated by the receptor under study. For neurotransmitters such as dopamine, with marked regional variations in endogenous levels throughout the brain, the regional variations in receptor bindings should closely parallel endogenous transmitter content. In the case of dopamine, receptor binding sites are highly concentrated in the corpus striatum, nucleus accumbens, and olfactory tubercle, with very low or negligible levels of binding in other brain areas (4).

Bearing all these considerations in mind, extensive studies in our own laboratory (4,5,6), as well as those of Seeman (7,8), have established that butyrophenones such as ^{3}H-spiroperidol and ^{3}H-haloperidol, as well as agonists such as ^{3}H-dopamine and ^{3}H-apomorphine, can label selectively dopamine receptors under appropriate conditions. It must be emphasized that the characterization of dopamine receptor binding for a ligand under one set of conditions does not imply that the ligand will label dopamine receptors in other situations. For example, ^{3}H-spiroperidol labels dopamine receptors in the striatum, but also labels serotonin receptors in the cortex. Although ^{3}H-dopamine labels dopamine receptors in the calf striatum, we have been unable to demonstrate specific dopamine receptor binding of ^{3}H-dopamine in the rat striatum by filtration assay. These techniques have permitted us to examine the relationship between dopamine receptor binding and the pathophysiology of tardive dyskinesia.

The notion that tardive dyskinesia is caused by dopamine receptor supersensitivity assumes that deprivation of dopamine from its receptors after a period of time induces receptor supersensitivity. One direct means of obtaining a preparation in which striatal dopamine receptors are deprived of dopamine is to lesion the nigrostriatal dopamine pathway. Selective lesions of this pathway can be obtained by microinjections of 6-hydroxydopamine into the substantia nigra, which contains cell bodies of dopamine neurons projecting to the corpus striatum. Since the nigrostriatal dopamine pathway is uncrossed, such lesions can be performed unilaterally, so that the unlesioned side of an animal can provide a control.

Behavioral evidence suggests receptor supersensitivity after such lesions (9). In normal rats, apomorphine stimulates postsynaptic striatal dopamine receptors. Thus, if receptor sensitivity is not altered following nigrostriatal lesions, apomorphine should affect lesioned and unlesioned sides to the same extent. If receptor sensitivity is changed following the lesion, one would anticipate motoric asymmetry. Indeed, following unilateral nigrostriatal lesions, apomorphine elicits rotation in a direction opposite to the side of the lesion (9,10). The fact that rotation contralateral to the lesions is due to supersensitivity of receptors on the side of the lesion is confirmed by experiments examining the influence of amphetamine in the same animals. Amphetamine acts by releasing dopamine from nerve terminals. Following the lesions, one would expect a great reduction in dopamine release from the lesioned side, so that dopamine receptors on the unlesioned side would be stimulated to a much greater extent than those on the lesioned side. This is opposite to what occurs with apomorphine receptor supersensitivity following nigrostriatal lesions. In animals with these lesions, amphetamine induces rotation, but in the direction ipsilateral to the side of the lesion, opposite to that elicited with apomorphine.

What might be the cause of apparent behavioral supersensitivity of dopamine receptors after unilateral nigrostriatal lesions? Alterations could occur at several levels, including changes in nondopaminergic neurons or metabolic changes within cells postsynaptic to dopamine neurons. Such changes might include alterations in cyclic AMP or energy metabolism. One might also anticipate changes in dopamine receptors themselves. We found a marked enhancement of ^{3}H-haloperidol binding following unilateral nigrostriatal lesions (11).

It has been established that the extent of behavioral supersensitivity can be monitored by the amount of rotation. We observed a correlation between the augmentation of ^{3}H-haloperidol binding and the amount of rotation in animals following nigrostriatal lesions (Fig. 1), which suggests strongly that the increase in binding can explain the behavioral supersensitivity. By evaluating different concentrations of ^{3}H-haloperidol, we ascertained whether increased binding was due to a change in the affinity of dopamine receptors for ^{3}H-haloperidol or to an increase in the number of binding sites. We found no alteration in affinity, but a 50% increase in the number of receptor sites (Table 1).

In absolute terms, the extent of behavioral supersensitivity, as measured by the number of rotations provoked by a fixed dose of apomorphine, is greater than the 50% increase in the number of dopamine receptors. This could mean that other mechanisms are responsible in part for the behavioral alterations. Alternatively, it is conceivable that comparing rotation with receptor binding is like comparing apples and oranges. Perhaps changes in receptor numbers are amplified in some fashion within the corpus striatum, so that a 50% increase in receptors elicits a substantially greater behavioral change.

Properties of dopamine receptor sites as labeled by ^{3}H-agonists and ^{3}H-antagonists differ (4–6). Agonists are more potent in competing for the binding of ^{3}H-agonists such as ^{3}H-dopamine and ^{3}H-apomorphine, whereas antagonists are relatively more potent in influencing the binding of ^{3}H-antagonists such as ^{3}H-spiroperidol and ^{3}H-haloperidol. Apparently, agonist and antagonist interact with different, but possibly interconverting, states of the dopamine receptor. Alternatively, there may exist distinct agonist and antagonist favoring receptors. The dopamine-sensitive adenylate cyclase is presumably associated with dopamine receptor sites. Response to drugs by the cyclase parallel more closely effects upon ^{3}H-dopamine than upon ^{3}H-spiroperidol binding. Destruction of neuronal cells in the corpus striatum by microinjections of kainic acid induces a profound depletion of dopamine-sensitive adenylate cyclase in the tissue, with only a 40% reduction in ^{3}H-haloperidol binding (12; See also Table 2). Cerebral cortex ablation depletes much of the remainder of ^{3}H-haloperidol binding sites, indicating that these sites are probably located on nerve terminals of neurons that project from the cerebral cortex to the corpus striatum (Fig. 2). Thus, certain of the ^{3}H-haloperidol binding sites are distinct entities from the dopamine-sensitive adenylate cyclase.

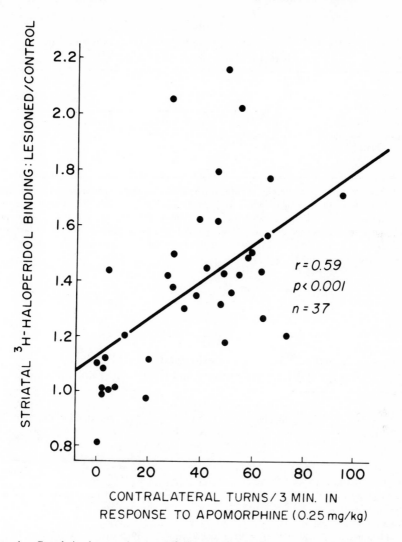

Figure 1.   Correlation between increased [³H]haloperidol binding in the lesioned striatum and behavioral supersensitivity to apomorphine following unilateral nigrostriatal 6-hydroxydopa-mine lesion. Rotational behavior to apomorphine (0.25 mg/kg s.c.) was measured between 2 and 7 months after unilateral injection of 6-hydroxy-dopamine into the substantia nigra. Striatal [³H]haloperidol binding was assayed in the lesioned and control striatum of each rat separately between 1 and 10 weeks later and is expressed as the mean ratio of specific c.p.m. [³H]haloperidol bound in the lesioned/control striatum at 4 concentrations of [³H]haloperidol (0.4-4.0 nM). Each data point represents an individual rat.

Table 1
Effect of Unilateral Nigro-Striatal 6-Hydroxydopamine Lesions on Rat [³H]Haloperidol Binding Parameters

		K_D, nM	pmol/g wet wt. tissue
Control Striatum	(n=24)	0.69 ± 0.08	16.1 ± 1.1
Lesioned Striatum	(n=24)	0.75 ± 0.07	22.7 ± 1.2
Paired Differences		0.06 ± 0.08	6.6 ± 1.2
		NS	$p < 0.001$

Rats were injected unilaterally with 6-hydroxydopamine in the substantia nigra, and the left and right striata of each rat were assayed separately at least 2 months following lesion with 4 concentrations of [³H]haloperidol between 0.4 and 4 nM. The K_D and B_{MAX} values were calculated from Scratched plots of [³H]haloperidol binding data and analyzed by t-tests (two-tailed) of the paired differences between the lesioned and control striatum of each rat. (NS = Not Significant.)

Table 2
Effect of Kainic Acid Lesion and Cortical Ablation on Rat Striatal Enzyme Activity and [³H]Haloperidol Binding

	[³H]Haloperidol Binding	Tyrosine Hydroxylase Activity	Choline Acetyltransferase Activity	Glutamic Acid Decarboxylase Activity
		% Control ± SEM		
Kainate 22 day postlesion	64 ± 3* (n = 6)	97 ± 6† (n = 6)	49 ± 4† (n = 6)	42 ± 7 (n = 6)
Cortical ablation 5 day postlesion	68 ± 5† (n = 22)	101 ± 3 (n = 22)	73 ± 5† (n =16)	99 ± 7 (n = 12)
Kainate and cortical ablation	30 ± 5† (n = 9)	120 ± 9 (n = 9)	39 ± 6† (n = 9)	41 ± 6† (n = 8)

Rats received an intrastriatal injection of kainic acid (2 µg) or cortical ablation or kainate injection, followed by cortical ablation, as described in the text. The striata were assayed for the activities of tyrosine hydroxylase, choline acetyltransferase, and glutamate decarboxylase, and specific binding of [³H]haloperidol. Results are presented in terms of percent (± S.E.M.) of the level in the contralateral nonlesioned striata that did not differ significantly from those in unlesioned rats. Absolute values for the contralateral striatum expressed in terms of mg tissue: [³H]haloperidol binding 15 fmoles (710 cpm/sample) tyrosine hydroxylase, 230 pmoles hr.⁻¹; choline acetyltransferase, 20 nmoles-hr.⁻¹; glutamic acid decarboxylase 13 nmoles-hr.⁻¹. The number of separate preparations is indicated in parentheses.

*p < 0.005   †p < 0.001

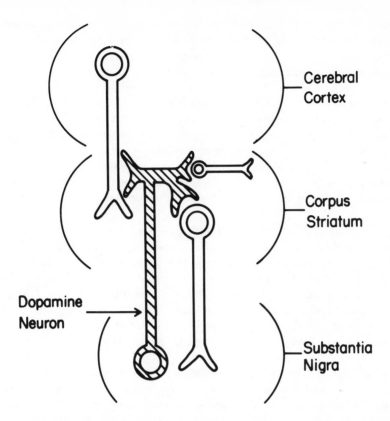

Figure 2.   Diagram of different populations of dopamine receptors in rat corpus striatum.
Receptors associated with the dopamine-sensitive adenylate cyclase are localized almost solely
to neuronal cells intrinsic to the corpus striatum. Dopamine receptors labeled by ^{3}H-haloperidol
occur to a similar extent on neurons intrinsic to the striatum and on axons and/or terminals of
neuronal projections from the cerebral cortex.

CHRONIC NEUROLEPTIC TREATMENT ENHANCES DOPAMINE RECEPTOR BINDING

Does the behavioral supersensitivity and alteration in dopamine receptors
following nigrostriatal lesion relate to tardive dyskinesia? In animal models of
tardive dyskinesia, researchers have administered neuroleptics for about 3
weeks and then evaluated alterations in the behavioral effects of apomorphine.
After 3 weeks of treatment with a variety of neuroleptics and a 5-day interval in
which drug administration is terminated to permit ''washout'' from the body,
rats do indeed become hypersensitive to certain behavioral effects of apomorphine (13, 14). Large doses of apomorphine in normal rats elicit a stereotyped

pattern of sniffing, licking, and gnawing. After chronic neuroleptic administration, this stereotyped behavior can be elicited by lower doses of apomorphine than it can in naive rats. Using this experimental paradigm, we evaluated
dopamine receptor binding in such animals (15). Following chronic treatment
with the butyrophenone haloperidol or the phenothiazine fluphenazine, increases of about 20%–25% in ^{3}H-haloperidol binding occurred (Table 3).
Reserpine, an effective neuroleptic antischizophrenic agent, which produces
parkinsonian effects by depleting dopamine, also elicited about a 25% increase
in receptor binding. By contrast, treatment for three weeks with a substantially
higher dose of the phenothiazine promethazine, which lacks antischizophrenic
neuroleptic activity, failed to affect ^{3}H-haloperidol. Treatment with the
stimulant amphetamine for three weeks did not change receptor binding significantly.

To evaluate the dose characteristics and time course of the changes in
receptor binding, we compared the effects of two doses of haloperidol, 0.5 and
5.0 mg/kg, given daily for 1 to 3 weeks. We measured ^{3}H-haloperidol binding
5, 12, and 17 days after terminating drug treatment (Table 4). The augmentation of binding was as great with the lower as with the higher dose. Likewise,
the increase in binding after 1 week of haloperidol treatment was similar to that
after 3 weeks. Twelve days after haloperidol treatment was terminated, the
increased binding was less apparent than at 5 days, while at 17 days no increase
was detected.

To determine whether enhanced receptor binding is attributable to an increased number of binding sites or to a change in affinity, we measured binding
of various concentrations of ^{3}H-haloperidol and analyzed the data by Scatch-

Table 3
Effect of Chronic Drug Treatments on [^{3}H]Haloperidol
Binding in the Rat

Injected Drug	Haloperidol	Reserpine	Fluphenazine	Promethazine	Amphetamine
Percentage change	19 ± 4 (21)	23 ± 7 (10)	27 ± 12 (6)	3 ± (12)	−2 ± 4 (5)
Relative to control	p < .0005	p < .005	p < .05	NS	NS

Rats were injected subcutaneously with haloperidol (Haldol®, 0.5 mg/kg), reserpine
(Serpasil®, 0.25 mg/kg), fluphenazine (Prolixine®, 0.5 mg/kg), promethazine (Phenergan®, 2.5
mg/kg), or d-amphetamine sulfate (5 mg/kg) daily for three weeks and killed 5–7 days later.
Freshly removed corpora striata were assayed for binding with 3 concentrations of
[^{3}H]haloperidol (0.2-1.4 nM). Results for the 3 concentrations were averaged for each rat. Data
for each treated rat were expressed as the percentage change in bound radioactivity relative to that
in a matched, uninjected control rat assayed in parallel. The tabulated results give the means ±
S.E.M. for the indicated number of rats. The p values are by the one-tailed t-test, (NS = Not
Significant.)

Table 4.
Time Course and Dose Dependence of Increase in [³H]-
Haloperidol Binding, Following Chronic Haloperidol
Treatment

Injection period Drug-free period		1 wk 5d	3 wk 5d	3 wk 12d	3 wk 17d
Daily dose	[³H]Halo conc.	Percentage increase (n = 5)			
0.5 mg/kg	0.4 nM	19±5 $p < .01$	25±2 $p < .001$	13±14 NS	0±6 NS
	0.8 nM	36±11 $p < .025$	24±9 $p < .05$	18±6 $p < .05$	8±5 NS
5 mg/kg	0.4 nM	27±7 $p < .01$	17±6 $p < .025$	—	—
	0.8 nM	15±9 NS	31±7 $p < .005$	—	—

Rats were injected daily for 1 or 3 weeks with 0.5 or 5 mg/kg haloperidol as in Table 1 and were killed 5–17 days later. Freshly removed striata were assayed for binding with 0.4 nM and 0.8 nM [³H]haloperidol. Each result is the mean (±S.E.M.) of 5 pairs of rats, paired in order of assay. The p values were calculated by the one-tailed t-test. [³H]Haloperidol binding in control striata was equivalent to 5 pmol/g tissue (0.4 nM) or 8 pmol/g tissue (0.8 nM). (NS = Not Significant)

ard plots. Following 21 days of treatment with haloperidol and a five-day washout, we could not detect any alteration in the affinity of binding, but did observe a consistent 20%–25% increase in the number of binding sites.

Like denervation supersensitivity of dopamine receptors, the increase in receptor binding sites following chronic neuroleptic treatment is less than the apparent behavioral supersensitivity. Conceivably, postreceptor components are involved in the increased behavioral response. The activity of a dopamine-sensitive adenylate cyclase in the corpus striatum is not altered in mice treated chronically with neuroleptics (16). Moreover, the ability of apomorphine to elevate striatal cyclic AMP concentrations in vivo is not changed in these mice (14). The apparent discrepancy between increased receptor binding, reflecting the recognition sites of the dopamine receptor, and adenylate cyclase activity accords with other data indicating that receptor binding sites and adenylate cyclase may be distinct entities. Interestingly, the behavioral supersensitivity to apomorphine as well as the increase in the number of receptor sites is more pronounced after lesions of the nigrostriatal pathway than after chronic treatment with neuroleptic drugs.

In summary, chronic treatment with neuroleptic drugs enhances dopamine receptor binding, which could explain the symptoms of tardive dyskinesia. It should be emphasized that rats are treated for a period of only 3 weeks with neuroleptics in these experiments, while humans developing symptoms of tardive dyskinesia have usually received the drugs for much longer periods of time. Of course, one cannot directly compare drug treatment in rats and man. Also, the behavioral sensitivity to apomorphine as well as the increase in the number of dopamine receptors in rats is reversible. In humans, the symptoms of tardive dyskinesia are also reversible, provided that drug treatment has not been for a prolonged period of time. In humans treated for a year or more with neuroleptics, symptoms of tardive dyskinesia sometimes appear to be irreversible.

REFERENCES

1. Snyder, S.H., Pasternak, G.W., Pert, C.B. Opiate receptor mechanisms. In *Handbook of Psychopharmacology*, vol. 5, Iversen, I.I., Iversen, S.D., Snyder, S.H., (eds.). New York: Plenum Press, pp. 329–360, 1975.
2. Davis, J.N., Strittmatter, W.J., Hoyler, E., Lefkowitz, R.J. [^{3}H]Dihydroergocryptine binding in rat brain. *Brain Res., 132*:327–336, 1977.
3. Enna, S.J., Bennett, J.P., Jr, Burt, D.R., Creese, I., U'Prichard, D.C., Greenberg, D.A., Snyder, S.H. Stereospecificity and clinical potency of neuroleptics. *Nature, 267*:183–184, 1977.
4. Creese, I., Burt, D.R., Snyder, S.H. The dopamine receptor: differentiation of agonist and antagonist states with ^{3}H-dopamine and ^{3}H-haloperidol. *Life Sci., 17*:993–1002, 1975.
5. Burt, D.R., Creese, I., Snyder, S.H. Characteristics of ^{3}H-haloperidol and ^{3}H-dopamine binding associated with dopamine receptors in calf brain membranes. *Mol. Pharmacol., 12*:800–812, 1976.
6. Creese, I., Burt, D.R., Snyder, S.H. Biochemical actions of neuroleptic drugs: focus on the dopamine receptor. In *Handbook of Psychopharmacology*, vol. 10, Iverson, I.I., Iversen, S.D., Snyder, S.H., (eds.). New York: Plenum Press, pp. 37–89, 1978.
7. Seeman, P., Chau-Wong, M., Tedesco, J., Wong, K. Brain receptors for antipsychotic drugs and dopamine: direct binding assays. *Proc. Natl. Acad. Sci. USA, 72*:4376–4380, 1975.
8. Seeman, P., Lee, T., Chau-Wong, M., Tedesco, J., Wong, K. Dopamine receptors in human and calf brains using [^{3}H]apomorphine and an antipsychotic drug. *Proc. Natl. Acad. Sci. USA, 73*:4354–4358, 1976.
9. Ungerstedt, U., Arbuthnott, G.W. Quantitative recording of rotational behavior in rats after 6-hydroxydopamine lesions of nigrostriatal dopamine system. *Brain Res., 24*:485–493, 1970.
10. Creese, I., Iversen, S.D. Behavioral sequelae of dopaminergic supersensitivity: postsynaptic supersensitivity? In *Pre- and Postsynaptic Receptors*. Usdin, E., Bunney, W.E., Jr., (eds.). New York: Dekker, pp. 171–190, 1975.
11. Creese, I., Burt, D.R., Snyder, S.H. (eds.). Dopamine receptor binding enhancement accompanies lesion-induced behavioral supersensitivity. *Science, 197*:596–598, 1977.
12. Schwarcz, R., Creese, I., Coyle, J.T., Snyder, S.H. Dopamine receptors localized on cerebral cortical afferents to rat corpus striatum. *Nature*, 1978. (In press.)
13. Tarsy, D., Baldessarini, R.J.: Behavioral supersensitivity to apomorphine following chronic treatment with drugs which interfere with the synaptic function of catecholamines. *Neuropharmacology, 13*:927–940, 1974.

14. Moore, K.E., Thornburg, J.E. Drug-induced dopaminergic supersensitivity. In *Advances in Neurology*, vol. 9, Calne, D., Chase, T.N. Barbeau, A., (eds.). New York: Raven Press, pp. 93–104, 1975.

15. Burt, D.R., Creese, I., Snyder, S.H. Antischizophrenic drugs: chronic treatment elevates dopamine receptor binding in brain. *Science, 196*:326–328, 1977.

16. Von Voigtlander, P.E., Losey, E.G., Triezenberg, H. Increased sensitivity to dopaminergic agents after chronic neuroleptic treatment. *J. Pharmacol. Exp. Ther., 193*:88–94, 1975.

12

Receptor-Cell Sensitivity Modification (RSM) as a Model for Pathogenesis and Treatment of Tardive Dyskinesia

ARNOLD J. FRIEDHOFF
HELEN ROSENGARTEN
and KENNETH BONNET

INTRODUCTION

We have been carrying out a series of basic and clinical studies of tardive dyskinesia based on the supersensitivity model of this syndrome. According to this paradigm, tardive dyskinesia, at least in part, results from the development of supersensitivity of the postsynaptic dopaminergic receptor cells as a result of chronic neuroleptic treatment (1–5).

Neuroleptic agents have potent dopamine-blocking properties. After chronic blockade (usually years in man), it is believed that the postsynaptic cells compensate for the loss of specific agonist at the receptor by becoming more sensitive. Evidence from human studies supporting this view has thus far been largely circumstantial. It consists principally of the observation that tardive symptoms frequently emerge when neuroleptics are withdrawn, and disappear, at least transiently, if neuroleptics are readministered. It is believed that this sequence occurs because the withdrawal of the blocking agent exposes the supersensitive receptor cell to the full effect of the transmitter, in this case dopamine, resulting in overactivity of this system. Readministering the blocker will at least transiently shield the supersensitive cell, and thus relieve the symptoms.

From the teleological standpoint, it appears that the chronic administration of antipsychotic agents—that is, dopamine blockers—induces the postsynaptic cell to become more sensitive in an attempt to overcome the blockade. Why this should first occur, often after ten or more years, is not clear, since the blockade is very complete after several weeks of treatment.

Observations from earlier animal studies are also supportive of the supersensitivity model. It has been shown that if rats are treated chronically with antipsychotic agents followed by washout, the rats become supersensitive to the effects of dopaminergic agents such as apomorphine (6). However, in rats the compensatory increase in sensitivity occurs after several weeks.

These changes in receptor-cell sensitivity may occur at one or more loci. There may be changes that occur in front of the receptor, for instance, involving a change in the access of ligand to receptor or through the masking or unmasking of existing receptors. Alternatively, there may be changes in the receptor itself. These could involve a change in the conformation of the receptor, resulting in a modification of the affinity of the ligand for the receptor. Another possibility is a change in the influence of one receptor on an adjacent one. This interaction of receptors (cooperativity) may be positive or negative. Also at the level of the receptor, there may be a change in receptor number and/or density.

In back of the receptor a number of changes may occur that can also influence the "sensitivity" of the receptor-cell response (see Fig. 1). These include electrolyte flux, particularly Ca^{++}. This ion is believed to be involved in the activation of a protein that in turn activates the enzyme adenylate cyclase. This enzyme, responsible for the generation of cyclic AMP, is activated by a specific dopamine-receptor interaction via the activator protein. Thus, factors affecting the level or state of adenylate cyclase, or the degradation of cyclic AMP, can be important in determining the level of cyclic AMP resulting from dopamine stimulation. The cyclic AMP formed is involved in activating protein kinases, enzymes that are responsible for phosphorylation of proteins, including membrane proteins in some cases. This may be a means by which the receptor-ligand interaction is translated into a more enduring modification of the cell via the phosphorylation of elements of the cell membrane which influence cell response.

Some or all of these chemical changes are believed to be involved in modulating the nervous activity of the cell; however, the exact relationship between the chemical events and the electrical activity of the cell is unclear.

At the functional level, the net effect of the underlying neuronal events is to modify behavior. One would predict that behaviors strongly regulated by dopaminergic centers would become more responsive to the effects of dopaminergic agents when the dopamine receptors were supersensitive, and less responsive when subsensitive.

In the studies described here, supersensitivity of the dopamine system has been defined in an operational sense to be that state which results in increased specific dopamine binding to dopamine receptors; in increased response of

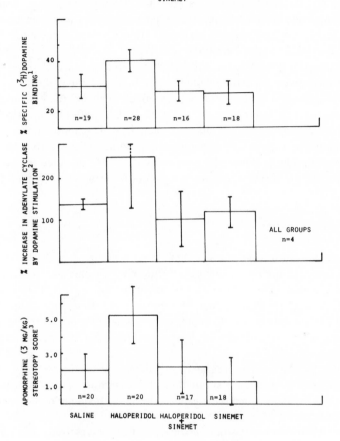

Figure 1.

[1] Specific (^{3}H)-dopamine binding defined as percent of total (^{3}H)
binding displaced by (+) butaclamol
[2] Adenylate cyclase activity defined as the amount of cAMP formed
in 0.3mm striatal slices in the presence of Ro 20-1724
[3] Sterotopy scores were taken 30' after injection of apomorphine

* A COMBINATION OF L-DOPA AND CARBIDOPA

dopamine-specific adenylate cyclase; and in increased behavioral response
(stereotypy) to dopaminergic agents.

METHODS

In these studies, 4 groups of rats were treated. Groups I (saline) and IV (sinemet—a combination of carbidopa and levodopa) were treated with physiological saline i.p. for 28 days. Groups II (haloperidol) and III (haloperidol + sinemet) received haloperidol, 2.5 mg/kg i.p. for 28 days to produce supersensitivity of striatal dopamine receptors. Subsequently, Groups I and II received saline for 10 days. In order to produce a reversal of haloperidol-induced supersensitivity, Group III rats subsequently received sinemet (L-dopa, 50 mg/kg, and carbidopa, 5 mg/kg) p.o. for 10 days. Group IV rats also received the 10-day sinemet treatment. At the end of the 10-day period in all groups, all treatments were stopped to permit the elimination of residual sinemet in Groups III and IV. On the fifth day after termination of all treatments (forty-third day), all rats were sacrificed. Dopamine receptor binding and adenylate cyclase responses were determined in the corpus striata as previously described (7). Stereotypy scores (6) were determined in additional animals from all groups 30 minutes after apomorphine injection (3 mg/kg i.p.).

Results and Discussion

The results of these studies are summarized in Figure 2. It can be seen that specific dopamine binding is increased following chronic haloperidol treatment and washout. This increase is reversed by subsequent treatment with sinemet followed by washout. A similar increase is seen in dopamine-specific adenylate cyclase activity and in apomorphine-induced behavioral stereotypy. The increase in the latter two responses is also reversed by sinemet treatment and washout.

The ability of the sinemet treatment to produce subsensitivity in previously normosensitive rats was also studied. In this case only trends can be seen, without clear evidence that normosensitive cells respond to an increased supply of dopamine by a reduction in sensitivity.

The ability to reverse the manifestations of supersensitivity of dopamine receptors by treatment with sinemet may have potential as a treatment for tardive dyskinesia. If tardive dyskinesia is the result of compensatory supersensitivity following prolonged dopamine-receptor blockade, then group II in this study may be a model of this syndrome. The fact that sinemet is capable of reversing this state has led us to undertake a therapeutic trial of these compounds in patients with tardive dyskinesia (2). Initial results are encouraging, but the studies are still underway.

REFERENCES

1. Klawans, H.L. The pharmacology of tardive dyskinesias. *Am. J. Psychiatry, 130*:82–86, 1973.

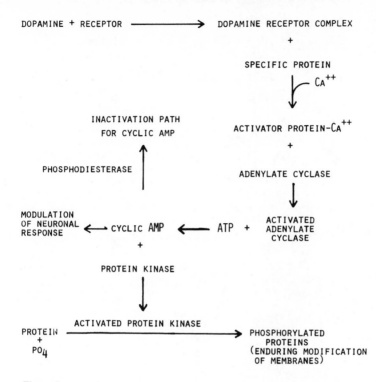

Figure 2.

2. Friedhoff, A.J. Receptor sensitivity modification—a new paradigm for the potential treatment of some hormones and transmitter disturbances. In *Psychopathology and Brain Dysfunction*. Shagass, C., Gershon, S., Friedhoff, A.J. (eds.). New York: Raven Press, pp. 139–148, 1977.

3. Moore, K.E., Thornburg, J.E. Drug-induced dopaminergic supersensitivity. In *Advances in Neurology*, vol. 9. Calne, D., Chase, T.N., Barbeau, A. (eds.). New York: Raven Press, pp. 93–104, 1975.

4. Muller, P., Seeman, P. Increased specific neuroleptic binding after chronic haloperidol in rats. *Neuroscience Abstracts, 2*:874, 1976.

5. Burt, D.R., Creese, I., Prado, J., Coyle, J.T., Snyder, S.H. Dopamine receptor binding: influences of age, chronic drugs and specific lesions. *Neuroscience Abstracts, 2*:775, 1976.

6. Tarsy, D., Baldessarini, R.J. Behavioral supersensitivity to apomorphine following chronic treatment with drugs which interfere with the synaptic function of catecholamines. *Neuropharmacology, 13*:927–940, 1974.

7. Friedhoff, A.J., Bonnet, K.A., Rosengarten, H. Reversal of two manifestations of dopamine receptor supersensitivity by administration of L-dopa. *Res. Commun. Chem. Pathol. Pharmacol., 16*:411–423, 1977.

13

Biochemical and Behavioral Studies of Neuroleptic-Induced Dopamine Hypersensitivity

ANA HITRI,
PAUL CARVEY,
WILLIAM J. WEINER
and HAROLD L. KLAWANS

Tardive dyskinesia is a choreiform movement disorder (1,2) related to chronic neuroleptic therapy (3–7). The pathogenesis of tardive dyskinesia is felt to be related to the chronic dopamine receptor blockade produced by neuroleptic therapy (1,2). This chronic receptor-site blockade is thought to alter the subsequent receptor-site responsiveness, resulting in receptor-site hypersensitivity, which plays a primary role in the pathophysiology of the abnormal movements (1). This proposal has received considerable support from animal models of tardive dyskinesia, which have employed altered behavioral response to the dopamine agonist apomorphine following chronic neuroleptic treatment (8–10). In a recent attempt to provide biochemical evidence of hypersensitive dopamine receptors following chronic haloperidol, Burt et al. (11) reported an increase in the number of dopamine receptor sites when receptor binding was assayed with the tritiated dopamine antagonist H^3-haloperidol. A similar observation was reported by Muller et al. In this study dopamine receptors were assayed with a dopamine agonist H^3-apomorphine (12).

The present study investigated whether or not there is an alteration in dopamine receptor binding following chronic haloperidol administration in rats. Dopamine receptor binding was assayed with the tritiated, naturally occurring agonist H^3-dopamine. Since haloperidol is not just a dopamine antagonist, but also has activity at norepinephrine (13) and muscarinic (14) receptor sites, and since it is possible that haloperidol receptor sites may also exist, haloperidol binding should not be expected to be identical to or necessarily representative of dopamine binding. The alteration in the dopamine receptor site is, of course, the crucial one for any theory of receptor-site hypersensitivity in tardive dyskinesia.

Dopamine binding was studied in both the striatum and the nucleus accumbens. The former area is thought to be the area involved in tardive dyskinesia, while the nucleus accumbens is a dopamine-rich area that many investigators feel may play a role in the pathophysiology of schizophrenia.

METHODS

White male rats and guinea pigs received haloperidol (0.5 mg/kg) for 14 days, and after a 7-day drug-free period, were sacrificed. The caudate-putamens and nucleus accumbens were dissected out and homogenized in Tris buffer. Brain homogenates were then incubated with radiolabeled dopamine at 4°C, and bound radioactivity was collected by rapid ultrafiltration technique.

RESULTS AND DISCUSSION

Fourteen days of haloperidol pretreatment followed by a 7-day drug-free interval were associated with increased dopamine binding in the striatum. In order to determine accurately the number of binding sites and the affinity constants for the binding sites, the data was represented in a Scatchard plot (15) in Figure 1. The slope on the Scatchard plot represents the binding-site affinity, while the intercept on the abscissa represents the number of receptor sites. The Scatchard plot demonstrates that the above treatment regime results in a significant (p = 0.01) increase in H^3-dopamine binding sites (67%) as well as a significant (p = 0.005) increase in binding affinity (ninefold).

In striatal membranes of animals sacrificed on the last (fourteenth) day of chronic haloperidol treatment, there was a threefold increase in affinity, but the number of binding sites was significantly reduced (12%) as compared to control striatal membranes. The decrease in the number of available H^3-dopamine binding sites is felt to be due to persistent occupation of striatal dopamine receptor sites in these animals that received haloperidol on the day of sacrifice.

These results support previous behavioral studies that have concluded that chronic neuroleptic treatment alters striatal dopamine receptor-site responsiveness (9,10,16). These results also support the studies of Burt *et al.* (11) and Muller *et al.* (12), who demonstrated that striatal dopamine receptor-site binding is altered following chronic neuroleptic treatment. However, dopamine receptor-site binding was assayed in these studies by the use of H^3-haloperidol, a dopamine antagonist, or H^3-apomorphine, an artificial

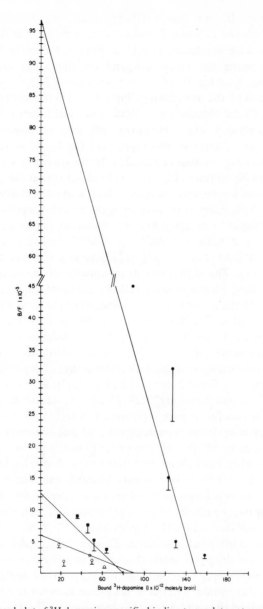

Figure 1.   Scatchard plot of ^{3}H dopamine specific binding to caudate putamen membranes derived from control rat brains 0—0, chronic haloperidol-treated rat brains without a drug-free interval■——■, and after a 7-day drug-free interval ●——●. Specific ^{3}H dopamine binding was measured as excess over blank tubes containing 100 micromolar cold dopamine. Each point is the mean value of two separate experiments, with the binding assays performed in duplicate. The slope of the lines obtainind by linear regression analysis represents the affinity of the binding site for ^{3}H dopamine (K_a). The point at which the straight line intercepts the x axis represents the number of binding sites.

dopamine agonist. In our study, H^3-dopamine, the naturally occurring agonist, was employed to assay dopamine receptor-site binding. These studies were conducted at $4°C$ in order to minimize MAO activity (17) and to preserve the receptor-ligand complex. Previous reports of dopamine receptor binding (18,19) were conducted at $37°C$, and MAO activity was minimized by the use of pargyline (an MAO inhibitor). At $37°C$ the rate of receptor-ligand association is rapid, and equilibrium is achieved after 10 minutes' incubation (18). However, the rate of dissociation of the dopamine-receptor complex is also rapid, and the ligand separates from its receptors in a matter of seconds (19,20,21). In our studies at $4°C$, equilibrium was reached after 40 minutes (22). This indicates a slower rate of association and dissociation at lower temperatures, which may reflect greater receptor-ligand stability. This delay in separation of the receptor-ligand complex may make actual changes in receptor binding easier to determine. Our studies demonstrate a 67% increase in striatal dopamine binding sites, as compared to a 20% increase in Burt et al.'s study (11), and to a 40% increase in Muller et al.'s study (12). The difference in magnitude of the altered dopamine receptor-site binding characteristics following chronic haloperidol may be attributed in part to the use of the agonist instead of the antagonist to measure binding characteristics. The natural agonist may well be more specific for dopamine receptors. In addition, the binding of haloperidol to other sites (haloperidol, muscarinic, and/or acceptor) could also influence the results.

The observations that agonist and antagonist assays of dopamine binding are altered differently by chronic haloperidol may also be explained by the "two state" model of receptor function (23,24,25,26). According to this theory, the receptor exists in two forms with differential, selective high affinity for the agonist and antagonist. It has been demonstrated that dopamine agonists have about 50 times greater affinity for dopamine than haloperidol sites, whereas dopamine antagonists have about 100 times greater affinity for haloperidol than dopamine sites (18). It is certainly possible that chronic neuroleptic treatment alters the two forms of the dopamine receptor differently.

Figure 2 contrasts the results of chronic haloperidol pretreatment with and without a drug-free interval on H^3-dopamine specific binding in the nucleus accumbens (Scatchard plot). Fourteen days of haloperidol administration followed by a 7-day drug-free interval resulted in a slight increase in binding sites and in affinity, which were not significant (standard deviation overlap). Haloperidol administration without a drug-free interval resulted in a 72% reduction in binding sites and a fourfold increase in affinity.

Chronic haloperidol treatment without a drug-free interval affects dopamine receptor-binding characteristics in both the striatum and the nucleus accumbens. The increased affinity constant seen in both striatal and accumbens dopamine receptors, and the decreased number of dopamine receptor sites seen in both the striatum and nucleus accumbens, may reflect either the acute effect

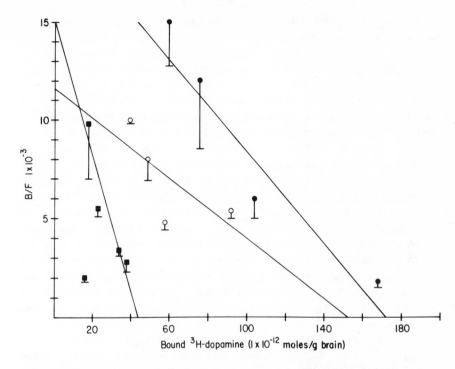

Figure 2.   Scatchard plot of ^{3}H dopamine specific binding to nucleus accumbens membranes derived from control rat brains 0—0, chronic haloperidol treated rat brains without a drug-free interval ■——■, and with a 7-day drug-free interval ●—●. Specific ^{3}H dopamine was obtained as the excess over blank tubes containing 100 micromolar cold dopamine. The straight lines were obtained by linear regression analysis. Each point is the mean value of two separate experiments, with the binding assays performed in duplicate.

of the last dose of haloperidol on receptor membranes or a combination of acute and chronic effects. In these animals the drug was administered up to and including the day of sacrifice, and no time was allowed for loss of acute drug effects.

The decrease in the number of binding sites, when compared to controls, is significant in both brain regions after chronic haloperidol followed by a drug-free interval. The increased affinity constants may reflect, at least in the striatum, a combination of the increased affinity caused by chronic haloperidol (and seen best after withdrawal) and acute affects of the haloperidol. It is more difficult to explain the observation that not only did chronic haloperidol itself result in increased affinity in the accumbens, but that after a drug-free period the affinity was essentially unchanged. This suggests that we may be dealing with two types of receptors. One set is blocked by chronic haloperidol, leaving only a small number of unblocked nucleus accumbens dopamine receptors that either have or develop higher affinity, and a large number that became available for binding only after haloperidol is discontinued.

It has been postulated that dopamine receptor characteristics may vary regionally within the central nervous system (27,28,29). Our results support such speculations, since we have demonstrated a differential alteration in dopamine receptor-binding characteristics in the striatum versus the nucleus accumbens following chronic haloperidol treatment. Striatal dopamine receptors were clearly supersensitive following haloperidol withdrawal, whereas dopamine receptors in the nucleus accumbens were not. This differential effect on the two sets of dopamine receptors may have clinical significance. Tardive dyskinesia is a choreiform disorder, and as such should reflect altered striatal physiology (1,2). The fact that haloperidol induced altered binding characteristics of striatal dopamine receptors may explain in part, at least, the mechanism behind neuroleptic-induced tardive dyskinesia. These results, then, are consistent with the hypothesis that chronic neuroleptic therapy does induce striatal dopamine receptor hypersensitivity, which could be the major factor in the pathophysiology of tardive dyskinesia.

The hypothesis that antagonist-induced "denervation hypersensitivity" may be related to the increased number of dopamine receptors gains fuller support by the recent work of Snyder et al. (30), which demonstrates that there is a correlation between the alteration in rotational behavior induced by unilateral lesions of the nigrostriatal pathway and increased numbers of striatal dopamine receptors. This should not be surprising, since denervation hypersensitivity in the periphery has long been thought to be related to increased numbers of receptor sites.

The fact that chronic haloperidol treatment did not permanently alter nucleus accumbens binding is consistent with the observation that tardive dyskinesia occurs without alteration of the underlying psychiatric state for which the patient is receiving neuroleptics. It has been suggested that dopamine acting at dopamine mesolimbic receptors of the nucleus accumbens plays a major role in the pathophysiology of schizophrenia (31,32). If this is true, then neuroleptic-induced alterations in dopamine receptor-site binding in the nucleus accumbens should worsen schizophrenia. The fact that these characteristics were unchanged in the nucleus accumbens may explain why the development of tardive dyskinesia is not related to any worsening of the underlying schizophrenia.

Our most recent study investigated whether this neuroleptic-induced dopamine receptor-site hypersensitivity in the striatium is a permanent phenomenon or a transient one that is reversible with time. In this study young male guinea pigs were administered haloperidol 0.5 mg/kg i.p. for 21 days, after which the neuroleptic was discontinued. The first group of the animals was decapitated after a 7-day drug-free period, while the second group was sacrificed 3 weeks, and the third group 6 weeks, after the cessation of the haloperidol treatment. The corresponding control animals received i.p. saline injections for 3 weeks, and they were decapitated, together with the haloperidol-treated animals.

Figure 3 demonstrates the behavioral response of the haloperidol-treated guinea pigs as compared to controls at various times after discontinuation of the haloperidol treatment. The animals exhibited an increased behavioral response to subthreshold doses of the dopamine agonist apomorphine 1 week and 3 weeks after haloperidol therapy, as can be seen from the increased intensity and duration of the stereotyped behavior. However, this increased behavioral responsiveness diminishes 6 weeks after the cessation of haloperidol. These results indicate that the neuroleptic-induced increased behavioral response to a dopamine agonist in animals is reversible with time. In order to correlate these behavioral results with the biochemical findings, we studied the ^{3}H dopamine stereospecific binding in the guinea pig striatum as the function of time after the discontinuation of the neuroleptic treatment.

Figure 4 represents the effect of chronic haloperidol treatment, 1 week after cessation of the treatment, on tritiated dopamine stereospecific binding to the guinea pig striatal membranes, as presented in Scatchard plot. As can be seen, there was a dramatic tenfold increase in the number of binding sites after haloperidol treatment, while the affinity of the stereospecific binding remained unchanged.

Figure 5 demonstrates that there was no effect of chronic haloperidol treatment 6 weeks after the cessation of the treatment. The Scatchard analysis revealed two distinct binding sites in the striatal membranes of the 15-week-old control animals. One of the regression lines is described by the slope of 5 x 10^9M, which represents the association constant (K_a). This binding line intercepts the abscissa at 22 pmoles/g, indicating the dopamine receptor-site density at this high affinity binding site. The low affinity binding site is characterized by an association constant of 8 x 10^7M and by receptor-site concentration of 200 pmoles/g. Six weeks after the cessation of the chronic haloperidol treatment, there was no change in ^{3}H dopamine stereospecifi‿ binding characteristics at either of the binding sites.

As indicated in Figure 4, there is only one binding line present for H^3-dopamine stereospecific binding in the 9-week-old guinea-pig striatal membranes. The striata from the animals of the same age group pretreated with chronic haloperidol also displayed only one binding site. This site had the same affinity as the control animals, but there was a tenfold greater receptor-site density. This finding may suggest that the receptors appearing after the chemical denervation by haloperidol may have the same binding properties as the normal striatal receptors.

The difference between the results obtained from the rat striatal ^{3}H dopamine binding and those obtained from the guinea pig brain studies may be partly attributed to species differences or to the fact that the stereospecific ^{3}H

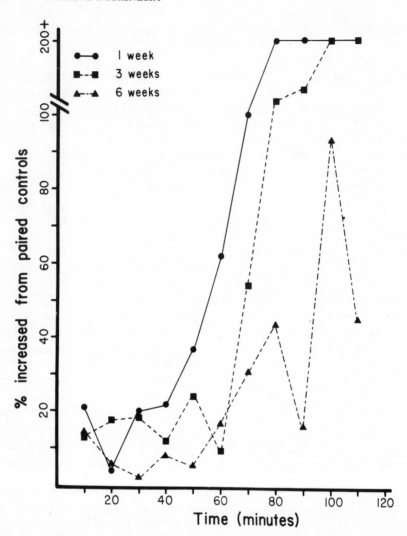

Figure 3.   Effect of chronic haloperidol treatment on the behavioral response of guinea pigs to subthreshold doses of apomorphine 1 week, 3 weeks, and 6 weeks after the discontinuation of the treatment. Data are expressed as percent increase over the paired controls.

dopamine binding studied in the guinea pig striatum may be a more accurate measurement of dopamine receptor binding than the specific binding that was studied in the rat brains under the same experimental conditions.

At this point it is not clear whether the newly proliferated dopamine receptor sites are caused by an increased receptor synthesis or induced by chronic haloperidol administration or by some other yet unknown mechanism.

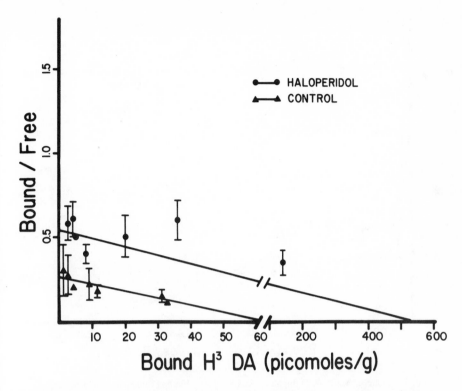

Figure 4.   Effect of chronic haloperidol pretreatment on stereospecific ^{3}H dopamine binding
to the striatal membranes of young guinea pigs (Scatchard plot). The stereospecific ^{3}H
dopamine binding was determined as the excess over blank tubes containing 1 micromolar (+)
butaclamol, the clinically effective enantiomer of the new antipsychotic drug (11,18,19,20).
Each point is the mean value of duplicate binding assays.

The fact that six weeks after the cessation of the chronic haloperidol
treatment the dopamine receptor binding characteristics were returned to
normal control values may imply that in a 6-week drug-free period the
hypothetical neuroleptic-induced enhanced dopamine receptor synthesis returned to its normal rate.

The appearance of the second binding site for dopamine in the guinea pig
striatal membranes in the 15-week-old animals is felt to be a maturational
phenomenon, since there is only one binding site present in the younger
animals. This finding is consistent with the previously reported results from
our laboratory. When the effects of chronic d-amphetamine (33) and L-dopa
(34) on dopamine receptor binding characteristics in the striatum were investigated in the guinea pigs of the same age group, two distinct dopamine binding
sites were also detected.

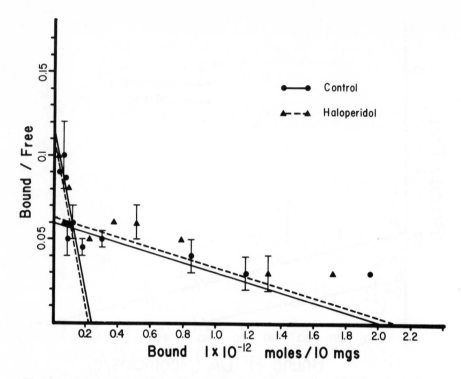

Figure 5. Scatchard plot of ^{3}H dopamine stereospecific binding to the mature guinea pig striatal membranes. Two binding lines were resolved by a stepwise linear regression analysis of the data. Each point is the mean of quadruplicate binding assays.

The observation presented above, that a 6-week drug-free interval returned the dopamine receptor binding characteristics to normal control values may have significant clinical implications, in spite of the fact that there are obvious differences between the animals studied here and patients with tardive dyskinesias. The behavioral and binding changes in animals occur within weeks of the initiation of neuroleptic therapy, while tardive dyskinesias usually take years to develop (1,3). Both behavioral and binding changes are seen in all animals, while only a minority of patients receiving neuroleptics chronically develop tardive dyskinesias (3), and finally, none of these animals demonstrate spontaneous abnormal movements, which are, of course, the *sine qua non* of tardive dyskinesia. Despite these difficulties, it is our belief that these observations may help to explain the pathophysiology of neuroleptic-induced tardive dyskinesia.

The finding that the dopamine receptor hypersensitivity is reversible with time may have two significant clinical implications:

1. This finding supports the concept that early detection and drug withdrawal may be an effective form of therapy for tardive dyskinesia.
2. These results also suggest that prolonged drug holidays may prevent permanent receptor-site alterations. Studies are now underway on the effect of more long-term haloperidol treatment on receptor-site hypersensitivity.

SUMMARY

It has been suggested on the basis of animal behavioral studies that the neuroleptic-induced dyskinesias result from denervation hypersensitivity of striatal dopamine receptors. Chronic pretreatment of laboratory animals with neuroleptics followed by a 7-day drug-free period resulted in a 67% increase in the number of specific striatal ^{3}H dopamine sites in the rats, and a tenfold increase in the number of stereospecific striatal ^{3}H dopamine sites in guinea pigs. The increased behavioral response of the animals 1 week and 3 weeks after the discontinuation of the haloperidol treatment diminished 6 weeks after the cessation of the treatment. This finding is supported by the fact that the dopamine receptor characteristics returned to normal control values in a 6-week drug-free period. These results indicate that the neuroleptic-induced increased dopamine receptor responsiveness in animals is reversible with time.

REFERENCES

1. Klawans, H.L. The pharmacology of tardive dyskinesias. *Am. J. Psychiatry, 130*:82–86, 1973.
2. Tarsy, D., Baldessarini, R.J. The tardive dyskinesia syndrome. In *Clinical Neuropharmacology*, vol. 1. Klawans, H.L. (ed.). vol. 1, New York: Raven Press, pp. 29–61, 1976.
3. Crane, G.E. Tardive dyskinesias in patients treated with major neuroleptics: a review of the literature. *Am. J. Psychiatry, 124*:40–48, 1968.
4. Faurbye, A. The structural and biochemical basis of movement disorders in the treatment with neuroleptic drugs in extrapyramidal diseases. *Compr. Psychiatry, 11*:205–224, 1970.
5. Faurbye, A., Rasch, P.J. Neurologic symptoms in the pharmacology of psychoses. *Acta Psychiatr. Scand., 40*:10–26, 1964.
6. Rodova, A., Hanunek, K. Persistent dyskinesias after phenothiazines. *Cesk Psychiatr., 60*:250–254, 1964.
7. Degwitz, R., Wenzel, W. Clinical observations of extrapyramidal hyperkinesia following long-term neuroleptic therapy. *Nervenarzt, 37*:368–370, 1966.
8. Fjalland, B., Møller-Nielsen, I. Enhancement of methylphenidate-induced stereotypies by repeated administration of neuroleptics. *Psychopharmacologia, 34*:105–109, 1974.
9. Gianutsos, G., Drawbaugh, R.B., Hynes, M.D., Lal, H. Behavioral evidence for dopamine supersensitivity after chronic haloperidol. *Life Sci., 14*:887–898, 1974.
10. Klawans, H.L., Rubovits, R. An experimental model of tardive dyskinesia. *J. Neural Transm., 33*:235–246, 1972.

11. Burt, D.R., Creese, I., Snyder, S.H. Antischizophrenic drugs: chronic treatment elevates dopamine receptor binding. *Science, 196*:326–327, 1977.

12. Muller, P., Bowles, J., Seeman, P. Dopaminergic and cholinergic receptors in striatal and limbic regions after chronic haloperidol. *Soc. Neurochem. Absts. III*, abst. No. 1466, 1977.

13. Ohta, M. Haloperidol blocks and alpha adrenergic receptor in the reticulo cortical inhibitory input. *Physiol. Behav., 16*:505, 1976.

14. Snyder, S.H., Greenberg, D., Yamamura, H. Antischizophrenic drugs and brain cholinergic receptors. *Arch. Gen. Psychiatry, 31*:58–61, 1974.

15. Scatchard, G. The attraction of proteins for small molecules and ions. *Ann. N.Y. Acad. Sci., 51*:660–672, 1949.

16. Tarsy, D., Baldessarini, R.J. Behavioral supersensitivity to apomorphine following chronic treatment with drugs which interfere with the synaptic function of catecholamines. *Neuropharmacology, 13*:927–940, 1974.

17. Fillion, G., Fillion, M.P., Spirakis, C., Bakers, J.M., Jacob, J. 5-hydroxytryptamine binding to synaptic membranes from rat brain. *Life Sci., 18*:65–74, 1975.

18. Creese, J., Burt, D.R., Snyder, S.H. Dopamine receptor binding: differentiation of agonist and antagonist states with ³H-dopamine and ³H-haloperidol. *Life Sci., 17*:993–1002, 1975.

19. Seeman, P., Chau-Wong, M., Tedisco, J., Wong, K. Brain receptors for antipsychotic drugs and dopamine: direct binding assays. *Proc. Natl. Acad. Sci. USA, 72*:4376–4380, 1975.

20. Burt, D.R., Enna, S.J., Creese, J., Snyder, S.H. Dopamine receptor binding in the corpus striatum of mammalian brain. *Proc. Natl. Acad. Sci. USA, 72*:4655–4659, 1975.

21. Seeman, P., Lee, T., Chau-Wong, M., Tedesco, J., Wong, K. Dopamine receptors in human and calf brains, using ³H-apomorphine and an antipsychotic drug. *Proc. Natl. Acad. Sci. USA, 83*:4354–4358, 1976.

22. Hitri, A., Weiner, W.J., Borison, R.L., Diamond, B.I., Nausieda, P.A., Klawans, H.L. Dopamine binding following prolonged haloperidol pretreatment. *Ann. Neurology.* (in press.)

23. Karlin, A. On the application of "a plausible model" of allosteric proteins to the receptor for acetylcholine. *J. Theor. Biol., 16*:306–320, 1967.

24. Changeux, J.P. Response of acetylcholinesterase from Torpedo mormorata to salts and curarizing drugs. *Mol. Pharmacol., 2*:369–392, 1966.

25. Changeux, J.P., Podleski, T.R. On the excitability and cooperation of electroplex membrane. *Proc. Natl. Acad. Sci. USA, 59*:944–950, 1968.

26. Neurotransmitter and drug receptors in the brain. *Biochem. Pharmacol., 24*:1371–1374, 1975.

27. Costall, B., Naylor, R.J., Neumayer, J.L. Differences in the nature of stereotyped behavior induced by apomorphine derivatives in the rat and in their actions in extrapyramidal and mesolimbic brain area. *Eur. J. Pharmacol., 31*:1–16, 1975.

28. Shellenberger, M.K., Gordon, J.H. Regional differences in responses to displacement and inhibition of synthesis of catecholamines in the cat brain. *Biol. Psychiatry, 9*:131–145, 1974.

29. Cools, A.R. Basic consideration on the role of concertedly working dopaminergic, GABA-ergic, cholinergic, and serotonergic mechanisms within the neostriatum and nucleus accumbens in locomotor activity, gnawing, turning, and dyskinetic activities. *Adv. Behav. Biol., 21*:97–141, 1975.

30. Snyder, S. H., Creese, I., Burt, D.R. Dopamine receptor binding in brain: relevance to psychiatry. In *Neuroregulators and Psychiatric Disorders*, Usdin, E., Hamburg, D.A., Barchos, J.D. (eds.). New York: Oxford University Press, pp. 526–537, 1977.

31. Klawans, H.L., Goetz, C., Westheimer, R. The pharmacology of schizophrenia. In *Clinical Neuropharmacology*, vol. 1, Klawans, H.L. (ed.). Vol. 1, New York: Raven Press, pp. 1–28, 1976.
32. Stevens, J.R. Anatomy of schizophrenia. *Arch. Gen. Psychiatry, 29*:177–189,
33. Klawans, H.L., Hitri, A., Carvey, P., Nausieda, P.A., Weiner, W.J. The effect of chronic d-amphetamine exposure on striatal dopamine receptors. (Submitted for publication.)
34. Klawans, H.L., Hitri, A., Carvey, P., Nausieda, P.A., Weiner, J.W. The effect of chronic levodopa administration on striatal ^3H dopamine binding. (Submitted for publication.)

14

Regional Brain Manganese Levels in an Animal Model of Tardive Dyskinesia

WILLIAM J. WEINER
PAUL A. NAUSIEDA
and HAROLD L. KLAWANS

Chronic manganese poisoning in man often produces a progressive permanent neurologic disorder, which includes a variety of abnormal involuntary movements (1,2). The extrapyramidal motor manifestations of chronic manganese poisoning include dystonia, tremor, choreoathetoid movements, and lingual-facial-buccal dyskinesias. Many of these movements are reminiscent of the abnormal movements seen in tardive dyskinesia (3,4). The pathophysiology of choreatic movement in all movement disorders including Huntington's chorea (5), tardive dyskinesia (6), and levodopa-induced dyskinesia (5,7,8), is felt to involve striatal dopaminergic mechanisms.

A previous report that chlorpromazine resulted in increased basal ganglia manganese level (9) raised the possibility that manganese toxicity could play a role in the neuroleptic-induced alterations in striatal physiology that occur in tardive dyskinesia. In order to further investigate this possibility, we have investigated the effect of chronic chlorpromazine administration on regional brain manganese concentrations in guinea pigs.

METHODS

Male guinea pigs with an average weight of 250 to 275 g were housed in large cages with free access to food and water. Chlorpromazine (10 mg/kg, subcutaneously) was administered daily for 10 days. Control animals received equal-volume saline injections. On the completion of chlorpromazine administration, there was a 2-day drug-free period. The animals were sacrificed by cervical fracture. The whole brain was removed and dissected into frontal cortex, caudate nucleus, and cerebellar hemisphere for further analysis. Caudate nucleus dissection was accomplished by anterior-posterior-directed serial coronal sections through each hemisphere until the anterior head of the caudate nucleus located immediately lateral to the ventricular system was reached. The caudate nucleus could then be easily separated from surrounding brain tissue. The tissue was prepared for atomic absorption spectrophotometry by a slight modification of the volume method of Jackson et al. (10). Each 30-100 mg sample, wet-tissue weight, was digested by 1cc Soluene for 48 hours at room temperature. This resulted in a clear homogenous-appearing liquid suitable for aspiration and placement in the graphite furnace. Standard curves for copper, iron, and manganese were prepared on the day of the experimental tissue determination by the use of a metal standard in a Soluene matrix. All samples were analyzed in a Perkin-Elmer Model 306 flameless atomic absorption spectrophotometer, using instrument settings suggested by the manufacturer and adjusted slightly in our own laboratory to provide the highest absorbance readings.

RESULTS

Chronic chlorpromazine administration resulted in a significant increase in caudate nucleus and cerebellar hemisphere manganese concentration, but there was no change in the frontal cortex manganese concentration (Table 1).

Table 1
Manganese (ng/g) ± S.E.M.

	Caudate Nucleus	Frontal Cortex	Cerebellar Hemisphere
Control (n = 16)	214.64 ± 9.03	187.98 ± 9.99	265.50 ± 24.56
Chlorpromazine Pretreated (n = 12)	286.50 ± 13.18	198.36 ± 9.92	442.28 ± 34.13
	$p < .005$	$p > .40$	$p < .005$

DISCUSSION

The increased concentration of manganese in the caudate nucleus that accompanies chronic chlorpromazine administration may have implications for the pathogenesis of tardive dyskinesia. Since 1837 (11), it has been noted that exposure to manganese can result in neurologic symptomatology of an extrapyramidal nature. More recently, toxic exposure to manganese resulting in manganese madness with typical extrapyramidal manifestations has been studied extensively in manganese miners and industrial workers exposed to this ore (12–15). This clinical experience has been reproduced successfully in the laboratory, in that animals exposed to chronic manganese develop extrapyramidal neurologic syndromes (16,17). The neuropathologic findings in these animals involve not only the basal ganglia, but also the Purkinje cells of the cerebellum. There are also definite central nervous system biochemical changes that occur in animals exposed to chronic manganese. In rats and rabbits, chronic manganese exposure leads to depletion of whole brain dopamine and serotonin (18,19). In monkeys, the decreased dopamine concentration is most marked in the caudate nucleus, and the degree of caudate dopamine depletion correlates well with the degree of clinical toxicity as measured by the extent of induced extrapyramidal dysfunction (20). These biochemical changes have been noted to occur in the absence of any marked neurotoxic phenomena observable by light microscopy.

Bird and colleagues (9) have demonstrated that chronic administration of another phenothiazine, prochlorperazine, results in increased manganese in the basal ganglia of monkeys. The present finding that chlorpromazine also increases caudate nucleus manganese concentration in guinea pigs confirms the associated increase in brain manganese following phenothiazine administration, and extends the range of phenothiazines involved.

Neuroleptic-induced altered dopamine receptor-site responsiveness has been proposed as a possible model of tardive dyskinesia (21). In this model, prolonged neuroleptic administration in animals leads to increased behavioral responsiveness on subsequent exposure to amphetamine or apomorphine (21–23). The theory most commonly advanced to explain the altered responsiveness to dopamine following prolonged phenothiazine exposure is the production of denervation hypersensitivity secondary to blockage of the receptor site by the phenothiazine. However, as demonstrated here, chronic phenothiazine administration results in increased manganese in the caudate nucleus. Increased central nervous system manganese concentration profoundly effects dopamine and serotonin metabolism. Alteration in these neurotransmitters is known to be related to extrapyramidal dysfunction. Since chronic chlorpromazine administration raises caudate nucleus manganese, it is possible that the alterations in dopamine responsiveness produced by chronic chlorpromazine may in part be related to increased manganese concentration. It is altered responsiveness of striatal dopamine receptor sites following prolonged neuroleptic administration in patients that is believed to be a possible etiologic factor in the induction of neuroleptic-induced tardive dyskinesia (5). It may be that part of the alteration in striatal function following prolonged chlorpromazine is related to increased manganese concentration in the basal ganglia. If this were shown to be the case, then metal chelation therapy administered with neuroleptics might prove of value in preventing or reversing tardive dyskinesia.

SUMMARY

Chronic chlorpromazine pretreatment was associated with significant increases in manganese concentrations in the caudate nucleus and cerebellar hemisphere. The drug-induced alterations in caudate manganese levels could be a factor in the pathogenesis of tardive dyskinesia.

ACKNOWLEDGMENTS

This work was supported by grants from the United Parkinson Foundation and the Boothroyd Foundation, Chicago, Illinois.

REFERENCES

1. Mena, I.J., Court, S., Fuenzolida, P.S., Papavasiliou, P.S., Cotzias, G. Modification of chronic manganese poisoning. *N. Engl. J. Med., 282*:5–10, 1970.
2. Cook, D.G., Fahn, S., Brait, K.A. Chronic manganese intoxication. *Arch. Neurol., 30*:59–65, 1974.
3. Paulson, G.W. "Permanent" or complex dyskinesia in the aged. *Geriatrics, 23*:105–110, 1968.
4. Grane, G.E., Naranjo, E.R. Motor disorders induced by neuroleptics. *Arch. Gen. Psychiatry, 24*:179–184, 1971.
5. Klawans, H.L., Weiner, W.J. The pharmacology of choreatic movement disorders. *Progress in Neurobiology, 6*:48–80, 1976.
6. Klawans, H.L., Ilahi, M.M., Shenker, D. Theoretical implications of the use of L-dopa in parkinsonism. *Acta Neurol. Scand., 46*:409–441, 1970.
7. Klawans, H.L. The pharmacology of dyskinesia. *Am. J. Psychiatry, 130*:82–86, 1973.
8. Klawans, H.L., Goetz, C., Nausieda, P., Weiner, W.J. Levodopa-induced dopamine receptor hypersensitivity. *Ann. Neurol., 2*:125–129, 1977.
9. Bird, E.D., Collins, G.H., Dodson, M.H., Grant, L.G. The effect of phenothiazines on the manganese concentration in the basal ganglia of sub-human primates. In *Progress in Neuro-Genetics*, vol. 1. Proceedings of the 2nd International Congress in Neuro-Genetics and Neuro-Ophthalmology, Montreal, Amsterdam: Excerpta Medica, 1967.
10. Jackson, A.J., Michael, L.M., Schumacher, H.J. Improved tissue solubilization for atomic absorption. *Anal. Chem., 44*:1064–1065, 1972.
11. Couper, J. On the effects of black oxide of manganese when inhaled into the lungs. *Br. Ann. Med. Pharmacol., 1*:41–42, 1837.
12. Rodier, J. Manganese poisoning in Moroccan miners. *Br. J. Ind. Med., 12*:21–35, 1955.
13. Mena, O.M., Fuenzalida, S., Cotzias, G.C. Chronic manganese poisoning: clinical picture and manganese turn over. *Neurology, 17*:128–136, 1967.
14. Rosenstock, Simons, D.G., Meyer, J.S. Chronic manganism. *JAMA, 217*:1354–1358.
15. Greenhouse, A.H. Manganese intoxication in the United States. *Trans. Am. Neurol. Assoc., 96*:248–249, 1971.

16. Mella, H. The experimental production of basal ganglia symptomotology in Macacus rhesus. *Arch. Neurol. Psychiatr.*, *11*:405–417, 1924.
17. Von Bogaert, L., Dallemgne, M.J. Approches experimentales des troubles nerveux in manganisme. *Mschr. Psychiatr. Neurol.*, *111*:60, 1945–46.
18. Mustafa, S.J., Chandra, S.V. Levels of 5-hydroxytryptamine, dopamine, and norepinephrine in whole brain of rabbits in chronic maganese toxicity. *J. Neurochem.*, *18*:931–933, 1971.
19. Bonilla, Diez-Ewald, M. Effect of L-dopa on brain concentration of dopamine and homovanillic acid in rats after chronic manganese chloride administration. *J. Neurochem.*, *22*:297–299, 1974.
20. Neff, N.H., Barrett, R.E., Costa, E. Selective depletion of caudate nucleus dopamine and serotonin during chronic manganese dioxide administration to squirrel monkeys. *Experientia*, *25*:1140–1141, 1969.
21. Klawans, H.L., Rubovits, R. An experimental model of tardive dyskinesia. *J. Neural Transm.*, *33*:235–246, 1972.
22. Tarsy, Baldessarini, R.J. Behavioral supersensitivity to apomorphine following chronic treatment with drugs that interfere with the synaptic function of catecholamines. *Neuropharmacology*, *13*:927–940, 1974.
23. Smith, R.C., Davis, J.M. Behavioral evidence for supersensitivity after chronic administration of haloperidol, clozapine, and thioridazine. *Life Sci.*, *19*:725–732, 1976.

15

The Effect of Lithium on Haloperidol-Induced Super-sensitivity to D-Amphetamine and Apomorphine

HAROLD L. KLAWANS
PAUL A. NAUSIEDA
and WILLIAM J. WEINER

Based upon clinical observations and analogies to other human chorieform movement disorders, Klawans *et al*. suggested that the abnormal involuntary movements of neuroleptic-induced tardive dyskinesia were mediated by the activity of dopamine at striatal dopamine receptors (1). They suggested that hypersensitivity of the striatal dopamine receptors played a key role in the pathophysiology of these movements and that this hypersensitivity was the result of prolonged dopaminergic receptor blockade produced by prolonged neuroleptic treatment (2,3). Thus, a pharmacologically induced denervation hypersensitivity of striatal dopamine receptors was hypothesized as the basic neural alteration in tardive dyskinesia (2,3,4).

As a direct result of this physiological insult, the striatal neurons respond in an abnormal manner to any dopamine that is able to act upon their altered receptors. The movements seen in tardive dyskinesia are thus the overt manifestation of the abnormal response of such neurons.

Over the last several years we have studied the effect of chronic neuroleptic pretreatment on stereotyped behavior (SB) as a model of tardive dyskinesia. Stereotyped behavior elicited by amphetamine and apomorphine is felt to be directly related to dopamine agonism at striatal dopamine receptors (4,5,6). It has been shown that prolonged administration of neuroleptic agents induces an apparently prolonged decrease in the threshold for both amphetamine- and apomorphine-induced stereotyped behavior (4,7,8). This suggests that chronic neuroleptic pretreatment does result in increased dopamine receptor-site responsiveness, and that this model may be analogous to human tardive dyskinesia.

Recent reports of the possible efficacy of lithium in the treatment of tardive dyskinesia (9–12) led us to use this model to study the efficacy of lithium in the prevention and treatment of neuroleptic-induced alterations in the threshold for d-amphetamine- and apomorphine-induced stereotyped behavior.

The use of this model makes it possible to differentiate between the preventive and therapeutic effects of any treatment regime. A preventive regime would be one that influences the pathogenesis of TD (i.e., the development of postsynaptic receptor-site hypersensitivity), while a therapeutic regime could either prevent the behavioral expression of this hypersensitivity without altering the hypersensitivity or could actually decrease the hypersensitivity.

METHODS

White male guinea pigs weighing between 250 and 300 grams were stored, 12 to a cage, at 24°C with a light-dark cycle of 0700 to 1600 hours on, and 1600 to 0700 hours off. Animals being treated with lithium were given a diet containing 2.79% lithium chloride and free access to both tap water and saline. In preliminary experiments, this was found to produce a stable blood level of lithium that was within the human therapeutic range. Animals treated with haloperidol (McNeil) were given daily subcutaneous injections of 0.5 mg/kg in 0.5 ml normal saline. Control animals received an injection of 0.5 ml normal saline daily.

The experimental groups consisted of the following: (a) control—normal diet, saline injections for 3 weeks; (b) haloperidol pretreated—normal diet, 0.5 mg/kg haloperidol for 3 weeks; (c) haloperidol and lithium treated—lithium diet and 0.5 mg/kg haloperidol for 3 weeks. For all the above groups, the diet and injections were stopped one week prior to further testing. The fourth experimental group was (d) haloperidol pretreated, lithium treated—normal diet and 0.5 mg/kg haloperidol for 3 weeks. After the 0.5 mg/kg haloperidol injections were stopped, the animals were placed on the lithium diet for 1 week and then given amphetamine or apomorphine.

On the morning of each experiment, animals were removed, placed 4 per wire mesh testing cage, and denied access to food or water. The d-amphetamine (Smith Kline & French) was diluted for injection on the morning of use. Apomorphine (Merck) was stored at 4°C and dissolved for injection in distilled water not more than 5 minutes prior to injection to minimize the possibility of oxidation. All injections were given simultaneously via the subcutaneous route.

All animals were observed continuously for the first half-hour following the injection and at 15-minute intervals thereafter for a maximum of 3 hours, or until the animals ceased stereotyped behavior. Rating of behavior was performed according to the method of Ernst, slightly modified: 0, no stereotyped behavior; 1+, occasional licking of the grid and exploration; 2+, occasional biting and gnawing at the grid, easily distracted by movement or sound in the room; 3+, persistent and intense gnawing at one location, without locomotion, distracted by loud noises only; 4+, persistent, continuous gnawing at one location, without locomotion, not distracted by noises (13,14). Scoring of the animals was performed during each 15-minute period and expressed as the maximum rating attained by each animal during that period of observation. The maximal behavior produced in each animal was then recorded and used in all calculations. Threshold for stereotyped behavior was considered to be a rating of 3+ or greater.

RESULTS

The effect of lithium given as a treatment following prolonged haloperidol pretreatment is shown in Table 1. The 3 mg/kg d-amphetamine is a subthreshold dosage, which does not induce fully developed SB behavior in control animals. This dosage did induce SB in haloperidol-pretreated animals, and lithium treatment did not prevent this increased response. Similarly, 0.15 mg/kg apomorphine did not induce SB in control animals, but did induce it in animals pretreated with haloperidol; once again, lithium treatment did not prevent this increased response.

The effect of lithium given simultaneously with haloperidol on the subsequent response to d-amphetamine and apomorphine is shown in Table 2. As before, prolonged haloperidol pretreatment resulted in increased behavioral response to both d-amphetamine and apomorphine. The prophylactic use of lithium during the phase of haloperidol pretreatment prevented this increased behavioral responsiveness to both d-amphetamine and apomorphine.

DISCUSSION

The data presented above suggest that chronic haloperidol administration decreases the threshold to both amphetamine- and apomorphine-induced stereotyped behavior. Lithium given concurrently with haloperidol prevents this drug-induced alteration, but the subsequent administration of lithium appears to have no effect.

Interest in lithium in the treatment of human choreatic disorders began with several brief reports of its efficacy in Huntington's chorea (11,15,16). Several preliminary reports have claimed at least partial efficacy for lithium in

Table 1
The Effect of Lithium As a Treatment on Haloperidol-Induced Decreased Threshold for Stereotyped Behavior

Group	N	Dosage of d-amphetamine	Dosage of apomorphine	Number developing SB	Significance
Control	12	3mg/Kg		0	
Haloperidol	6	3mg/Kg		6	p<0.05
Haloperidol followed by lithium	6	3mg/Kg		6	p<0.05
Control	12		0.15mg/Kg	0	
Haloperidol	6		0.15mg/Kg	6	p<0.05
Haloperidol followed by lithium	6		0.15mg/Kg	6	p<0.05

Table 2
Effect of Concurrent Lithium Prophylaxis on Haloperidol-Induced Decreased Threshold for Stereotyped Behavior

Group	N	Dosage of d-amphetamine	Dosage of apomorphine	Number developing SB	Significance
Control	12	3mg/Kg		0	
Haloperidol	6	3mg/Kg		6	p<0.05
Haloperidol & lithium	6	3mg/Kg		0	
Control	12		0.15mg/Kg	0	
Haloperidol	6		0.15mg/Kg	6	p<0.05
Haloperidol & lithium	6		0.15mg/Kg	0	

ameliorating the abnormal movements of tardive dyskinesia (9,12). Since neuroleptic-induced decrease in the threshold for stereotyped behavior appears to have the same physiologic basis as human tardive dyskinesia, the failure of lithium to reverse the former suggests that lithium will probably not be an effective treatment for tardive dyskinesia once the movements are present.

The successful prevention of haloperidol-induced hypersensitivity by the simultaneous ingestion of lithium suggests that lithium might be able to prevent the development of tardive dyskinesia. No human data is available on this issue.

Since tardive dyskinesia should be viewed as a progressive disorder (17), it remains possible that lithium may, however, have some role in the management of patients who are already manifesting some features of this disorder.

The concept that tardive dyskinesia is a progressive disorder is based on several clinical observations. First, there is the epidemiologic evidence that the incidence of tardive dyskinesia is related to the duration of therapy. This suggests that the longer the pathogenesis persists, the more frequently the physiology is disrupted, to the point where clinical abnormalities appear. The observation that the disease is progressive in many individuals is more cogent. Tardive dyskinesia does not begin in most patients as a full-blown, generalized choreatic disorder. It usually begins as an asymptomatic sign, with mild lingual-facial-buccal dyskinesias, and only later does it become more severe and more generalized. This increase in clinical manifestation represents two types of progression: (1) increase in the severity of the movements in those areas already involved, and (2) increase in the number of areas involved. The results presented here—that lithium given concurrently with haloperidol prevents haloperidol-induced dopamine receptor hypersensitivity from developing—raise the possibility that lithium treatment might prevent the progression of tardive dyskinesia without necessarily decreasing the movements already present.

SUMMARY

The chronic administration of neuroleptics results in a decreased threshold for both amphetamine- and apomorphine-induced stereotyped behavior. This prolonged drug-induced dopamine receptor-site hypersensitivity is a workable model of tardive dyskinesia. In this model the simultaneous administration of lithium prevents the development of haloperidol-induced decreased threshold for amphetamine- and apomorphine-induced stereotyped behavior. The subsequent administration of lithium does not have this effect. These results suggest that lithium will not be an effective treatment for tardive dyskinesia once the disorder has become manifest, but may play a role in preventing the appearance or progression of this disorder.

ACKNOWLEDGMENTS

This work was supported by grants from the United Parkinson Foundation and the Boothroyd Foundation, Chicago, Illinois.

REFERENCES

1. Klawans, H.L., Ilahi, M.M., Shenker, D. Theoretical implications of the use of L-dopa in parkinsonism. *Acta Neurol. Scand.*, 46:409–441, 1970.
2. Klawans, H.L. The pharmacology of tardive dyskinesia. *Am. J. Psychiatry*, 130:82–86, 1973.

3. Klawans, H.L. *Pharmacology of Extrapyramidal Movement Disorders.* Basel: S. Karger, 1973.
4. Klawans, H.L., Rubovits, R. The pharmacology of tardive dyskinesia and some animal models. In *Proceedings of the IX Congress of the Collequim Internationale Neuropsychopharmacologicum*, J.R. Bossier, H. Hippius, and P. Pichot (eds.). Amsterdam: Excerpta Medica, pp. 58–67, 1975.
5. Munkvad, I., Pakkenberg, H., Randrup, A. Aminergic systems in basal ganglia associated with stereotyped hyperactive behavior and catalepsy. *Brain Behav. Evol.,* *1*:89–101, 1968.
6. Rubovits, R., Klawans, H.L. Implications of amphetamine induced stereotyped behavior as a model of tardive dyskinesia. *Arch. Gen. Psychiatry, 27*:502–507, 1972.
7. Klawans, H.L., Rubarts, R. An experimental model of tardive dyskinesia. *J. Neural Transm., 33*:235–246, 1972.
8. Gianutsos, G., Drawbaugh, R.B., Hynes, M.D., Lal, H. Behavioral evidence for dopamine supersensitivity after chronic haloperidol. *Life Sci., 14*:887–898, 1974.
9. Simpson, G.M. Tardive dyskinesia. *Br. J. Psychiatry, 122*:618, 1973.
10. Prange, A., Wilson, I.C., Morris, C.E., Hall, C.D. Preliminary experience with tryptophan and lithium in the treatment of tardive dyskinesia. *Psychopharmacol. Bull., 9*:36–37, 1973.
11. Dalen, P. Lithium therapy in Huntington's chorea and tardive dyskinesia. *Lancet, 1*:936, 1973.
12. Reda, F.A., Scanlon, J.M., Kemp, K., Escobar, J.I. Treatment of tardive dyskinesia with lithium carbonate. *N. Engl. J. Med., 291*:850, 1974.
13. Ernst, A.M. Relation between the action of dopamine and apomorphine and their O-methylated derivative upon the CNS. *Psychopharmacologia, 7*:391–399, 1965.
14. Klawans, H.L., Weiner, W.J., Nausieda, P.A. The effect of lithium on an animal model of tardive dyskinesia. *Prog. Neuro-psychopharmac, 1*:53–60, 1977.
15. Mattson, B. Huntington's chorea and lithium therapy. *Lancet, 1*:718–719, 1973.
16. Aminoff, M.J., Marshall, J. Treatment of Huntington's chorea with lithium carbonate. *Lancet, 1*:107–109, 1974.
17. Klawans, H.L. Therapeutic approaches to neuroleptic-induced tardive dyskinesia. In *Basal Ganglia Disorders*, Yahr, M.D. (ed.). New York: Raven Press, pp. 447–457, 1976.

16

Modulation of Chlorpromazine Toxicity in Mice by Cesium Chloride: Implication for Research in Tardive Dyskinesia

F.S. MESSIHA

Considerable evidence suggests that chronic administration of certain psychotropic drugs, such as the neuroleptic chlorpromazine (CPZ), may produce extrapyramidal dysfunction, which in some patients resembles parkinsonism and in others a choreiform dyskinesia or late-appearing dyskinesia such as the tardive dyskinesia (1–4). Several investigators have used animal models to study the mechanism(s) underlying the neuroleptic-produced disorder of movements (5–9) to provide a pharmacotherapeutic rationale for the development of novel therapeutic agents. The ability of rats to tolerate acute lethal dosages of CPZ after chronic administration, and their subsequent development of hyperkinesia following acute withdrawal of CPZ (10), coupled with the clinical trials with lithium carbonate in tardive dyskinesia (11–14) and the evidence for cesium chloride (CsCl) antagonism to certain CPZ-evoked responses in rodents (15), provided the basis for the present study. Accordingly, it was decided to study the effect of CsCl on some aspects of CPZ-mediated behavioral and toxic manifestations in mice.

METHODS

Albino male Swiss-Webster mice, 10–13 weeks old, were obtained from Sprague-Dawley Company, Madison, Wisconsin. All animals were fed Purina pellet food and water ad libitum and were maintained at 23 to 25°C in a room with 12-hour light and dark cycles.

In the first series of experiments, CsCl was administered, 5.0 mEq/kg once daily for 7 consecutive days. Mice were sacrificed by decapitation 1,3,6, or 12 days after last injection of CsCl. Blood specimens were collected over anticoagulant, their volumes measured, deproteinized by 6% trichloracetic acid, extracted, and centrifuged. The supernatants obtained were measured for their volume and saved for the determination of their content of Cs^+. The mice brains were quickly removed, blotted with filter paper, and dissected into cerebral cortex, striatum, hippocampus, brain stem, diencephalon, and cerebellum. The brain regions were weighed, homogenized individually in ice-cold 0.4% $HClO_4$ to yield a 10% homogenates (w/v), extracted, and centrifuged for 30 minutes at 20,000 x g. The resulting pellets were resuspended into $HClO_4$, re-extracted twice, recentrifuged, and both supernatants' washes were combined with the initial corresponding supernatants' fluid. The volumes of combined supernatants were recorded for each sample. The quantitative determinations of Cs^+ and electrolytes were made by atomic absorption spectroscopy and flame emission spectroscopy, respectively. The concentrations of Cs^+, K^+, and Na^+ in the brain regions are expressed as mEq/kg wet tissue. The endogenous concentrations of these ions obtained from the controls were subtracted from the corresponding values of the experimental groups.

In the second series of experiments, the effect of short-term administration of CsCl on motility of mice treated with saline or CsCl, 2.5 mEq/kg/day for 5 days prior to the administration of CPZ, 2.0 mg/kg, or reserpine (RES), 2.0 mg/kg, or saline was studied. All drugs were injected 30 minutes post the fifth dose of CsCl. Motility was measured in groups of 3 mice by means of selective-activity meter device in the vertical mode of operation (Columbus Institute, Ohio). The motor activity counts were recorded for 45 minutes for CPZ, and for 120 minutes for RES, after 10 minutes of drug injection. The results are expressed as mean ± SE counts recorded as a function of time.

In the third series of experiments, the effect of gradual dosage build-up of CPZ alone or coadministered with CsCl, 1.0 mEq/kg, i.p., on CPZ-caused reduced motility and morbidity were studied. Two groups of mice were administered CPZ alone or combined with CsCl. Each group consisted of 30 mice divided into 10 subgroups of 3 mice each. CPZ was injected once daily in gradual dose build-up from 3 mg/kg/day to 50 mg/kg/day, as shown in Figure 4. The highest dose of CPZ used was maintained during a 12-day period prior to abrupt discontinuation of drug treatment. The daily CsCl dose was maintained at 1.0 mEq/kg/day throughout the 48 days of combined administration of CPZ with CsCl. Death occurring in animals, probably due to CNS depression as a function of CPZ dose given, was recorded and expressed as % morbidity from initial number of animals receiving the respective type of treatment at the beginning of the experiment. The motor activity was recorded during the 24-hour and 40-hour period of drug withdrawal and expressed as counts/2h.

All drugs were dissolved in saline, kept in brown containers, and injected intraperitoneally (i.p.). The significance of the results was evaluated by student t test for independent means.

RESULTS

Figure 1 shows the distribution and retention profiles of exogenously administered Cs^+ in specific brain regions in mice pretreated with CsCl, 5.0 mEq/kg/day for 7 days, and sacrificed 1,2,6, or 12 days after discontinued CsCl treatment. Measurable amounts of Cs^+ were present in all brain regions studied. Cs^+ were evenly distributed through the brain and tended to increase during the initial 6 days of discontinued CsCl administration, and then declined rapidly during a subsequent 6-day period. Whole blood Cs^+ contents amounted to 1.9 ± 0.2 mEq/L at day 1, 2.8 ± 0.5 mEq/L at day 6, and 0.6 ± 0.2 mEq/L at day 12, subsequent to termination of the CsCl treatment.

Figure 2 shows the effect of equal mEq dosages of the alkali metal salts LiCl, RbCl, or CsCl, 5.0 mEq/kg/day for 7 days, on whole mouse brain content of endogenous K^+ and Na^+ for the 24-hour and 72-hour periods post administration of the chloride salt solution of the alkali metal ions. Rb-treated mice showed a significant ($p < 0.001$) reduction in brain K^+ concentration from controls, concomitant with a similar moderate reduction ($p < 0.05$) in blood K^+ levels. Conversely, Li-treated mice showed a moderate increase ($p < 0.05$) in brain K^+ levels. Cs-treated mice showed no marked changes in brain or blood contents of the electrolytes measured.

Figure 3 shows the effect of short-term administration of CsCl on spontaneous locomotor activity and on CPZ- and RES-produced behavioral depression in mice. Administration of CsCl, 2.5 mEq/kg/day for 5 days, resulted in 62.5% ($p < 0.02$) and 51.5% ($p < 0.05$) increase in locomotor activity from saline controls during 45 minutes and 120 minutes of drug injection, respectively. Treatment with CsCl prior to administration of a single dose of CPZ, 2.0 mg/kg, i.p., counteracted CPZ-mediated decrease in motility during the initial 45 minutes of CPZ injection. However, a 120-minute period post to the administration of RES 2.0 mg/kg to Cs-treated mice was required to show a significant ($p < 0.02$) antagonism of RES-produced effect by CsCl.

Figure 4 shows the effect of increasing daily dosage of CPZ alone or combined with CsCl, 1.0 mEq/kg/day. On CPZ-caused toxicity in mice, mice treated with CPZ displayed approximately 8% mortality during the 30 mg/kg daily dosage of CPZ, while no death occurred in mice injected with the combination of CPZ and CsCl. There was approximately 47% death in animals receiving CPZ at 50 mg/kg/day, with additional 7% occurring during the 24 hour period following abrupt withdrawal of CPZ. This is contrasted with no fatality recorded for mice treated with identical daily dosage of CPZ, but combined with CsCl.

The changes of motility occurring 24h after drug withdrawal is shown in

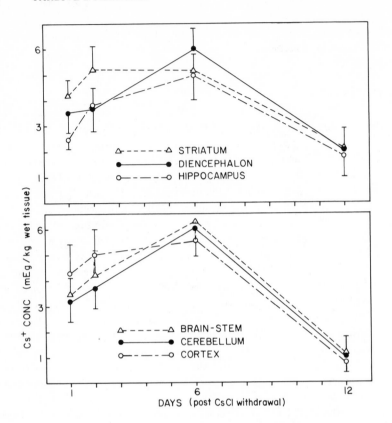

Figure 1.   The retention profile of exogenously administered Cs⁺ in distinct brain regions of
the mouse. Obtained after administration of CsCl 5 mEq/kg/day for 7 consecutive days.
Values are for means ± SD of at least 8 independent experiments for each given time intervals.

Figure 5. There were no major changes in motility scores of both groups of
mice tested for the period between 24 hours and 36 hours of drug withdrawal.
However, the groups of mice receiving the combined treatment of CPZ and
CsCl tended to display faster recovery in their motility than the groups of mice
treated with CPZ alone. There was approximately 23% ($p < 0.02$) greater
counts recorded for mice treated with CPZ and CsCl combined than that
measured for mice treated with CPZ alone at the end of the experiment.

DISCUSSION

Little is known on the precise mechanism of action of Cs⁺. However, there
is some indirect evidence to suggest that the action of Cs salts contrasts with

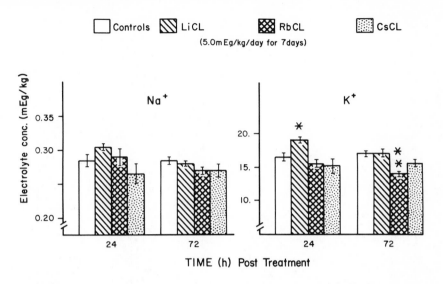

Figure 2.   The effects of equimiliequivalent concentration of LiC1, RbC1, or CsC1, 5.0 mEq/kg/day for 7 days, on endogenous whole brain content of Na^+ (left panel) and K^+ (right panel). Values obtained 24h and 72h post termination of treatments. Electrolyte concentrations are expressed as mEq/kg wet tissue. Values represents means ± SE of at least 5 independent experiments.
**$p<0.001$

that of the neuroleptics, i.e., CPZ. For example, CPZ and other neuroleptics reduce spontaneous locomotor activity in rodents (16), compared to enhancements of motility by Cs salts (17,18). CPZ increases the central action of ethyl alcohol (19), while Cs^+ decreases ethanol-mediated narcosis in experimental animals (20). Similarly, the central stimulant action of d-amphetamine is inhibited by CPZ (21), while Cs^+ potentiates d-amphetamine-produced enhancements of the cerebral activity (22). The present pharmacokinetic study shows that Cs is slowly absorbed, penetrates the brain, and reaches equal distribution in all parts of the brain studied after short-term administration. Thus, exogenously administered Cs^+ is retained over greater periods of time in cerebral tissue than is Li^+ (18,23–25). This may suggest far greater T ½ for Cs^+ than other alkali metal ions (26). Consequently, the prolonged retention of Cs^+ in cerebral tissue may result in changes in electrolytes balance, which may lead to alterations in cell membrane excitability. It is conceivable that such changes may influence intraneuronal uptake, storage, and release of certain putative neurotransmitters involved in the mode of action of CPZ-produced extrapyramidal side effects.

Evidence is accumulating that the management of the symptoms of tardive dyskinesia may be shared by a fairly wide spectrum of agents with various

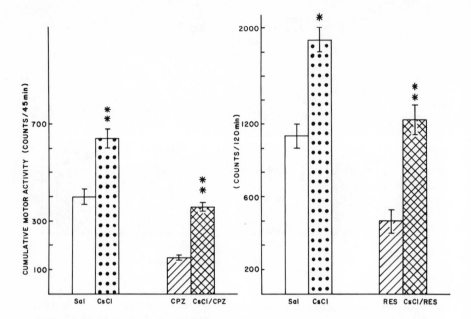

Figure 3.   The effect of pretreatment with CsCl on chlorpromazine-(CPZ) and reserpine-(RES) produced behavioral depression in mice. Mice were administered saline (sal) or CsCl, 2.5 mEq/kg/day for 5 consecutive days prior to the administration of CPZ, 2.0 mg/kg, i.p., or RES, 2.0 mg/kg, i.p., or RES, 2.0 mg/kg, i.p. Values are for means ± SE of 8–12 motility experiments.
$**p < 0.02$

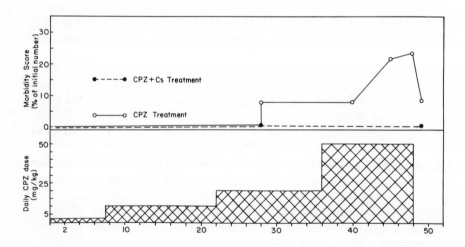

Figure 4.   The effect of chlorpromazine (CPZ) alone and combined with CsCl on morbidity score in mice. Percent of death occurring in mice treated with CPZ is plotted as a function of time and CPZ dose given.

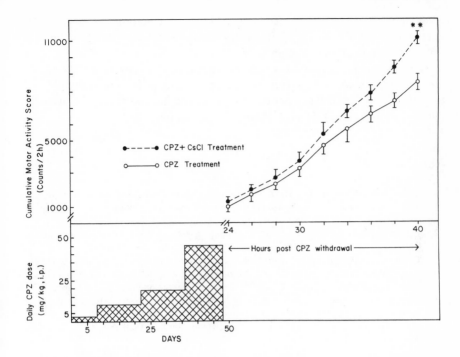

Figure 5.   The effect of CPZ alone or combined with CsCl on spontaneous locomotor activity after discontinued drug administration. Values are for means ± SE.
**$p < 0.02$

pharmacologic properties. It has been shown in several clinical trials that drugs possessing dopaminergic-blocking properties (i.e., thiopropazate [27,30]) and compounds acting by depleting central (i.e., tetrabenazine [31–33]) or central and peripheral (i.e., reserpine [34–35]) stores of biogenic amines can produce amelioration of the dyskinetic symptoms. Likewise, encouraging reports indicate the potential of certain alkali metal salts—i.e., lithium carbonate—in the treatment of certain naturally occurring and drug-produced extrapyramidal disorders, i.e., Huntington's chorea, tardive dyskinesia (11–14,36), Tourette's syndrome (37), and L-dopa-induced dyskinesia (38). However, the improvement of the latter by lithium therapy is controversial (39). Furthermore, an imbalance between acetylcholine and dopamine in the striatum has been implicated in various disorders of movements. For example, a predominance of striatal dopaminergic activity over cholinergic activity may underly involuntary movements of tardive dyskinesia. This hypothesis prompted clinical trials with drugs that potentiate cholinergic function in the management of tardive dyskinesia—i.e., choline (40) and physostigmine (41,42)—and that may increase cerebral acetylcholine and cholinergic activity. It is of interest to note that Cs^+ possesses weak cholinergic activity (43).

Thus, it seems that a further mechanism that may account for the observed Cs antagonism to CPZ-mediated responses studied involves possible modification of the cholinergic function by Cs^+. The foregoing observations on the potency of Cs^+ in negating CPZ-mediated responses studied suggest further evaluation of CsCl as a modifier of CPZ toxicity and in the management of extrapyramidal adverse reaction caused by chronic administration of high doses of neuroleptics.

REFERENCES

1. Sigwald, J., Bouttier, D., Raymondeaud, C. Quatre cas de dyskinesie facio-bucco-lingo-masticatirce a evolution prolongee secondaire a un traitement par les neuroleptiques. *Rev. Neurol., 100*:751–755, 1959.
2. Degkwitz, R., Luxemburger, O. Das terminale insuffizien bzw. Defektsyndrom infolge chronischer anwendung von neuroleptika. *Nervenarzt, 36*:173–175, 1965.
3. Crane, G.E. Dyskinesia and neuroleptics. *Arch. Gen. Psychiatry, 19*:700–703, 1968.
4. Fann, W.E. Tardive dyskinesia and neuroleptics. In *Animal Models in Psychiatry and Neurology*, Hanin, I., Usdin, E. (eds.). New York: Pergamon Press, pp. 457–466, 1977.
5. Deneau, G.A., Crane, G.E. Dyskinesia in rhesus monkeys tested with high doses of chlorpromazine. In *Psychotropic Drugs and Dysfunctions of the Basal Ganglia*, Crane, G.E., Gardner, J.R., Jr. (eds.). U.S. Public Health Service, Publ. No. 1938, Washington, D.C., pp. 12–14, 1969.
6. Paulson, G. Dyskinesias in monkeys. *Adv. Neurol., 1*:647–650, 1973.
7. Mones, R.J. Experimental dyskinesias in normal rhesus monkey. *Adv. Neurol., 1*:665–669, 1973.
8. Messiha, F.S. A study of biogenic amine metabolites in the cerebrospinal fluid and in urine of monkeys with chlorpromazine-induced dyskinesia. *J. Neurol. Sci., 21*:39–46, 1974.
9. Messiha, F.S. The relationship of dopamine excretion to chlorpromazine-induced dyskinesia in monkeys. *Arch. Int. Pharmacodyn. Ther., 209*:5–9, 1974.
10. Boyd, E.M. Chlorpromazine tolerance and physical dependence. *J. Pharmacol. Exp. Ther., 128*:75–78, 1960.
11. Dalen, P. Lithium therapy in Huntington's chorea and tardive dyskinesia. *Lancet, 1*:107–108, 1973.
12. Prange, A., Wilson, I.C., Morris, C.E., Hall, C.D. Preliminary experience with tryptophan and lithium in the treatment of tardive dyskinesia. *Psychopharmacol. Bull., 9*:36–37, 1973.
13. Simpson, G.M. Tardive dyskinesia. *Br. J. Psychiatry, 122*:618, 1973.
14. Gerlach, J., Thorsen, K., Munkvad, I. Effect of lithium on neuroleptic-induced tardive dyskinesia compared to placebo in a double-blind cross-over trial. *Pharmakopsychiatr. Neuropsychopharmakol., 8*:51–56, 1975.
15. Messiha, F.S. Cesium ion: antagonism to chlorpromazine and l-dopa-produced behavioral depression in mice. *J. Pharm. Pharmacol., 27*:873–874, 1975.
16. Kouzmanoff, S.P., Eckfeld, R., Tislow, R., Seifter, J. Meprobamate and phenothiazine antagonism to some morphine-induced phenomena in the mouse. *J. Pharmacol. Exp. Ther., 22*:40A, 1958.
17. Messiha, F.S., Krantz, J.C. Jr. Effect of cesium ion on cerebral activity of the mouse. *Am. J. Pharm., 145*:17–21, 1973.
18. Messiha, F.S. Alkali metal ions and ethanol preference: a psychopharmacological study of rubidium and cesium salts. *The Finnish Found. for Alcohol Studies, 24*:101–118, 1975.

19. Graham, R.C., Lu, F.C., Allmark, M.C. Combined effect of tranquilizing drugs and alcohol on rats. *Fed. Proc., 16*:302, 1957.
20. Messiha, F.S. Alkali metal ions and ethanol narcosis in mice. *Pharmacol., 14*:153–157, 1976.
21. Bradley, P.B., Hance, A.J. The effect of chlorpromazine and methopromazine on the electrical activity of the brain in the cat. *Electroencephalogr. Clin. Neurophysiol., 9*:191–215, 1957.
22. Messiha, F.S. Antidepressant action of cesium chloride and its modification of chlorpromazine toxicity in mice. (Submitted for publication.)
23. Messiha, F.S. Distribution and retention of exogenously administered alkali metal ions in the mouse brain. *Arch. Int. Pharmacodyn. Ther., 219*:87–96, 1976.
24. Messiha, F.S., Larson, J.W. A pharmacokinetic study of rubidium and cesium salts. *Proc. West. Pharmacol. Soc., 19*:108–112, 1976.
25. Messiha, F.S. Preclinical pharmacology of rubidium and cesium salts: modification of ethyl alcohol elicited responses. Revista del Inst. Nat. Neurol., Mexico (in press).
26. Hasanen, E., Rahola, T. The biological half-life of ^{137}Cs and ^{24}Na in man. *Ann. Clin. Res., 3*:236–240, 1971.
27. Roxburch, P.A. Treatment of persistent phenothiazine-induced oral dyskinesia. *Br. J. Psychiatry, 116*:277–280, 1970.
28. Singer, K., Cheng, M.N. Thiopropazate hydrochloride in persistent dyskinesia. *4*:22–25, 1970.
29. Carruthers, S.G. Persistent tardive dyskinesia. *Br. Med. J., 4*:572– 1971.
30. Curran, J.P. Tardive dyskinesia: side effect or not? *Am. J. Psychiatry, 130*:406–410, 1973.
31. Kazamatsuri, H., Chien, C., Cole, J. Treatment of tardive dyskinesia. II. Short-term efficacy of dopamine blocking agents haloperidal and thiopropazate. *Arch. Gen. Psychiatry, 28*:100–103, 1975.
32. Brandrup, E. Tetrabenazine treatment in persisting dyskinesia caused by psychopharmaca. *Am. J. Psychiatry, 118*:551–554, 1961.
33. Macullum, W.A.G. Tetrabenazine for extrapyramidal movement disorders. *Br. Med. J., 1*:760, 1970.
34. Wolf, S.M. Reserpine: cause and treatment of oral-facial dyskinesia. *Bull. Los Angeles Neurol. Soc., 38*:80, 1973.
35. Kobayashi, R.M. Drug therapy of tardive dyskinesia. *N. Engl. J. Med., 296*:257–260, 1977.
36. Mattsson, B. Huntington's chorea and lithium therapy. *Lancet, 1*:718–179, 1973.
37. Messiha, F.S., Erickson, H., Goggin, J. Lithium carbonate in Gilles de la Tourette's disease. *Res. Commun. Chem. Pathol. Pharmacol., 15*:609-612, 1976.
38. Dalen, P., Steg, G. Lithium and levodopa in parkinsonism. *Lancet, 1*:936–937, 1973.
39. Van Woert, M.H. Parkinson's disease. *Lancet, 1*:1390, 1973.
40. Davis, K.L., Berger, P.A., Hollister, L.E. Choline for tardive dyskinesia. *N. Engl. J. Med., 293*:152, 1975.
41. Fann, W.E., Lake, C.R., Gerber, C.J., McKenzie, G.M. Cholinergic suppression of tardive dyskinesia, *Psychopharmacologia, 37*:101-107, 1974.
42. Fann, W.E., Gerber, C.J. McKenzie, G.M. Physostigmine in rigid Huntington's disease. *Confin. Neurol., 35*:312-315, 1973.
43. Williams, R.J.P. The chemistry and biochemistry of lithium. In *Lithium: Its Role in Psychiatric Research and Treatment*. Gershon, S., Shopsin, B. (eds.). New York: Plenum Press, pp. 15-31, 1973.

17

The Pathophysiologic Basis of
Tardive Dyskinesia

ROSS J. BALDESSARINI
and DANIEL TARSY

It is now generally accepted that tardive (late) neurological disorders, including abnormal oral, facial, and tongue movements as well as choreoathetosis of the trunk and extremities, called tardive dyskinesias (TD), are associated with prolonged clinical exposure to neuroleptic-antipsychotic drugs. While the evidence for this association is mainly epidemiologic, it is quite compelling. With increased recognition in recent years, incidence rates have ranged as high as 40–50% of patients so treated, including outpatients as well as those in psychiatric institutions. The cause of this distressing condition, which challenges the current practice of almost routine prolonged "maintenance" therapy of chronically psychotic patients—mostly schizophrenics—is not known. The leading hypothesis is that dopamine (DA), as a synaptic neurotransmitter in the basal ganglia or limbic forebrain, may be overactive, either through increased availability or by increased efficacy, or possibly by way of postsynaptic receptor supersensitivity. Many of the details of the clinical neurologic, basic scientific, and experimental therapeutic aspects of this extremely puzzling and difficult to treat disorder are presented elsewhere in reviews by Tarsy and Baldessarini (1–4) and in a report by an American Psychiatric Association Task Force, edited by Baldessarini et al. (5). Those reviews should be consulted for full bibliographic support of the material summarized below.

Any hypothesis that attempts to explain the pathophysiology of this syndrome (or, possibly, series of related syndromes, varying in their timing, duration, and precise clinical manifestations) must take into account a number of salient clinical observations (1). These include a late onset after months of treatment with ordinary doses of neuroleptics, usually with some worsening on withdrawal of the drug; more rapid occurrence on abrupt discontinuation of unusually large doses; close similarity to dyskinesias induced during L-dopa therapy of parkinsonism, abuse of amphetamines, or the clinical use of stimulants in children with "minimum brain dysfunction"; worsening of TD by L-dopa or stimulants, but amelioration by small parenteral doses of the partial direct (possibly selectively presynaptic) DA agonist, apomorphine; at least partial and temporary suppression by DA antagonists, including receptor blockers (potent neuroleptics), storage blockers (reserpine, tetrabenazine), or a synthesis inhibitor (α-methyl-p-tyrosine); mild and variable effects of cholinergic agents (generally worsening with antimuscarinic-antiparkinson agents, and occasionally partial improvement with eserine, deanol, or choline, given to enhance the availability of acetylcholine) or agonists of GABA (γ-amino-butyric acid) or serotonin receptors. In short, the syndrome's differential pharmacology is strikingly opposite that of parkinsonism, a condition that almost certainly includes DA deficiency of the basal ganglia as an important contributing feature; moreover, it is very similar to that of other hyperkinesias, such as Huntington's chorea, which is believed to represent a state of relative, and possibly indirect (e.g., by loss of neurons, including GABA-secreting cells that modulate DA neurons), excess of DA function. Moreover, many of the clinical features of severe forms of TD are remarkably similar to those of Huntington's chorea.

Such a state of relative excess of DA function in TD, if indeed it is present, could come about through several mechanisms: (a) presynaptic dyscontrol of DA synthesis and release; (b) decreased availability of other modulating systems (including those using GABA or other neuroinhibitory amino acids, acetylcholine [ACh], serotonin, or substance P or other peptides); (c) increased quantity or effectiveness of postsynaptic DA receptors or "effectors" (mechanisms that mediate the postsynaptic effects of DA, including possibly a variety of protein-phosphorylating effects mediated by cyclic AMP, the synthesis of which can be stimulated by DA).

Regarding mechanism (a), animal data strongly indicate that the initial strong increase of DA turnover and metabolite (homovanillic acid, HVA) production induced by neuroleptics is short-lasting. The very "tolerance" involved in this response to prolonged neuroleptic treatment may be mediated by increased sensitivity to DA transmission postsynaptically or at proposed presynaptic "auto-receptors," believed to modulate DA synthesis and possibly also release. Human data on this point are confusing and inconsistent as increases, decreases, and no change have variously been reported in HVA levels in lumbar CSF of chronic schizophrenics, with a possible trend toward relatively low HVA levels in those with signs of TD (3). This phenomenon is opposite to the result predicted by a presynaptic hypothesis, but is possibly consistent with a mechanism involving DA receptor supersensitivity (see 3). There are also unconfirmed or conflicting reports that the enzyme converting

DA to norepinephrine (dopamine beta-hydroxylase, or DBH) may be de-creased, or that dopamine or HVA levels may be increased in the brains of chronic schizophrenic patients (not necessarily with TD) post-mortem (see 3 and 4).

It is difficult to comment on other transmitters since they have been much less intensively investigated than DA; furthermore, there are few potent and selective agonists or antagonists for many of these, and those that exist have weak or inconsistent clinical effects on TD (1,2). Data from recent post-mortem studies of brain tissue of chronic schizophrenics exposed to neurolep-tics (but not necessarily showing signs of TD) include increases and decreases of choline acetyltransferase (ChAc, the ACh-synthesizing enzyme) activity, but fairly consistent, if sometimes small, decreases in glutamic acid decarbox-ylase (GAD, the GABA-synthesizing enzyme), as has also been found in brains of patients with Huntington's disease (6). These results may possibly suggest neurotoxic effects of neuroleptics on GABA or ACh neurons that may have *indirect* DA-enhancing actions.

Evidence on the existence of DA receptor supersensitivity in animals is quite compelling. It includes direct and crossed tolerance to many behavioral (e.g., catalepsy) and biochemical (especially DA turnover-enhancing) effects of neuroleptics. Such effects are not seen with neuroendocrine responses to neuroleptics (e.g., prolactin release), suggesting differences in the regulation of hypothalamic versus forebrain DA systems. In addition, there is striking and consistently increased sensitivity to DA agonists on the same behavioral effects (but in the opposite direction) in many species, including primates, upon withdrawal from repeated treatment with neuroleptics, but not other central nervous system (CNS) depressants (3,7). Generally, these aspects of supersensitivity to DA agonists after neuroleptic treatment are short-lived (days to weeks), raising questions about their pertinence to long-lasting or even irreversible forms of TD, although some recent primate behavioral models provide more prolonged effects (8). Another paradox is that some DA agonists (including d-amphetamine, apomorphine, ergot alkaloids, and possi-bly also L-dopa) may also induce supersensitive behavioral responses to themselves or other DA agonists (direct and crossed "reverse tolerance"). Moreover, these paradoxical effects, (which may reflect presynaptic DA turnover *reducing* actions, which outlast their acute stimulant actions [9] and so lead to receptor "disuse supersensitivity"), as well as supersensitivity after neuroleptic treatment, have been described in several laboratories as following even a single dose of the agent in question (10).

Other results that derive from frank denervation of DA projections to forebrain strongly support the occurrence of DA receptor supersensitivity in laboratory animals. These examples of "denervation supersensitivity" in-clude strongly enhanced behavioral responses to DA agonists (see 7); inconsis-tent and small increases in the sensitivity of adenylate cyclase in striatal homogenates to DA (11); increased sensitivity of striatal neurons to iontophoretically applied DA agonists or stimulation of nigrostriatal neurons (12); and increases in the binding of ligands (^{3}H-DA and ^{3}H-neuroleptics), proposed to label "DA receptors" in brain tissue (13). Moreover, most of these observations have more recently been replicated in brain tissues of animals repeatedly treated with neuroleptic agents (14,15), and there is even an unconfirmed late report that the post-mortem binding of ^{3}H-neuroleptics is increased in brain tissue of chronic schizophrenics, possibly, or at least in part, as a consequence of prolonged exposure to neuroleptic agents (16).

For all these impressive scientific findings, there remain a number of serious problems and shortcomings of the DA receptor disuse supersensitivity hypothesis in TD. First, the duration of supersensitive responses in most animals is relatively *brief*, usually involving a return to baseline status within a few weeks, at most, after discontinuation of the neuroleptic agent (see 7), while clinical TD may be virtually irreversible. On the other hand, newer primate models are more promising in this regard, as long-lasting (months) supersensitivity to DA agonists and spontaneous dyskinesias have been produced, particularly in Cebus monkeys (8). Second, supersensitivity to DA agonists locally applied to DA-sensitive limbic regions of the forebrain of the neuroleptic-pretreated rat has recently been described (17). Since increasing psychosis following prolonged neuroleptic therapy ("tardive schizophrenia") is unknown clinically, this second phenomenon suggests either that DA-sensitive areas (such as the nucleus accumbens septi) that are supposedly limbic in function may actually contribute to extrapyramidal function, or that the popular "protothesis" that psychoses are mediated by excessive limbic DA function may be invalid or too simplistic. Third, most biochemical and behavioral manifestations of presumed DA receptor supersensitivity involve quantitatively *small* changes (typically 20–30% increases in receptor-ligand binding, and not more than 2- or 3-fold shifts in ED_{50} values for stimulation of iontophoretic responses, adenylate cyclase, or of behavior by DA agonists [11–16]). Moreover, these are rapidly reversible, adaptive, and plastic, sometimes developing and fading over times as brief as minutes to hours (10), and seemingly designed to restore DA function toward normal—that is, to subserve *homeostasis* of neurotransmitter function, rather than to lead to sustained unbalanced increases of function.

For long-lasting or even irreversible changes, one would expect visible neuropathologic changes, such as frank cell loss, although the available animal and human neuropathologic studies following prolonged exposure to neuroleptics do not support that prediction (see 1–3). Possibly, other as yet unknown functionally important but histologically so far invisible toxic metabolic or structural changes in DA-secreting or DA-sensitive cells or their membranes can occur. For example, there is one recent report of electron-microscopic evidence of a change in presynaptic vesicles after treatment with chlorpromazine (18).

In summary, the DA receptor supersensitivity hypothesis may help to explain some features of the pathophysiology of TD, and is most likely to contribute to its more rapidly reversible forms, such as acute "withdrawal" dyskinesias (19). Furthermore, the entertainment of this hypothesis has shed light on mechanisms only recently appreciated that evidently exert important regulatory effects on central synaptic function and that contribute to neuronal "plasticity" and adaptiveness in the CNS. Moreover, the hypothesis suggests new therapeutic strategies, such as the attempt to suppress supersensitive receptors by the restoration of agonist availability or through the induction of tolerance to agonists (20), as a way of moving beyond current attempts to suppress DA availability or function, which seem basically "anti-rational" or likely to aggravate the very condition being treated.

ACKNOWLEDGMENTS

Partially supported by U.S. PHS (NIMH) Research Grant MH-16674, Research Career Scientist Award MH-74370, and a grant from the Scottish Rite Schizophrenia Research Foundation, NMJ of the USA.

Based in part on a presentation for the ACNP Symposium on Tardive Dyskinesia, San Juan, Puerto Rico, December 14-16, 1977.

REFERENCES

1. Tarsy, D., Baldessarini, R.J. The tardive dyskinesia syndrome. *Clinical Neuropharmacology*, vol. 1, Klawans, H.L. (ed.). New York: Raven Press, pp. 29–61, 1976.
2. Baldessarini, R.J., Tarsy, D. Mechanisms underlying tardive dyskinesia. In *The Basal Ganglia*, Yahr, M. (ed.). New York: Raven Press, pp. 433–466, 1976.
3. Tarsy, D., Baldessarini, R.J. The pathophysiologic basis of tardive dyskinesia. *Biol. Psychiatry*, *12*:431–460, 1977.
4. Baldessarini, R.J., Tarsy, D. The pathophysiologic basis of tardive dyskinesia. *Int. Rev. Neurobiol.*, 1978 (in press).
5. Baldessarini, R.J. (ed.). Task Force Report on Late Neurological Consequences of Antipsychotic Drugs. American Psychiatric Association, Washington, 1978 (in press).
6. Bird, E.D., Barnes, J., Iversen, L.L. Increased brain dopamine and reduced glutamic acid decarboxylase and choline acetyl-transferase activity in schizophrenia and related psychoses. *Lancet*, *II*:1157–1159, 1977.
7. Tarsy, D., Baldessarini, R.J. Behavioral supersensitivity to apomorphine following chronic treatment with drugs which interfere with the synaptic function of catecholamines. *Neuropharmacology*, *13*:927–940, 1974.
8. Gunne, L.M., Barany, S. Haloperidol-induced tardive dyskinesia in monkeys. *Psychopharmacology*, *50*:237–240, 1976.
9. Segal, D.S. Behavioral and neurochemical correlates of repeated d-amphetamine administration. In *Neurobiological Mechanisms of Adaptation and Behavior*, Mandell, A.J. (ed.). New York: Raven Press, pp. 247–262, 1975.
10. Martres, M.P., Costentin, J., Baudry, Long-term changes in the sensitivity of pre- and

postsynaptic dopamine receptors in mouse striatum evidenced by behavioral and biochemical studies. *Brain Res., 136*:319–337, 1977.

11. Mishra, R.K., Gardner, E.L., Katzman, R. Enhancement of dopamine-stimulated adenylate cyclase activity in rat caudate after lesions in substantia nigra: evidence for denervation supersensitivity. *Proc. Natl. Acad. Sci., USA, 71*:3883–3887, 1974.

12. Feltz, P., DeChamplain, J. Enhanced sensitivity of caudate neurones for microiontophoretic injections of dopamine in 6-hydroxydopamine-treated rats. *Brain Res., 43*:601–605, 1972.

13. Creese, I., Burt, D.R., Snyder, S.H. Dopamine receptor binding enhancement accompanies lesion-induced behavioral supersensitivity. *Science, 197*:596–598, 1977.

14. Burt, D.R., Creese, I., Snyder, S.H. Antischizophrenic drugs: chronic treatment elevates dopamine receptor binding in brain. *Science, 196*:326–328, 1977.

15. Friedhoff, A.J., Bonnet, K., Rosengarten, H. Reversal of two manifestations of dopamine receptor supersensitivity by administration of L-dopa. *Res. Commun. Chem. Pathol. Pharmacol., 16*:411–423, 1977.

16. Lee, T., Seeman, P. Dopamine receptors in normal and schizophrenic human brains. *Proc. Soc. Neurosci., 4*:443–(Abs. No. 1414), 1977.

17. Jackson, D.M., Anden, N.-E., Engel, J., Liljequist, S. The effect of long-term penfluridol treatment on the sensitivity of dopamine receptors in the nucleus accumbens and the corpus striatum. *Psychopharmacologia, 45*:151–155, 1975.

18. Kaiya, H., Iwata, T., Moriuchi, I., Namba, M. Chlorpromazine induces population increase of synaptic vesicles in the rat hypothalamic ventromedial nucleus. *Biol. Psychiatry, 12*:323–330, 1977.

19. Jacobson, A., Baldessarini, R.J., Manschreck, T. Tardive and withdrawal dyskinesia associated with haloperidol. *Am. J. Psychiatry, 131*:910–913, 1974.

20. Alpert, M., Friedhoff, A.J. Receptor sensitivity modification in the treatment of tardive dyskinesia. *Clin. Pharmacol. Ther., 19*:103, 1976.

Part II

Studies in Man and Pharmacology of
Drugs Used in Treatment of
Tardive Dyskinesia

18

A Classification of the Neurologic Effects of Neuroleptic Drugs

GEORGE E. CRANE

The motor disorders induced by neuroleptics have been subdivided into acute dystonia, parkinsonism, akathisia, and akinesia; they are believed to subside as the result of drug withdrawal, dose reduction, the use of anticholinergics, or with the passage of time. Tardive dyskinesia has been added later. Its main characteristics have been described as follows: choreiform movements, late development, occurrence in older persons, irreversibility, and appearance upon drug withdrawal. A classification based on these facts is no longer complete or accurate. In the early stages of treatment, parkinsonism (Pk) is completely reversible, but as the exposure to drugs continues, patients become hypersensitive to neuroleptics and more susceptible to this disorder. The number of chronic schizophrenics in hospitals who exhibit tremors and impairment of associated movements is far in excess of what one may expect in a population of comparable age. It is not known how many persons continue to suffer from Pk after the complete withdrawal of drugs, but undoubtedly many features of this disorder are present in a high proportion of those who are treated with minimal amounts of neuroleptics and adequate doses of anticholinergics over long periods of time. Akathisia does not belong in a classification of involuntary motor disorders, since the major problem is a feeling of inner restlessness, which the patient tries to alleviate by pacing or shifting position. These are voluntary actions.

As for tardive dyskinesia (TD), enough has been learned in the last decade to necessitate major revisions of earlier concepts. The movements in this condition may be choreiform or athetoid, but their main features are involvement of specific areas and similarity with normal functions, such as chewing, masticating, and grasping; a slow rhythm; and modifications in intensity by

changes in attention and the performance of certain tasks. The typical dyskinesias are rather forceful and can be easily distinguished from the choreas,
which are scattered, sudden, and jerky, and from tremors, which consist of
rapid oscillations. A symptom that is seldom mentioned in rating scales is
hypotonia. It is found in various combinations with dyskinesias and causes an
exaggeration of associated movements. These may be confused with the
dyskinesias. Many neurological disorders are postural rather than motor and
should be referred to as dystonias.

To be sure, the distinction between the several types of abnormalities is not
always easy. For instance, the pill-rolling that is considered a typical parkinsonian feature has many characteristics in common with TD. The differential
diagnosis between Pk and TD has other problems. The two major classes of
symptoms may coexist. They usually occur in different parts of the body, but
in many instances they can be observed in the same areas, although not
simultaneously. A change in posture or in general activity may be sufficient to
cause a shift in the pattern of abnormal motility. Even more important are the
effects of drugs. Tremors tend to become slower and to acquire the characteristics of the dyskinesias after the withdrawal of neuroleptics, or less frequently,
after the administration of anticholinergics. Usually, within a week all Pk
features are replaced by manifestations consistent with TD. The reverse
phenomenon occurs when the administration of psychotropics is reinstituted
(1).

There is general agreement that TD is late in appearance, seldom before six
months of drug therapy, a fact that helps the differential diagnosis when the
symptomatology is ambiguous. Contrary to earlier beliefs, the disorder does
not affect the elderly only, as it is fairly common among young adults. The
irreversibility of TD has also been questioned. Recent reports seem to indicate
that signs of dyskinesia disappear if they are detected early and the use of all
drugs is discontinued promptly (2). A careful examination, however, reveals
residual motor abnormalities. Most likely, the reversible or transitory dyskinesias are incipient forms of the chronic variety, but for the time being they
should be considered as separate clinical entities. The patient's almost complete recovery from this disorder in the early stage of drug therapy is possible,
because the exposure to noxious agents has not been sufficient to cause
irreversible damage. Similarly, the dyskinesias of children and juveniles
subside after drug withdrawal, because of the greater resilience of their central
nervous systems.

The fact that TD emerges as the result of the discontinuation or the reduction
of medication is a phenomenon of considerable complexity and is also relevant
to a comprehensive classification of motor disorders. In juveniles, symptoms
appear mainly upon the withdrawal of neuroleptics, whereas in the adult
variety they can be observed while the patient is on drug therapy. It is
conceivable, however, that all manifestations disappear if doses are raised to

very high levels. Hence a distinction between dyskinesias that occur only in a drug-free status and those observed during treatment does not seem to be justified.

Most classifications of drug-induced motor disorders do not include the atypical syndromes simulating the naturally occurring diseases of the central nervous system. A condition resembling Huntington's disease is often misdiagnosed. This was particularly true at a time when the existence of TD was not known by many physicians. In addition to chorea, one finds ballismus, tics, and dystonia among these chemical encephalopathies. The last-named condition is fairly common, and its severity ranges from minimal to extreme; in rare instances it simulates dystonia muscolorum deformans. There is no evidence that the acute dystonias are forerunners of the chronic variety. The pathology underlying the two conditions does not seem to be the same, since anticholinergics are very effective in the acute but not the chronic form. The differential diagnosis between the encephalopathies caused by neuroleptics and those occurring for natural reasons is often very difficult. In my opinion, all extrapyramidal and systemic disorders developing in the course of treatment with neuroleptics should be attributed to chemotherapy unless a pharmacological etiology can be ruled out by definite clinical findings, a family history, and laboratory data.

It is possible to use pharmacological criteria to supplement a predominantly phenomenological classification of drug-induced motor disorders. Thus all these abnormalities can be subdivided into three broad categories: (1) Pk, acute dystonia, and akinesia, which are enhanced by neuroleptics and reduced by anticholinergics; (2) transitory, juvenile, and permanent dyskinesias, which are exaggerated or emerge as the result of the withdrawal of neuroleptics, and to a lesser extent, by the addition of anticholinergics; and (3) the encephalopathies and probably certain forms of late Pk, which do not respond to these drugs or respond only minimally. For instance, the rabbit syndrome, which disappears after the administration of anticholinergics (3), should not be included among the tardive dyskinesias.

A classification based on phenomenological and pharmacological considerations was proposed in a previous publication and with the permission of the publisher (4) is reproduced in Table I. Since the elements of this table are described in considerable detail in that paper, I will limit myself to a few comments and will suggest a few additions. There are eleven categories; they are arranged in the approximate order in which the symptoms develop in the course of drug treatment. In column II, I indicate whether or not the symptoms appear or disappear following drug withdrawal; the entries will have the opposite sign if one uses administration rather than withdrawal of neuroleptics. The table lists the pharmacological actions of only two substances— neuroleptics and anticholinergics. The effects of other agents, such as cholinergics or GABA agonists and antagonists, are not included, since their

Table 1
Neurologic Effects Induced by Neuroleptics

	Irreversible	Appearing upon Withdrawal	Effectiveness of Anticholinergics
1. Acute dystonia + tetanus, oculogyrus	−	−	+
2. Akinesia	−	−	+
3. Akathisia + tasikinesia	−	−	±
4. Rapid tremor	−	−	+
5. Acute parkinsonism (Tremor, bradykinesia, rigidity)	−	−	+
6. Dyskinesia, dysmetria, ataxia (Juvenile)	−	+	−
7. Transient dyskinesia	−	+	−
8. Dyskinesia + dystonia (Tardive)	+	±	−
9. Hypotonia	+	?	−
10. Encephalopathies (Chorea, dystonia, ballismus)	+	−	−
11. Tremor + loss of associated movement	+	−	±

actions on motor disorders are still under investigation. Some comments on specifications are discussed below.

Items 3 and 9: Akathisia, tasikinesia, and hypotonia are part of the classification, although they are not involuntary motor disorders, because the table lists all, or most, neurologic effects.

Item 8: Dyskinesias and postural abnormalities may be subdivided into (a) residual (see above), (b) latent, when masked or converted into tremor by drug use, and (c) tardive, which may be subdivided further according to the anatomical location of symptoms. I find it not necessary to place in separate categories dyskinesias of the mouth, of the extremities, and of the trunk. The types of movement and postural disorders in the various parts of the body are very similar if one makes allowance for differences in muscular organization.

Item 11: A complete picture of Pk is seldom observed in patients who receive only minimal or no medication; on the other hand, tremors, impaired associated movements, and some diminution of facial expression are fairly common.

For the sake of completeness, one may wish to add two more items to cover the infrequent brain syndromes with dementia and the convulsions due to excessive medication. The proposed classification can be expanded to include details on severity, disabling effects, subjective reactions, etc., and thus can be the basis for a rating instrument in clinical practice and research.

REFERENCES

1. Crane, G.E. Pseudoparkinsonism and tardive dyskinesia. *Arch. Neurol.*, 27:426–430, 1972.
2. Quitkin, F., Rifkin, A., Gochfeld, L., Klein, D.F. Tardive dyskinesia: are first signs reversible? *Am. J. Psychiatry, 134*:84–87, 1977.
3. Sovner, R., DiMascio, A. The effects of benztropine mesylate on the rabbit syndrome and tardive dyskinesia. *Am. J. Psychiatry, 134*:1301–1302, 1977.
4. Crane, G.E. Tardive dyskinesia and related neurologic disorders. In *Handbook of Psychopharmacology*, Vol. 10, Snyder, Iversen, and Iversen (eds.). New York: Plenum Publishing, pp. 185–216, 1977.

19

Dyskinetic and Neurological Complications in Children Treated with Psychotropic Medications

POLIZOES POLIZOS
and DAVID M. ENGELHARDT

INTRODUCTION

Drug-induced neurological complications associated with the administration of psychotropic medications in adults comprise a wide variety of neurological symptoms, which can be summarized under the following:

Disturbances of sensorium and sensory organs. Drowsiness and lethargy, excitement, confusion, euphoria, disorientation, blurred vision, diplopia, tinnitus, vertigo, and insomnia.

Disturbances of motor system—extrapyramidal symptoms.

a. Acute dystonic reactions: protrusion, arching, and rounding of the tongue, and clonic spasms of the masticatory muscles, with trismus, dysphagia, numbness, and aching of the muscles

b. Parkinsonism, manifested by rigidity, bradykinesia, slurred speech, tremor, increased salivation, and hyperhydrosis

c. Akathisia

d. Tardive dyskinesia (TD)

Convulsive disorders. With the exception of tardive dyskinesia, which has been reported in some cases to be irreversible in adults, the above symptoms are readily reversed with either dose adjustments or administration of counteractive medication, or both. The neurological complications occur, as a rule, primarily as a consequence of the administration of neuroleptics.

A variety of pathophysiologic mechanisms, including disturbances in the

193

dopaminergic systems and dopamine turnover in the basal ganglia, are presumed to be related to the etiology of the extrapyramidal symptoms, including tardive dyskinesia. The incidence of extrapyramidal reactions in adults is fairly high. Ayd reviewed 3,775 patients treated with neuroleptics of the group of the phenothiazines, and found that 1,472—that is, 38.9% of the patients—had developed extrapyramidal reactions consisting of parkinsonism, dystonic reactions, and akathisia (1).

There is no agreement as to the incidence of TD occurring in adults treated with neuroleptics, and a reliable percentile has not been clearly established. Reports in the literature indicate an incidence as high as 20% in chronic elderly patients who have been receiving high doses of neuroleptics for a long time, and as low as 3% to 6% in mixed psychiatric populations (2).

There is no known effective treatment for tardive dyskinesia. In some cases in adult populations, it has been reported to be irreversible (3). The treating physician must be familiar with the conditions where there is potential danger for the occurrence of TD, and take appropriate preventive measures.

Neurological complications, including tardive dyskinesia, also occur in children treated with neuroleptic medications. The literature, however, is inadequate with regard to the incidence and severity of neurological side effects in children receiving pharmacotherapy. The only review of adverse reactions in children receiving neuroleptics can be found in Shader and DiMascio's textbook on side effects. DiMascio and associates, in reviewing the literature, comment on the minimal attention that has been paid to this particular subject, and they find the literature on drug-induced side effects in children inadequate and nonsystematically documented (4). The various reports regarding children concentrate primarily on drug efficacy.

In this chapter, we will present our experience with regard to neurological complications occurring in children receiving neuroleptics (5). Our data are derived from drug studies that have been conducted at the Children's Psychopharmacology Research Unit at Kings County Psychiatric Hospital in Brooklyn, New York. The data, with the exception of two studies, are derived exclusively from single-blind studies. All the children who participated in the drug trials were outpatients, and they were a relatively homogeneous population, carrying the diagnosis of childhood schizophrenia with autistic features. The mean age of the children was 8.8 years; the majority were between the ages of 6 and 12. The ratio of boys to girls was 5 to 1, the girls being on the average 7 months younger than the boys. The most common presenting target symptoms of these children consisted of hyperactivity, severe stereotyped activity, labile and inappropriate affect, mood disturbances, severe disturbances of language development and communication, severe impairment of cognitive functioning, disturbances of sleep. Almost all children showed severe handicaps in self-management and functioned at a retarded level. Most of the drug trials tended to be long-term, 3 to 24 months, with an average of 8 months' duration of treatment. The data that will be presented in this chapter will be limited to side effects that emerged during the first 16 weeks of treatment.

Sample size per drug trial ranged from 12 to 42, with a mean of 28. Dosages were comparable to those used in adults.

The number of children studied represents an unusually large sample, considering the diagnostic category. Ten drugs were investigated, comprising 7 phenothiazines, 2 thioaxanthines and 1 butyrophenone.

The incidence of neurological side effects, which are reported in Table 1, is considered to be an underestimate of neurological complications likely to occur during neuroleptic treatment. Children are very poor informants and unreliable in reporting on subjective data. Most of them are uncommunicative, and our data was derived exclusively from direct observation of the child and information received from the parent(s). Akathisia, for instance, is a very difficult symptom to assess in children with the degree of hyperactivity that our population exhibited, and this particular side effect may have been overlooked because it was superimposed on the already existing hyperactivity.

Disturbances of sensorium and sensory organs (Table 1)

Drowsiness was a common side effect, which was observed in 19% of all children treated. It occurred 3 times as often in children treated with high-dose drugs as with those treated with low-dose drugs. The drug most implicated was chlorpromazine, with 91% of the children who developed side effects exhibiting drowsiness. There was a trend for drowsiness to appear more often in female children. Other disturbances of sensorium and sensory organs were reported only sporadically.

Disturbances of motor system—Extrapyramidal symptoms (Table 1)

a. Dystonic reactions were fairly common and were observed in 25% of the children who developed extrapyramidal symptoms. Dystonias were characterized by protrusion of the tongue, wide opening of the mouth, inability to swallow, usually associated with drooling and torticolis. Oculogyric crises were not observed in our children. There was only a trend for dystonic reactions to occur with greater frequency among low-dose-drug-treated children. Symptoms subsided promptly upon administration of parenteral counteractive medication.

b. Parkinsonism (tremor, rigidity, bradykinesia, etc.) was present in 23% of the children treated. These symptoms were twice as common in low-dose (29%) as in high-dose (15%) drug-treated children. There was no difference in incidence between male and female children. The most frequently observed neurological side effects were increased salivation, rigidity, tremor, bradykinesia, and mask-

Table 1
Incidence of Side Effects by Drug

Drug	N[a]	Mean Dosage (Mg/d)	% With Adverse Reactions	% With Drowsiness	% With EPS[b]
Chlorpromazine	42	196	55	50	14
Thioridazine	42	282	67	21	21
Mesoridazine	16	153	56	6	13
Chlorprothixene	24	203	33	25	4
Total High-Dose Drugs	124		55	30	15
Thiothixene	31	12.1	35	19	16
Haloperidol	30	10.0	67	17	40
Butaperazine	15	22.5	33	7	33
Trifluoperazine	40	20.8	43	13	35
Fluphenazine	32	10.4	44	13	31
Prochlorperazine	12	11.4	17	0	0
Total Low-Dose Drugs	160		43	11	29
Total All Drugs	284		48	19	23

[a]The actual number of children involved is 95 (i.e., many children participated in more than one drug study).
[b]Extrapyramidal symptoms.

Table 2
Incidence of Withdrawal Emergent Symptoms (WES) by Drug

Drug	N[a]	Mean Dosage (Mg/d)	Mean Weeks of Treatment Before Withdrawal	% Developing WES
Chlorpromazine	13	251	26	31
Thioridazine	15	378	45	33
Mesoridazine	14	174	19	50
Chlorprothixene	20	215	21	10
Total High-Dose Drugs	62		28	29
Thiothixene	32	16	22	50
Haloperidol	16	10	39	50
Butaperazine	13	29	21	62
Trifluoperazine	15	12	22	87
Fluphenazine	34	17	54	79
Prochlorperazine	12	11	14	25
Total Low-Dose Drugs	122		29	61
Total All Drugs	184		28	51

[a]The actual number of children involved is 53 (i.e., many children participated in more than one study).

like facies (parkinsonism). We cannot explain the absence of extrapyramidal symptoms in children who have been treated with prochlorperazine. (The study is still in the process of being analyzed.)

c. Akathisia was reported in only two children treated with thioridazine; however, as we mentioned above, this is a very difficult symptom to identify in children who already exhibit hyperactivity, restlessness, and stereotyped behavior. All extrapyramidal symptoms were very readily controlled with either dose adjustment or the administration of counteractive medication.

d. Tardive dyskinesia (TD) in adults may occur after prolonged treatment with high doses of neuroleptics in middle-aged and older patients. Most often it occurs after reduction or discontinuation of medication, and it may be masked by high doses of medication. In children, the appearance of TD and TD-like symptoms differ somewhat from that occurring in the adult. TD occurring *during* treatment in children treated with the neuroleptics is an extremely rare phenomenon. Over the past 11 years that we have been treating psychotic children with neuroleptics at the Psychopharmacology Unit, we observed only two cases of TD occurring in children *during* treatment. One occurred in a 9-year-old girl who was receiving fluphenazine for a total of approximately 17 months. For the first two months, she received an average of 10 mg daily; subsequently, she received 25 mg daily for a total of 12 months, and when the medication was increased to 35 mg of fluphenazine daily, she began exhibiting tongue movements similar to the ones we see in oral dyskinesia of adults. The medication then was gradually reduced by 5 mg per week. At the end of the fifth week, she was receiving only 10 mg of fluphenazine daily and the tongue movements completely disappeared.

The other case involved a 9-year-old boy who was receiving Mellaril for a total of 5 months. He was started on 150 mg of Mellaril daily, which was increased to 800 mg daily within 3 weeks, and at the eighth week of his treatment he developed typical oral dyskinesia, consisting of extremely rapid tongue movements associated with choreoathetoid movements and myoclonic jerks of the extremities. The medication was gradually decreased to 300 mg of Mellaril daily, and the tongue movements and the choreoathetoid movements decreased markedly within 2 weeks and disappeared completely during the subsequent 4 weeks of treatment. In both children, the dyskinetic phenomena subsided on reduction of medication only.

Convulsive disorders

These were not observed in our children. Tardive dyskinesia is a rare phenomenon in children. However, a dyskinetic syndrome is quite common after neuroleptic treatment has been discontinued (6). We have conducted a series of drug withdrawal studies at our unit and have observed that many children developed a neurological syndrome that resembles, in part, tardive dyskinesia. The syndrome consists of abnormal involuntary movements, ataxia, and on occasion, oral dyskinesia. We are referring to this syndrome as Withdrawal Emergent Symptoms (WES). Out of 184 cases withdrawn from neuroleptic treatment, 51% developed WES. Children withdrawn from low-dose, high-potency drugs are twice as likely to develop WES (61%) than those children withdrawn from high-dose, low-potency drugs (29%). (See Table 2.)

Forty-one percent of the children developed involuntary movements and ataxia. The involuntary movements were present in over 90% of the children affected and involved the extremities, head, and trunk. They were primarily choreoathetoid, but myoclonic and hemiballistic movements, posturing, and head-rocking movements were also occasionally observed. Oral dyskinesia, when present, was always mild; it was observed in less than 20% of the children, and it occurred only 6 times as the sole symptom. Ataxia, which was characterized by ataxic gait, dysmetria, terminal tremor on volition, and generalized hypotonia, was observed in 86% of the children involved, and it was always jointly present with involuntary movements.

In 80% of the children, dyskinetic symptoms appeared within 14 days after drug withdrawal. We were able to observe spontaneous remission in 35% of the children. The mean duration of the symptoms in these children was 15 days. In the majority of the children, active treatment had to be reinstituted within a week of drug discontinuation because of clinical deterioration. The WES disappeared within 2 weeks after active treatment was reinstituted.

As Table 2 indicates, children treated with low-dose drugs were twice as likely to develop WES as children receiving high-dose drugs. Children withdrawn from high-dose drugs were twice as likely to remit spontaneously as those withdrawn from low-dose drugs. There was no relationship between the incidence of WES and age, sex, dosage, or duration of treatment. There was no relationship between the occurrence of EPS during treatment and the development of WES following termination of treatment. Of the children who developed EPS during treatment, 52% developed WES, while 48% did not. The chemical class to which the drug belonged had no relevance with regard to the development of WES.

We chose to call these dyskinetic phenomena in children Withdrawal Emergent Symptoms (WES) to distinguish them from the true tardive dyskinesia of the adult. Our data, however, suggests that tardive dyskinesia may occur in children treated for long periods of time with high doses of neuroleptics, but it is extremely rare and it subsides quite readily with dose reduction. WES, on the other hand, is a much more frequently occurring syndrome in children. Whether this syndrome in children may represent an atypical, reversible form of tardive dyskinesia that has been masked by the use of neuroleptics and becomes apparent after discontinuation of medication is a difficult question to answer.

The determination of the reversibility of WES is complicated by the fact that administration of neuroleptics may mask the presence of dyskinetic phenomena. We are of the opinion that the dyskinetic phenomena observed in children are reversible. This is based in part on the brief duration and spontaneous remission of symptoms in those children whom we were able to maintain drug-free for at least 3 weeks. This belief is further supported by the findings of McAndrew *et al.* (7), which is the only reference in the literature with regard to dyskinetic phenomena in children treated with neuroleptics.

In summary, neurological complications do occur in children treated with neuroleptics. The neurological complications are similar to those occurring in adults, but their incidence seems to be lower than that of the adults. Tardive dyskinesia is a rare phenomenon in children, but a postwithdrawal dyskinetic syndrome, (WES), is quite frequent. In general, dyskinetic phenomena in children have a good prognosis, and they do not appear to be a serious complication of neuroleptic treatment.

ACKNOWLEDGMENTS

This study was supported in part by grants MH 18180 and MH 26960 from the National Institute of Mental Health, U.S. Public Health Service.

REFERENCES

1. Ayd, F.J., Jr. A survey of drug-induced extrapyramidal reactions. *JAMA*, *175*:1054–1060, 1961.
2. American College of Neuropsychopharmacology. Neurological syndromes associated with antipsychotic drug use: a special report. *Arch. Gen. Psychiatry*, *28*:463–467, 1973.
3. Crane, F. Tardive Dyskinesia in patients treated with major neuroleptics: a review of the literature. *Am. J. of Psychiatry, Suppl. 8*, *124*:40–48, 1968.
4. DiMascio, A., Soltys, J.J., Shader, R.L. In *Psychotropic Drug Side Effects*, Baltimore: Williams & Wilkins, chap. 23, 1970.
5. Engelhardt, D.M., Polizos, P. Adverse effects of pharmacotherapy in childhood psychosis. In *Psychopharmacology*, Lipton, M., DiMascio, A., Killam, K. (eds.). New York: Raven Press, p. 1463, 1978.
6. Polizos, P., Engelhardt, D.M., Hoffman, S.P., Waizer, J. Neurological consequences of psychotropic drug withdrawal in schizophrenic children. *J. Autism Child, Schizo.* *3*:247–253, 1973.
7. McAndrew, J.B., Case, Q., Treffert, D.A. Effects of prolonged phenothiazine intake on psychotic and other hospitalized children. *J. Autism Child. Schizo.*, *2*.1:75–91, 1972.

20

Problems in the Assessment of Tardive Dyskinesia

GEORGE GARDOS
and JONATHAN O. COLE

The present authors have recently developed a marked preoccupation, if not obsession, with the problems encountered in the accurate assessment of tardive dyskinesia. There are several unique features which make assessment more of a problem in tardive dyskinesia research than elsewhere in clinical psychiatry. There are major disagreements among experts on prevalence, course, prognosis, and the promise of effective treatment has so far remained a mirage. While the pathophysiology and treatment of tardive dyskinesia remain challenging problems, one should at least be able to resolve more mundane issues, such as (1) what constitutes tardive dyskinesia; (2) what is the prevalence; (3) what is the course of the syndrome; (4) what is the prognosis, and in particular, what percent become functionally impaired; and (5) what proportion of patients benefit when a drug is given.

The present article is directed towards the resolution of the last set of questions. The major problems of assessment are reviewed and possible remedies towards solving these problems are presented.

THE MEASUREMENT PROBLEM

The authors recently published a review of the available assessment techniques for tardive dyskinesia (1). A shortened and up-dated version is presented here.

Instrumentation

Techniques included under this heading lead to the graphic presentation of limb, face, and tongue movements. Electromyographic methods record activity from electrodes placed over selected muscles. Movements have been recorded from the bucco-lingual region (2), fingers (1,3,4), and the soleus muscle (5), but could be feasibly obtained from other sites, such as wrist, ankle, chin (6). Accelerometers have also been employed in recording movements (4,6). Denny and Casey (7) employed a pneumatic transducer connected to a small inflatable balloon inside the mouth. Hand movements were recorded from a pneumatic cannula placed between two fingers. Klawans and Rubovits (8) photographed excursions of a pocket flashlight produced by arm movements, leading to the visualization of choreiform dyskinesia. Assessment of vocal function has been employed in dyskinetic patients, since subtle dysarthria may be the first sign of tardive dyskinesia. Fann *et al.* (6) devised a 7-test speech assessment battery. The instrumental component is the Tonar-II device, which measures nasality.

EEG abnormalities have been shown to occur in some tardive dyskinesia patients. Jus *et al.* (2) were able to distinguish tardive dyskinesia from the "rabbit syndrome" through polygraph records obtained during sleep. Wegner *et al.* (9) found an unusually high incidence of the B-mitten EEG dysrhythmia in patients with tardive dyskinesia. This abnormal pattern is detected during sleep only and may have predictive value since it may be present before dyskinesia is seen clinically.

Frequency Counts

The basic assumption in these methods is that the severity of tardive dyskinesia is related to the frequency, intensity, or both, of the most conspicuous dyskinetic movements. A number of studies utilized frequency counts of bucco-linguo-facial movements, such as tongue protrusions, chewing, pursing of lips (10–17). Gerlach and Thorsen (18,19) devised a scoring system, taking into account both frequency and amplitude of oral dyskinesia. Longin *et al.* (20) employed behavioral techniques in reducing choreiform movement. Their criterion measure was "per cent time spent in choreic movements," which was recorded several times a day. Duration of tongue extension was a measure used by Klawans and Rubovits (8), based on the observation that dyskinetic patients are often unable to keep their tongue beyond the outer lip for more than a few seconds.

Rating Methods

Global ratings have a long and respectable history in clinical research. Numerous studies have utilized global ratings of dyskinesia; the format and complexity, however, vary a great deal.

In some studies (21,22,23), patients were dichotomized into those who did and those who did not have tardive dyskinesia. A simple classification in treatment studies involves placing patients into "improved," "worse," and "no change" categories. Other investigators used global ratings on 3–7 point scales (24–26). In psychometric terms, these constitute ordinal scales where each scale point denotes more or less dyskinesia than adjacent scale points. Several rating scales have been developed that consist of a number of global ratings, either of types of abnormal movement (e.g., choreiform [27,28]) or of movements by body regions (29). The Abnormal Involuntary Movements Scale, or AIMS (30), is probably the most widely used rating instrument. It consists of dyskinesia ratings of the face, lips, jaw, tongue, arm, leg, and trunk on 5-point scales. In addition, global severity, patient awareness, and incapacitation, as well as dental status, are recorded.

Multi-item rating scales attempt to present a comprehensive picture of tardive dyskinesia by recording each frequently observable dyskinetic movement separately. The earliest, and a relatively uncomplicated scale, was developed by Crane, who rated 11 symptoms (31), although he used different versions of this rating method in other studies (32–35). The scale was expanded by Smith (36,37) to include 11 items of extrapyramidal symptoms and 16 denoting dyskinesia. A 14-item scale, recording frequency and severity separately, has been developed at the St. Paul-Ramsey Hospital (38,39). Highly complex scales have been developed by a group of German investigators (40,41) and by a British group (42,43).

A rating scale was recently developed by Simpson (44). The original version consisted of 33 items of abnormal movements commonly seen in patients with tardive dyskinesia. The scale was employed by the present authors in several studies (45–48). It has been revised recently and the final version, consisting of 34 items, plus write-ins on 6-point scales, is awaiting publication.

Audio-Visual Methods

The videotaping of patients with tardive dyskinesia has gained increasingly wide application for such purposes as training raters, evaluating drug effects, and for educational and teaching purposes. Sequential filming often captures dramatically how a patient may change over time. Strictly speaking, audio-visual documentation is not by itself an assessment method, since the resulting tape has to be presented to observers who then have to make a quantitative evaluation, usually by means of a rating scale.

One of the major problems with the audio-visual technique is that by reducing three-dimensional movements to two dimensions, certain movements may be missed or are harder to see. Other problems are protecting patient privacy and the cost in obtaining high-quality audio-visual equipment and expertise. A particular asset of videotaping in treatment trials is the ease with which raters can be kept blind. An unexplored potential is the application of "instant replay" in slow motion of the tape to improve the accuracy of ratings.

Overview of Assessment Methods

Judging by the great variety of approaches, it becomes intuitively obvious that no single method approaches the ideal. Table I presents the relative strengths and deficiencies of the methods referred to above. It can be readily seen that no assessment method satisfies all criteria. Instrumental techniques tend to be precise and reliable, but may pose problems in applying them to unselected groups of patients. Validity may be doubtful and needs to be demonstrated. Frequency counts are also quite sensitive and reliable, but may only be applicable to patients with obvious and countable movements. The most promising of these methods appeared to be "duration of tongue extension" (8), since it does not have the drawback of restricted applicability. The present authors have employed the tongue extension method with rather disappointing results. It appeared that many patients with severe oro-facial dyskinesia were able to extend their tongue for the required 30 seconds, while other patients without apparent dyskinesia scored well below 30 seconds. Correlational analysis showed that duration of tongue extension scores did not correlate significantly with lingual dyskinesia ratings or other tardive dyskinesia scores, with the exception of akathisia (49). Therefore, the clinical value of this particular measure is limited to patients who show greatly reduced scores, where improvement in response to a particular treatment may yield a quantitative measure.

Global rating scales show good validity and are easy to administer. The demonstration of satisfactory reliability, however, is an absolute requirement. AIMS is emerging as the most widely employed scale of this type, and satisfactory interrater reliability coefficients have been reported recently (50). Reliability is also essential to document in multi-item rating scales, and several of the scales reported above have been shown to be reliable when used by trained raters (36,38,42,44,47). The unique value of multi-item scales appears to be their usefulness in leading to improved typology and thereby to a better understanding of the features of tardive dyskinesia.

The pragmatic question of which measures to employ in a given study can only be answered by considering the research questions asked. In general, coupling a rating method with one of the objective techniques may yield optimal results in that the validity and clinical relevance of the former may be complemented by the precision and sensitivity of the latter. Multi-item scales should be used in studies of prevalence and of etiological factors since the

Table 1

Comparison of Assessment Methods

	Instrumentation	Frequency Counts	Rating Methods	
			Global Judgments	Multi-Item Scales
Psychometrics				
Validity	Questionable, has to be demonstrated	Good face validity	Generally good, construct validity needs demonstration	Generally good, but may depend on scale items
Reliability	Excellent	Tends to be satisfactory	Poor, usually not reported. Essential to demonstrate	Variable. Essential to document
Sensitivity	Excellent	Excellent	Mostly poor	Variable. May be related to number of items
Clinical Features				
Amount of Training and Preparation	Extensive technical preparation and hardware needed	Brief practice required	Little or none required	Considerable, often requires prolonged training
Ease of Administration	Cumbersome, patients often have to go to lab	Patient may have to be rated	No problems	May be time-consuming
Patient Cooperation	Highly necessary, may be useless for uncooperative patients	Minor degrees of cooperation may be necessary	Not an essential requirement	Some degree of cooperation may be needed for some items (e.g. opening of month)
Applicability to Large Patient Groups	Limited to patients with the "right movements"	Frequency counts are restricted patients with easily countable movements	Universal	Universal
Comprehensiveness	Restricted, tends to assess only 1–2 types of movements	Only estimates frequency of most prominent movements	Too molar, does not assess individual movements	Tend to give the most comprehensive picture of dyskinesia

frequency distributions of different types of dyskinetic movements may be a key issue. Treatment studies can benefit from at least one highly sensitive measure, in addition to which a global rating ought to be included since any effective therapeutic agent should produce clinically evident changes. Patients with distinct oro-facial movements may be assessed by a frequency count method, and exceptionally cooperative or motivated dyskinetic patients could be followed by electromyography. Videotaping appears to be invaluable for educational purposes and for rater training.

THE PROBLEM OF DEFINITION

The tardive dyskinesia syndrome is commonly described as characterized by choreoathetosis of the bucco-linguo-facial region, trunk, and extremities, as well as tics, grimaces, and dystonia (51,52). The specificity of this concept has been criticized on the basis that schizophrenic stereotypies and mannerisms resemble many of the choreoathetoid movements of tardive dyskinesia, as do a number of neurological syndromes—Huntington's chorea, torsion dystonia, senile chorea, etc. (53). Skeptics continue to claim that the existence of a syndrome of drug-induced tardive dyskinesia has not been convincigly demonstrated (54). Even if these objections are disregarded, a number of problems in definition are encountered in real life.

Who Has Tardive Dyskinesia—Or, the Problem of Continuous Distribution

The authors have become keenly aware of the fact that there is hardly a patient who will not show up with one or two ratable abnormal movements during a 5-minute observation period. In fact, occasional tongue protrusion, puckering, foot tapping, choreiform finger movement, or a tic or grimace may also be observed in presumably normal fellow-raters. Thus, very low scores on a scale almost certainly do not indicate tardive dyskinesia.

The senior author has rated two large groups of chronic schizophrenics unselected for abnormal movements. In the first study, there was a suggestion of a bimodal distribution (46); in the second, the distribution more closely resembled a normal distribution, skewed to the right (55). The problem is that any cutoff point is purely arbitrary, and there does not appear to be an easy way in which it can be determined who has mild tardive dyskinesia, as opposed to mannerisms or stereotypies. We feel that the sidestepping of this very issue, i.e., the lack of establishing diagnostic criteria for tardive dyskinesia, is largely responsible for the widely divergent prevalence figures (10.5%–50%) in the literature for similar populations (1).

In order to make prevalence figures more meaningful, there should be specific operational criteria for defining tardive dyskinesia. By defining criteria, prevalence figures would have more specific meaning; furthermore, in treatment studies the percentage of patients becoming markedly improved could also be defined according to the original criteria. In surveys of tardive dyskinesia, prevalence rates could be expressed as a series of % figures, depending on different cutoff points. For instance, in a recent follow-up study completed by the authors, the prevalence rates for tardive dyskinesia could be expressed as follows:

Most experts would agree that the 24% of patients with at least one "moderate" score have tardive dyskinesia, and that the 17% of patients who do not have at least one "mild" rating do not have tardive dyskinesia. However, in the majority of patients (60%) who showed mild ratings, considerable disagreement may occur, and the disagreement may not be resolvable on the basis of AIMS scores alone. Using a similar approach, Smith *et al.* (50) carried out a tardive dyskinesia survey in an inpatient schizophrenic population. They reported a prevalence of 30% when tardive dyskinesia was defined as at least one "moderate" rating on the AIMS; and 60% when tardive dyskinesia was defined as one "mild" rating. From the above, one may conclude that rating-scale criteria may make prevalence figures more meaningful, but by themselves do not solve the problem of how to agree on the diagnosis of tardive dyskinesia.

Coexistence of Different Neurological Syndromes

Disagreement and uncertainty may arise when a patient manifests a variety of abnormal movements rather than the typical choreoathetosis of tardive dyskinesia. Recognition of a number of neurological entities which may mimic tardive dyskinesia, such as Huntington's chorea or torsion dystonia, is an

Table 2
Dyskinesia Scores (AIMS) of 83 Chronic
Schizophrenic Patients (55)

Criterion	# Patients	%
Score on items 1–7 at least . . .		
No score (0)	1	1.2
One minimal item	5	6.2
Two minimal (but no mild)	8	9.6
One mild	14	16.9
Two mild (but no moderate)	35	42.2
One moderate	9	10.8
Two moderate or one severe	11	13.2

obvious necessity (52). Since Fann and Lake (16) first called attention to the coexistence of tardive dyskinesia and drug-induced parkinsonism, the occurrence of both syndromes has been seen in many patients. This phenomenon may be based on a common pathological mechanism and may reflect a breakdown of feedback regulation of cholinergic and dopaminergic activity in the basal ganglia. The presence of akathisia may likewise create an assessment problem, since it has been described as a side effect of early neuroleptic treatment but has also been found quite frequently in tardive dyskinesia patients and is rated in scales such as Simpson's (44). The nature of akathisia, the necessity of a subjective component of distress, the underlying neurochemical mechanism, and its treatment are all unresolved issues.

The presence of additional movement abnormalities in a patient may give rise to difficulties in assessing tardive dyskinesia in a number of ways:

(1) Certain movements may be included in some tardive dyskinesia scales but not in others. For instance, AIMS specifically excludes all tremors, while other scales consider the possibility that certain tremors, such as tongue or eyelid tremor, may be indicative of early tardive dyskinesia. Similarly, akathisia may or not be included in a given rating scale. Electromyographic techniques have to distinguish between parkinsonian tremor and tardive dyskinesia movements, but this problem is apparently surmountable (3).

(2) Certain types of movements may become reclassified as new knowledge becomes available. For instance, the rabbit syndrome, which was originally to be a type of tardive dyskinesia, is now considered to be a form of parkinsonism. The rabbit syndrome can be distinguished from tardive dyskinesia by polygraph records (2), and it seems to respond to drugs which aggravate tardive dyskinesia (56).

(3) During trials of putative therapeutic agents, complex changes in movements may occur which defy simple explanations and may influence global judgement unpredictably. For instance, in a recently completed trial of papaverine, some patients showed alleviation of choreoathetosis, but developed parkinsonian tremor or rigidity (57).

THE VARIABILITY OF DYSKINESIA

A particularly troublesome problem in the assessment of tardive dyskinesia is the tendency for its manifestations to undergo extensive fluctuations, at times apparently spontaneously. It has been generally recognized that dyskinesia is not present during sleep and that its severity is influenced by emotional factors. There are, in addition, a number of other sources of variability which need to be discussed.

Shifting of Movements to Different Areas

The clinical observation that a particular dyskinetic movement, e.g., tongue protrusion, may cease apparently spontaneously to be replaced by a different movement, such as lip smacking or wiggling of toes or fingers, is not uncommon. However, an analysis of repeated measures of area scores on the Simpson scale revealed high consistency of movements at a given site, with the possible exception of upper-extremity scores, which tend to accompany ratings in other areas (58). These rather limited data suggest that while shifting of movements may be observed, it is not a major source of variation and may often occur within a limited area (e.g., tongue, lip and jaw movements appearing interchangeably).

Temporal Fluctuations

While many patients display constant and hardly varying patterns of dyskinesia, there are also patients who show marked fluctuation in movements from day to day or even at different times during a particular day. A recently completed longitudinal study of two tardive dyskinesia patients by the authors has provided relevant data (48). These patients were rated twice a week for 44 and 26 weeks. Tardive dyskinesia ratings underwent apparently spontaneous fluctuations, and varied as much as threefold on the same medication, with rater and set held constant. The degree of variation was greater than the apparent effect of cyproheptadine during a 6-week trial.

Arousal

The level of physiological arousal has a marked impact on the manifestations of tardive dyskinesia movements. During sleep, dyskinetic movements are abolished, which can be shown by polygraphic recording (2). Conversely, movements may also be inhibited in response to certain types of stress, such as a patient being stared at in a rating situation. Hence, the necessity for including a period of observation at rest before a standard examination is performed for ratings.

The corollary of the foregoing is that any factors, including diet, activity, and perhaps most importantly, medication, which affect arousal level may have an effect on the level of dyskinetic movements. Sedative compounds can be expected to have a suppressant effect on movements, while stimulating compounds are likely to show the reverse. In fact, many, if not most, drugs such as dopamine blockers, benzodiazepines, and barbiturates, which have been reported to show beneficial effects in tardive dyskinesia, do possess sedative effects. An apparent exception concerns deanol and other cholinergic compounds which do not generally produce sedation. Dopaminergic, anticholinergic compounds, and psychostimulants tend to produce increases in dyskinetic movements. The prevailing opinion suggests that the neuropharmacologic changes in the basal ganglia are more significant for dyskinesia than is arousal level. Nevertheless, in the evaluation of any compound for tardive dyskinesia, the influence of changes in arousal level have to be reckoned with.

Posture and Motility

Movements tend to be reduced in the sitting position. Trunk movements are more readily seen when the patient is standing. Hand and finger movements are best seen during walking, when the arms swing freely. Voluntary movements tend to inhibit dyskinesia in the proximity of the movement, but enhance it in areas far removed (51). For instance, speaking tends to reduce oral dyskinesia and writing suppresses hand and finger chorea. At the same time, distracting maneuvers, such as asking the patient to touch his thumb with each finger or to stand with eyes closed and outstretched hands, have been included in rating procedures to elicit oro-facial movements ("activated movements").

Recent and Current Drugs

Concurrent neuroleptic medication may have a powerful suppressant effect on the manifestations of tardive dyskinesia. Other types of psychotropic drugs may exercise a lesser, though still important influence on the level of manifest dyskinesia. The neurochemical basis for this relationship is that most psychotropic drugs influence central dopaminergic or cholinergic activity or affect arousal level. A special situation arises during withdrawal of neuroleptic compounds. Withdrawal-emergent dyskinesia or exacerbation of existing dyskinesia, usually lasting 1–6 weeks, at times longer, is often observed. Withdrawal dyskinesias have also been described for antidepressants, antihistamines, and narcotic analgesics. A resurgence of dopaminergic activity in the basal ganglia is believed to be an important mechanism in withdrawal dyskinesias (59).

Effect of Dose Schedules

In monkeys, haloperidol-induced bucco-lingual dyskinesia shows striking and consistent temporal relationship to the dose of haloperidol: movements are suppressed after each dose, but recur and become greatest just before the next dose (60).

In the longitudinal study carried out by the authors (48), significantly lower ratings were obtained in the morning about 1 to 2 hours after a regular daily dose of 20 mg haloperidol than in the afternoon. Unfortunately, an attempt to replicate this work with different raters in the same patient failed. Furthermore, the observed difference may have been due to diurnal variation rather than to short-term suppression of movements by haloperidol.

In the same project, we also studied the relationship between tardive dyskinesia ratings and the timing of depot fluphenazine injections. In a patient previously without neuroleptics, the introduction of fluphenazine decanoate produced a dramatic decrease in movements following the first two injections, followed by a rebound lasting until the next injection. However, after a steady state level of fluphenazine had been reached, these changes were no longer observed: average ratings completed during the 5 days before injections were not significantly different from ratings obtained during the 5 postinjection days.

METHODS OF REDUCING VARIABILITY

Just as in other areas of research, the elimination of major sources of error variance is an important design requirement. This is an especially important task in tardive dyskinesia research because drug effects are often modest, and the variability of ratings is quite large. In the light of the foregoing discussion on the identifiable sources of variance, a number of measures can be taken to minimize error variance.

Exclude the "Fluctuating Patient" from Drug Trials

Any unselected group of patients with dyskinetic movements probably includes a few whose dyskinetic movements undergo extensive fluctuations over time. The presence of such patients in a treatment trial increases the within-group variance and reduces the likelihood of demonstrating drug effects. Alternately, fluctuating patients may themselves be responsible for false positive results in drug trials when spontaneous remission coincides with drug administration. The solution to the "fluctuating tardive dyskinesia patient" is to study them separately and over a prolonged period of time, but to exclude them from drug trials when groups of patients are compared.

Control for Confounding Variables

Some of the well-recognized sources of variability can be eliminated by keeping the evaluation set constant. Thus, raters, time of day, and assessment site should be kept constant. Variations in arousal and activity levels can be reduced to some extent by attention to factors such as recent ingestion of alcohol, coffee, heavy meals, or smoking, and by standardizing the behavior of the evaluator. Rating scales should have precise instructions to raters, which are to be strictly adhered to. In addition, some estimate of arousal level needs to be recorded at the time of the rating, as by Smith's Tardive Dyskinesia Scale (36).

Adequate Experimental Controls

Placebo-controlled studies are clearly the optimal solution to control for confounding variables. When such is not feasible, it is advisable to include an adequate baseline observation period as well as a post-treatment observation period. If the above precautions are not observed, apparent improvement will often be erroneously attributed to the drug given. In many cases, the reason for this error lies in the not-too-well appreciated fact that patients tend to enter drug trials when they are at or near their worst, and are therefore likely to show spontaneous remission, irrespective of the treatment given. An ABA or ABAB design with on-and-off treatment periods would also tend to overcome this problem.

REFERENCES

1. Gardos, G., Cole, J.O., La Brie, R. The assessment of tardive dyskinesia. *Arch. Gen. Psychiatry, 34*:1206–1212, 1977.
2. Jus, K., Jus, A., Villeneuve, A. Polygraphic profile of oral tardive dyskinesia and of rabbit syndrome. *Dis. Nerv. Syst., 34*:27–32, 1973.
3. Alpert, M., Diamond, F., Friedhoff, A. Tremographic studies in tardive dyskinesia. *Psychopharmacol. Bull., 12*:5–7, 1976.
4. Young, R.R., Growdon, J.H., Shahani, B.T. Beta-adrenergic mechanisms in action tremor. *N. Engl. J. Med., 293*:950–953, 1975.
5. Crayton, J.W., Smith, R.C., Klass, D., Chang, S., Ericksen, S.E. Electrophysiological (H-Reflex) studies of patients with tardive dyskinesia. *Am. J. Psychiatry, 134*:775–781, 1977.
6. Fann, W.E., Stafford, J.R., Malone, R.L., Frost, J.D., Jr., Richman, B.W. Clinical research techniques in tardive dyskinesia. *Am. J. Psychiatry, 134*:759–762, 1977.
7. Denny, D., Casey, D.E. An objective method for measuring dyskinetic movements in tardive dyskinesia. *Electroencephalogr. Clin. Neurophysiol., 38*:645–646, 1975.
8. Klawans, H.L., Jr., Rubovits, R. Effects of cholinergic and anticholinergic agents on tardive dyskinesia. *J. Neurol. Neurosurg. Psychiatry, 37*:941–947, 1974.
9. Wegner, J.T., Struve, F.A., Kane, J.M. The B-Mitten EEG pattern and tardive dyskinesia: a possible association. *Am. J. Psychiatry, 134*:1143–1145, 1977.
10. Kazamatsuri, H., Chien, C-P, Cole, J.O. Treatment of tardive dyskinesia: I. Clinical efficacy of a dopamine-depleting agent, tetrabenazine. *Arch. Gen. Psychiatry, 27*:95–99, 1972.

11. Kazamatsuri, H., Chien, C-P, Cole, J.O. Treatment of tardive dyskinesia: II. Short-term efficacy of dopamine-blocking agents haloperidol and thiopropazate. *Arch. Gen. Psychiatry, 27*:100–103, 1972.

12. Kazamatsuri, H., Chien, C-P, Cole, J.O. Treatment of tardive dyskinesia: III. Clinical efficacy of a dopamine competing agent, methyldopa. *Arch. Gen. Psychiatry, 27*:824–827, 1972.

13. Kazamatsuri, H., Chien, C-P, Cole, J.O. Long-term treatment of tardive dyskinesia with haloperidol and tetrabenazine. *Am. J. Psychiatry, 130*:479–483, 1973.

14. Davis, K.L., Berger, P.A., Hollister, L.E. Choline for tardive dyskinesia. *N. Engl. J. Med., 293*:152, 1975.

15. Roxburgh, P.A. Treatment of persistent phenothiazine induced oral dyskinesia. *Br. J. Psychiatry, 116*:277–280, 1970.

16. Fann, W.E., Lake, R. On the coexistence of parkinsonism and tardive dyskinesia. *Dis. Nerv. Syst., 35*:324–326, 1974.

17. Growdon, J.H., Hirsch, M.J., Wurtman, R.J., Wiener, W. Oral choline administration to patients with tardive dyskinesia. *N. Engl. J. Med., 297*:524–527, 1977.

18. Gerlach, J., Thorsen, K. The movement pattern of oral tardive dyskinesia in relation to anticholinergic and antidopaminergic treatment. *Int. Pharmacopsychiatry, 11*:1–7, 1976.

19. Gerlach, J. The relationship between parkinsonism and tardive dyskinesia. *Am. J. Psychiatry, 134*:781–784, 1977.

20. Longin, H.E., Kohn, J.P., Macurik, K.M. The modification of choreal movements. *J. Beh. Ther. Exp. Psychiat., 5*:263–265, 1974.

21. Crane, G.E., Paulson, G. Involuntary movements in a sample of chronic mental patients and their relation to the treatment with neuroleptics. *Int. J. Neuropsychiat., 3*:286–291, 1966.

22. Brandon, S., McClelland, H.A., Protheroe, C. A study of facial dyskinesia in a mental hospital population. *Br. J. Psychiatry, 118*:171–184, 1971.

23. Laterre, E.C., Foretemps, E. Deanol in spontaneous and induced dyskinesias. *Lancet, 1*:1301, 1975.

24. Pryce, I.G., Edwards, H. Persistent oral dyskinesia in female mental hospital patients. *Br. J. Psychiatry, 112*:983–987, 1966.

25. Edwards, H. The significance of brain damage in persistent oral dyskinesia. *Br. J. Psychiatry, 116*:271–275, 1970.

26. Crane, G.E., Smeets, R.A. Tardive dyskinesia and drug therapy in geriatric patients. *Arch. Gen. Psychiatry, 30*:341–343, 1974.

27. Villeneuve, A., Lavallee, J-C, Lemieux, L-H. Dyskinesie tardive post-neuroleptique. *Laval. Med., 40*:832–837, 1969.

28. Villeneuve, A., Boszormenyi, Z. Treatment of drug-induced dyskinesias. *Lancet, 1*:353–354, 1970.

29. Gerlach, J., Reisby, N., Randrup, A. Dopaminergic hypersensitivity and cholinergic hypofunction in the pathophysiology of tardive dyskinesia. *Psychopharmacologia, 34*:21–35, 1974.

30. Abnormal Involuntary Movement Scale: HEW, Alcohol Drug Abuse and Mental Health Administration, Washington, D.C., 1974.

31. Crane, G.E., Ruiz, P., Kernohan, W.J. Effects of drug withdrawal on tardive dyskinesia. *Act. Nerv. Super., 11*:30–35, 1969.

32. Crane, G.E. Tardive dyskinesia in schizophrenic patients treated with psychotropic drugs. *Aggressologie, 9*:209–217, 1968.

33. Crane, G.E. High doses of trifluoperazine and tardive dyskinesia. *Arch. Neurol., 22*:176–180, 1970.

34. Crane, G.E., Naranjo, E.R. Motor disorders induced by neuroleptics. *Arch. Gen. Psychiatry, 24*:179–184, 1971.

35. Crane, G.E. Pseudoparkinsonism and tardive dyskinesia. *Arch. Neurol., 27*:426–430, 1972.
36. Smith, R.C., Tamminga, C.A., Haraszti, J., Pandey, G.N., Davis, J.M. Effects of dopamine agonists in tardive dyskinesia. *Am. J. Psychiatry, 134*:763–768, 1977.
37. Tamminga, C.A., Smith, R.C., Ericksen, S.E., Chang, S., Davis, J.M. Cholinergic influences in tardive dyskinesia. *Am. J. Psychiatry, 134*:769–774, 1977.
38. Reda, F.A., Scanlon, J.M., Kemp, K.F. Treatment of tardive dyskinesia with lithium carbonate. *N. Engl. J. Med., 291*:850, 1974.
39. Escobar, J.I., Kemp, K.F. Dimethylaminoethanol for tardive dyskinesia. *N. Engl. J. Med., 292*:318, 1975.
40. Hippius, H., Logemann, G. Zur Wirkung von dioxyphenylalanin (L-dopa) auf extrapyramidalmotorische hyperkinesen nach langfristiger neuroleptischer therapie. *Arzneim. Forsch, 20*:894–895, 1970.
41. Heinrich, K., Wegener, I., Bender, H-J. Späte extrapyramidale hyperkinesen bei neuroleptisher langzeitherapie. *Pharmakopsychiatr. Neuropsychopharmakol., 1*:169–195, 1968.
42. Kennedy, P.F., Hershon, H.I., McGuire, R.J. Extrapyramidal disorders after prolonged phenothiazine therapy. *Br. J. Psychiatry, 118*:509–518, 1971.
43. Hershon, H.I., Kennedy, P.F., McGuire, R.J. Persistence of extrapyramidal disorders and psychiatric relapse after withdrawal of long-term phenothiazine therapy. *Br. J. Psychiatry, 120*:41–50, 1972.
44. Simpson, G.M., Zoubok, B., Lee, H.J. An early clinical and toxicity trial of Ex 11-582A in chronic schizophrenia. *Curr. Ther. Res., 19*:87–93, 1976.
45. Gardos, G., Cole, J.O. Papaverine for tardive dyskinesia? *N. Engl. J. Med., 292*:1355, 1975.
46. Gardos, G., Sokol, M., Cole, J.O. Eye color and tardive dyskinesia. *Psychopharmacol. Bull., 12*:7–9, 1976.
47. Gardos, G., Cole, J.O., Sniffin, C. An evaluation of papaverine in tardive dyskinesia. *J. Clin. Pharmacol., 16*:304–310, 1976.
48. Gardos, G., Cole, J.O., Sokol, M. Pitfalls in the assessment of tardive dyskinesia. Presented at VIth World Congress of Psychiatry, Honolulu, Hawaii, September 1977.
49. Gardos, G., Cole, J.O. Unpublished data.
50. Smith, J.M., Oswald, W.T., Kucharski, L.T., Waterman, L.J. Tardive dyskinesia: age and sex differences in hospitalized schizophrenics. *Psychopharmacology.* In press.
51. Crane, G.E. Tardive dyskinesia: A review. *Neuropsychopharmacology,* Amsterdam: Excerpta Medica, International Congress, 359, 346–354, 1974.
52. American College of Neuropsychopharmacology, Food and Drug Administration Task Force: Neurological syndromes associated with antipsychotic drug use. *Arch. Gen. Psychiatry, 28*:463–467, 1973.
53. Marsden, C.D., Tarsy, D., Baldessarini, R.J. Spontaneous and drug-induced movement disorders in psychotic patients. In *Psychiatric Aspects of Neurologic Disease,* Benson, D.F. and Blumer, D. (eds.). New York: Grune and Stratton, pp. 219–266, 1975.
54. Turek, I.S. Drug induced dyskinesia: reality or myth? *Dis. Nerv. Syst., 36*:397–399, 1975.
55. Gardos, G., Cole, J.O. Unpublished data.
56. Gardos, G., Cole, J.O. A pilot study of cyproheptadine in tardive dyskinesia. *Psychopharmacol. Bull.* In press.
57. Gardos, G., Granacher, R.P., Cole, J.O., Sniffin, C. Modest effects of papaverine in tardive dyskinesia. Submitted for publication.
58. Gardos, G., Cole, J.O. Unpublished data.
59. Gardos, G., Cole, J.O., Tarsy, D. Covert dyskinesia. Submitted for publication.
60. Gunne, L-M, Barany, S. Haloperidol-induced tardive dyskinesia in monkeys. *Psychopharmacology, 50*:237–240, 1976.

21
Tardive Dyskinesia and Other Drug-Induced Movement Disorders

WILLIAM E. FANN

INTRODUCTION

Current theories of pseudoparkinsonism and tardive dyskinesia postulate an alteration in striatal transmitter amine function. Parkinsonism involves a deficit in dopamine activity, and tardive dyskinesia an excess of dopamine in the brain. Alternatively, excessive amounts of ACh in the brain could create clinical symptoms of parkinsonism, while deficits of ACh could be responsible for tardive dyskinesia. It is generally accepted that the movement disorders involve insult to the striatal neuronal mechanisms by administered neuroleptics, and seem to be at the opposite end of a continuum in their pathoneurophysiology. Pseudoparkinsonism is most commonly found early in the treatment with neuroleptics, while tardive dyskinesia, as its name indicates, is a late-onset condition usually following at least one year of therapy with higher doses of neuroleptics.

Complicating the picture is the fact that other transmitter amines, such as serototin, GABA, and substance P, have also been implicated in motor disorders, and that all of the currently marketed neuroleptics have some effect on these substances. Pharmacological manipulations of these neurotransmitter substances have been reported to exert some effect on both tardive dyskinesia and parkinsonism. However, for the purpose of this discussion we will examine the more clearly defined roles of dopamine and acetylcholine.

TARDIVE DYSKINESIA AND ANTIPSYCHOTICS

It has generally been assumed that the antipsychotic properties of the neuroleptics are correlated with disturbances in extrapyramidal function. Neuroleptics are thought to render their antipsychotic properties by blockade of dopamine receptor sites accompanied by enhanced turnover of striatal dopamine, but the resulting relative cholinergic dominance in the striatal portion of the brain is probably the origin of extrapyramidal side effects (1,2). Consequently, antischizophrenic effects and extrapyramidal symptoms seem to be inextricably linked.

In a study of 64 psychotic patients treated with haloperidol for up to 2 years, Man (3) noted that the sooner the patient developed extrapyramidal symptoms, the sooner psychotic symptoms improved. If the patient did not develop side effects, even at a high dose, the chances were that he would not improve or would show only minimal improvement. The author stated that by watching for the development of extrapyramidal symptoms, one could predict whether or not a patient would improve. Extrapyramidal symptoms occurred in 76.5% of the sample; 78% showed improvement in their psychosis. All symptoms were controlled with antiparkinsonian agents or reduction in dosage (3).

Though it is a concept not currently accepted, Haase's statement in 1965 is worthy of note: "The more affinity a drug possesses for the extrapyramidal system as shown by the production of extrapyramidal psychokinetic inhibitions, the higher is its neuroleptic potency" (4). Ayd also found a correlation between the absolute frequency of drug-induced extrapyramidal reactions and the milligram potency of the phenothiazines: the more potent the drug, the more frequent the occurrence of striopallidal symptoms. Thirty-five percent of patients treated with chlorpromazine, 44% of patients treated with thiopropazate, and 52% of patients prescribed fluphenazine developed extrapyramidal reactions (5).

Among the extrapyramidal reactions which might occur are akinesia, acute dystonia, akathisia, and parkinsonism. These side effects generally occur early in treatment and usually respond to a reduction in dosage or addition of a corrective medication (5,6,7). More recently, another syndrome, tardive dyskinesia, has been associated with antipsychotic drug use. Tardive dyskinesia generally occurs late in the course of treatment and often after discontinuation of neuroleptic administration; symptoms may persist for months or years and sometimes are permanent and irreversible; the condition shows poor response to any type of therapy (6,8,9). Tardive dysinesia should be distinguished from the other drug-induced extrapyramidal side effects; therefore, a brief description of each reaction follows.

The most frequent extrapyramidal reaction to neuroleptics is akinesia, a condition characterized by weakness, muscular fatigue, and apathy. The patient is constantly aware of fatigue in limbs used for ordinary motor acts, such as walking or writing, and in advanced form, may complain of aches and pains in the muscles in the affected limbs. Because of these symptoms, there is often a reduction in voluntary activity (5).

Acute dystonic reactions are of abrupt onset and consist of bizarre muscular spasms, facial grimacing and distortions, retrocollis, torticollis, dysarthria, and labored breathing. Oculogyric crises—spasm of the external ocular muscles with painful upward gaze persisting for minutes or hours—may also occur. Because of the unusual symptoms, dystonic reactions have been misdiagnosed as tetany, seizure, or hysteria (5,6,7). They occur more often in males than females and in young rather than old patients; occurrence appears to be a matter of individual sensitivity as well as dose and type of antipsychotic (6). Dystonic reactions can be relieved promptly by parenteral administration of a variety of agents such as antiparkinsonian agents, barbiturates, and antihistamines (5,6,7).

Akathisia or motor restlessness refers to a subjective desire to be in constant motion; patients complain of an inability to sit or stand still. Akathisia may be mistaken for psychotic agitation, leading to a further increase in dose, which invariably worsens the patient's condition. Parenteral antiparkinsonian agents may produce immediate response. Oral dose may also allay the restlessness, often without lowering the dose of neuroleptic. However, akathisia is generally the most difficult extrapyramidal reaction to manage, and the condition may not respond adequately to antiparkinsonian drugs. It is frequently necessary to lower dosage of the neuroleptic or to add a sedative agent, such as diazepam, diphenhydramine, or small doses of a barbiturate (5,6).

Drug-induced parkinsonism may be clinically indistinguishable from idiopathic or postencephalitic types. Cases of moderate severity will display mild rigidity, tremor, and a slowing of movement (bradykinesia). More severe cases will involve stooped posture, a marked pill-rolling tremor, masklike fixed facies, increased salivation with drooling, cog-wheeling rigidity, and an involuntary tendency to shorten steps and increase speed in walking (*marche petit pas*) (6,10,11). Treatment includes reduction of dose or addition of a conventional antiparkinsonian agent. It is generally preferable to add oral antiparkinsonian agents, since this permits uninterrupted neuroleptic therapy and avoids the risk of loss of therapeutic benefit. The clinician should be aware, however, that while anticholinergic agents mask drug-induced parkinsonism, they may also increase the intensity and duration of tardive dyskinesia in the patient (11,12,13).

INCIDENCE OF EXTRAPYRAMIDAL REACTIONS

Extrapyramidal reactions occur in about 1% of general medical patients treated with phenothiazines or tricyclic antidepressants. Depending upon dosage and duration of treatment, between 21% and 79% of psychiatric patients receiving long-term phenothiazine therapy have been reported to develop extrapyramidal symptoms (14).

Ayd surveyed 3,775 psychiatric patients treated with phenothiazines, and reported that 38.9% developed extrapyramidal symptoms: 2.3% developed dyskinesia; 15.4% developed parkinsonism; 21.2% developed akathisia. Of the patients exhibiting these side effects, 63% were women. Akathisia and parkinsonism occurred twice as often in women as men; dyskinesia, however, occurred twice as often in men (5).

Patients who have blood relatives with naturally occurring parkinsonism are more apt to have a neuroleptic-induced extrapyramidal reaction. Young patients are more likely to develop dystonic reactions or oculogyric crises. The older the patient, the more likely the development of parkinsonian symptoms (15).

Studies have suggested that older patients (6,8,16), females (5,6,8,15,17), and individuals with organic brain disorders (6,8), are more susceptible to development of extrapyramidal symptoms. Ayd, however, suggests that striopallidal symptoms due to neuroleptics are a matter of individual susceptibility even more than a matter of chemical structure, milligram potency, dosage, or duration of treatment, pointing to the fact that 61.9% of the patients in his survey never had a neurologic reaction to neuroleptics (5).

TARDIVE DYSKINESIA

Tardive dyskinesia (TD) has been observed with increasing frequency since it was first reported in the late 1950's. The syndrome was initially controversial. In 1968 Kline challenged the fact that the syndrome existed at all, stating that the incidence of side effects had been misrepresented and that TD should not be regarded as a significant danger in therapy with neuroleptics (18). As recently as 1973 the relationship between the administration of neuroleptics and the occurrence of tardive dyskinesia has been questioned with the suggestion that acceptance of a cause-effect relationship might be premature (19). Two studies in 1968 attempted to ascertain the prevalence of TD in institutionalized patients who never received neuroleptic drugs. Crane studied chronic psychiatric patients in the U.S. and Turkey, the two sample groups being comparable except for their exposure to drugs. Whereas no symptoms of dyskinesia were observed in the 97 Turkish patients, only 4 of whom had received neuroleptics, a considerable number of patients in the U.S. exhibited TD, the difference reaching statistical significance (20). Greenblatt et al. conducted a survey of geriatric patients in a nursing home. Only 2 of 100 untreated patients exhibited dyskinesia; 20 of 52 patients receiving neuroleptics were afflicted (21). In 1973 the American College of Neuropsychopharmacology took a firm stand in the controversy, declaring that the etiologic relationship between neuroleptic administration and tardive dyskinesia was sufficiently probable to urge caution in the routine prolonged use of these drugs (22). Tardive dyskinesia is now considered a well-defined neurologic entity and a major iatrogenic disease. The practice of maintaining literally millions of chronically psychotic patients on neuroleptics has currently been challenged (23), and clinicians are urged to use caution when prescribing these drugs on a long-term basis.

At the present time the pathogenesis of TD remains a matter of conjecture, although it is probable that a variety of pathophysiological factors is involved. Because TD is similar to the hyperdopaminergic disease Huntington's chorea, (both conditions are improved by dopamine-blocking agents, and both are exacerbated by drugs that enhance CNS catecholamine action and by anticholinergic compounds, such as antiparkinsonian agents) (10,13,24,25) it has been speculated that TD is also due to a hyperdopaminergic state resulting from long-term neuroleptic administration. It is postulated that prolonged dopaminergic blockade eventually induces a chemical denervation of dopaminergic receptors, rendering the receptors supersensitive to dopamine. If dopamine blockade is diminished by reduction in dosage or discontinuation of the neuroleptic, the system responds in an exaggerated manner to what would ordinarily be a normal level of dopamine input. This relative excess of dopamine is thought to underlie the clinical manifestations of tardive dyskinesia (2,6,9,11,13,24,25).

Clinical features of the syndrome include the following: (1) Symptoms become manifest after neuroleptics are significantly reduced or withdrawn; (2) symptoms are masked or disappear when neuroleptics are reinstated or dose is significantly increased; (3) anticholinergic drugs do not relieve and often worsen the symptoms of TD (6,8,9,13).

The classic symptom of TD is a bucco-facial-lingual triad consisting of involuntary movements of the lips, jaws, and tongue. Characteristic manifestations include smacking and sucking movements of the lips, thrusting, rolling, and "fly-catching" movements of the tongue, lateral jaw movements, and puffing of the cheeks. These symptoms often worsen under emotional tension and disappear during sleep (6,9).

TD is identified by sight alone, and unlike most disorders, the symptoms are best observed when the examiner does not appear to be examining. The dyskinesias may be inhibited by the patient when he is alerted, but can be seen while the patient is walking, sitting, or conversing (7). Tongue and mouth movements, generally the most common manifestation, seem to be less altered by voluntary control (24).

In addition to oral-facial dyskinesia, the extremities may show choreiform movements (variable, purposeless, involuntary quick movements) or athetoid movements (continuous, arhythmic, wormlike slow movements) in the distal parts of the limbs (6,9). Circular movements of the big toe are frequently noted in resting patients (7). Severe dystonia involving muscles controlling balance of the body may be painful and greatly reduce the patient's activity. These symptoms also disappear during sleep (6,9).

It has been suggested, but not established, that fine vermicular (wormlike) movements of the tongue may be one of the earliest signs of the development of tardive dyskinesia. Periodic examination of the tongue provides a simple and convenient early detection technique (9).

PARKINSONISM AND TARDIVE DYSKINESIA

The relationship between acute pseudoparkinsonism and TD in not clear. Though their pathophysiology are at opposite ends of the DA-ACh spectrum, they could affect one another in one or several of the following ways: (1) Pseudoparkinsonism demonstrates a susceptibility of the striatum to alteration of function by neuroleptics; (2) pseudoparkinsonism may be treated with potent antimuscarinic agents, which enhance putative ACh deficits in TD; (3) the blockade of striatal DA receptor sites in pseudoparkinsonism may lead to supersensitivity of the postsynaptic DA neuron, yielding the putative hyperdopaminergic state in TD.

We have attempted to determine the incidence of pseudoparkinsonism by history in a group of hospitalized patients with TD, comparing them with a group of matched controls without TD. The patients were examined and interviewed, the old hospital records reviewed, and where possible, family members were interviewed for reports of a past history of pseudoparkinsonism.

Results show a significantly greater incidence of pseudoparkinsonism in patients with TD than those without dyskinetic symptoms ($p < 0.05$; see Fig. 1).

Symptoms of parkinsonism may coexist with tardive dyskinesia, making diagnosis difficult. Because it appears that these two conditions are reciprocal in their pathophysiology, treatment for one condition may aggravate the other (25).

Since drug-induced parkinsonism is symptomatically equivalent to the idiopathic or postencephalitic types of Parkinson's disease, clinicians have reasoned that the atropine-like agents which are effective in the treatment of Parkinson's disease might also reverse the drug-induced phenomena, and it had become standard practice to prescribe antiparkinsonian drugs prophylactically at the onset of neuroleptic therapy. However, not all patients started on neuroleptics develop drug-induced parkinsonism, and these atropinelike agents may increase the patients' risk of developing TD. Furthermore, in patients with tardive dyskinesia the institution of an anticholinergic regimen has been found to worsen the condition. It is important to note this because many patients with extrapyramidal symptoms are treated with anticholinergic agents, although the efficacy of anticholinergic therapy has been demonstrated only with parkinsonian syndrome. It is recommended that physicians prescribe antiparkinsonian drugs only after the development of extrapyramidal symptoms rather than prophylactically (25,26,27).

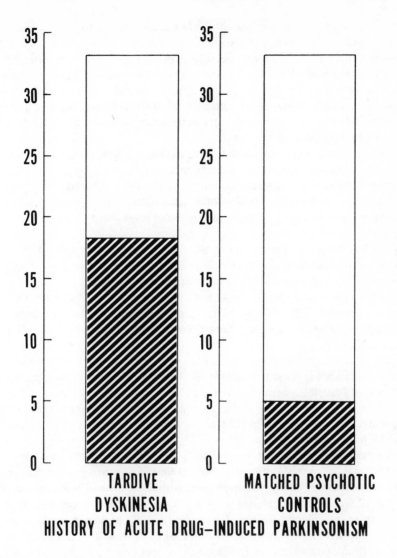

TARDIVE   MATCHED PSYCHOTIC
DYSKINESIA   CONTROLS
HISTORY OF ACUTE DRUG—INDUCED PARKINSONISM

Figure 1.   Comparison of past history of parkinsonism in 32 hospitalized psychiatric patients
with tardive dyskinesia to a group of matched control patients without tardive dyskinesia.
Difference in values between the two groups significant by t-test (p<0.05).

INCIDENCE AND EPIDEMIOLOGY OF TD

Our own survey of a V.A. and a state mental hospital population found that
36% of chronic patients manifested the tardive dyskinesia syndrome. The
reaction was slightly more prevalent in females, occurring in 44% as compared
to 33% of the males, but the difference was not statistically significant (28).

In a sample of 332 chronic patients, TD was present in 56%. There was a highly significant difference between age groups: Prevalence of TD was 46% among patients under 49 years of age; 60% in patients between 50 and 70 years; and 75% in patients older than 70 years. The appearance of TD is probably related to individual susceptibility, which might increase with the changes of dopamine metabolism that occur with aging. No significant difference by sex was reported, except that significantly more choreoathetoid movements occurred in females than in males (16).

Twelve psychiatric patients with tardive dyskinesia were observed from the inception of the syndrome. The authors reported that first symptoms rarely persisted if antipsychotics were discontinued. They concluded that the length of time symptoms have persisted prior to drug discontinuation, not patient's age at onset, may be a major variable determining reversibility of the syndrome (29).

There has been no clear evidence that TD is specifically related to any particular drug (30), dosage level (28,30), duration of treatment (30), or to the presence of brain damage (23,28). Neuroleptics are capable of evoking TD in nonspychotic as well as psychotic patients in the absence of obvious organic, metabolic, or neurological factors (23,31), and the continued use of neuroleptics in nonpsychotic patients has been deemed inappropriate by some physicians (32).

Crane suggests that patients who do not exhibit parkinsonian features while on neuroleptics are less likely to develop TD upon withdrawal of the drug (33); another study did not confirm this finding (16). Good (34) and Fann and Lake (25), on the other hand, suggest that persons who develop acute neurological symptoms, such as dystonia, akathisia, and parkinsonism, may be at high risk to develop TD (see Table 1).

An epidemiological study of tardive dyskinesia reported two interesting findings. (1) TD was significantly more frequent in schizophrenic patients with an insidious beginning than in patients with acute onset. (2) Prevalence of TD was lower if treatment began at a younger age; the mean age at the beginning of neuroleptic treatment was significantly higher in patients who subsequently developed TD than in those who did not. Paradoxically, the mean duration of treatment and total amount of drugs were less in patients who began treatment at a more advanced age. This study did not show a simple correlation between mean total amount of administered neuroleptic and TD (30), in disagreement with Crane, who reported that risk of TD rose with total quantity of drug and duration of treatment (8).

ATYPICAL CASES OF TARDIVE DYSKINESIA

Classically, TD develops after prolonged use of neuroleptics, usually more than 2 years, and especially in patients prescribed high doses. However, there are reports in the literature of patients developing TD following short-term, low-dose therapy with neuroleptic drugs. TD symptomatology developed in a patient treated for 30 weeks with haloperidol that never exceeded 10 mg/day. After medication was discontinued, symptoms lessened significantly within 4 weeks and had completely abated by 12.5 weeks (35). A 17-year-old woman maintained for 2 years on haloperidol began experiencing tremulousness in the hands, which was unresponsive to benztropine mesylate. Symptoms worsened, to include facial tics, grimacing, and head bobbing so severe that the patient had to use her hands to support her head. Haloperidol was discontinued, and the patient was prescribed 100 mg thioridazine. Dyskinesias lessened considerably with the disappearance of facial tics and grimacing, but a slight head bobbing remained (36). Crane described the case of a 41-year-old female who was treated with neuroleptics for less than 1 year and who developed TD. TD subsided in a matter of days after withdrawal of all medication (37). Jacobsen *et al*. reported 4 cases of TD associated with haloperidol at doses of 4–20 mg/daily. Two of the cases involved temporary oral-facial dyskinesias, and the other two exhibited a more persistent, complex mixture of neurological features (38). A 19-year-old male given relatively low doses of neuroleptic for less than 6 months developed tardive dyskinesia. The patient exhibited severe oral-facial dyskinesia, including protrusion of tongue, chewing movement, movement of the chin, and contraction of the upper lip exposing upper teeth. Mouth movements greatly improved 4 months after the discontinuation of medication, and by the sixth drug-free month symptoms had cleared completely (39). Crane and Smeets studied 39 geriatric patients who had had no previous exposures to neuroleptics. Moderate to moderately severe dyskinesia was detected only in persons treated for at least 7 months with a minimum daily dose of at least 72 mg chlorpromazine or equivalent, and a total dose of at least 14,000 mg (17). Marcotte reported that a patient who received 900 mg of mesoridazine in 72 hours became dysarthric, restless, and agitated, with gross tremor. After medication was discontinued, the patient developed lip smacking, protrusion of the tongue, and grimacing, which persisted 5 days after cessation of mesoridazine (40).

DRUG COMBINATIONS OR DISEASE INFLUENCING THE DEVELOPMENT OF EXTRAPYRAMIDAL SIDE EFFECTS

Although the high incidence of extrapyramidal side effects from moderate to high doses are well documented, complications occurring with low doses of neuroleptics necessitate the study of precipitating pathophysiological circumstances. One such factor may be the use of alcohol. Seven young patients treated with neuroleptics had a sudden occurrence of drug-induced akathisia and dystonia after imbibing ethyl alcohol. In 6 cases, symptoms subsided promptly with the administration of benztropine mesylate, biperiden HCl, or biperident lactate. One untreated case persisted for 36 hours. The author suggests that "it is possible that so-called neuroleptic nonreactors precipitate extrapyramidal side effects though brain dysfunction induced by alcohol or other means"(41). Lutz also described 4 cases of short-lasting akathisia during combined ECT and phenothiazine therapy (42).

A toxic neurological reaction following the combined use of lithium and haloperidol occurred in 7 patients with bipolar mania. None of the patients had a prior indication of TD or any other state of receptor hypersensitivity, and in all patients the extrapyramidal symptoms persisted longer than would be expected with haloperidol alone. Antiparkinsonian agents had a limited effect and even exacerbated the condition of one patient. In all patients, symptoms were reversible (43).

The rate of extrapyramidal reactions in patients taking neuroleptics or antidepressants increases when prednisone is given concomitantly. However, the finding is complicated by the fact that of 8 patients who received both trifluoperazine and prednisone, 4 had systemic lupus erythematosus (SLE). Three patients with SLE developed extrapyramidal reactions, whereas none without SLE developed side effects (14).

Good described a patient who presented with facial grimacing, myoclonus, and catatonialike symptoms associated with gluthemide discontinuance and antihistamine use. It is likely that additive or interactive effects of gluthemide and antihistamine led to significant alteration in the metabolism of dopamine and reduction in its intracellular concentration. This activity would account for the neuromotor signs. The catatonialike phenomena may be related to prior inhibition of dopamine reuptake by striatal neurons, with subsequent receptor hypersensitivity or hyperstimulation (34).

Altered thyroid states may influence the effect of psychotropic drugs. Lake and Fann report a case of neurotoxic rigidity apparently due to haloperidol in a hyperthyroid patient. The reaction was extreme, far greater than would be experienced from the dose, and was temporally related to the waxing and waning of the patient's hyperthyroid state; haloperidol was well tolerated, with no unusual response in the euthyroid state (44).

A patient with untreated hypoparathyroidism developed a severe dystonic reaction following IM prochlorperazine for nausea. Subsequently, the authors studied the effect of prochlorperazine in 5 untreated hypothyroid patients. All 5 had a severe dystonic reaction within 5 to 31 hours, indicating a striking phenothiazine sensitivity in the disease. The authors speculate that the extrapyramidal reaction may be related to the vascular and perivascular calcification of the basal ganglions that frequently occurs in hypoparathyroidism, or to the generalized increased excitability of the nervous system caused by hypocalcemia (45).

OTHER DRUGS CAUSING EXTRAPYRAMIDAL SIDE EFFECTS

Although the neuroleptics are the most common drug type to cause extrapyramidal reactions, other drug classes have been implicated in these neurologic conditions. Sympathomimetic vasoconstrictive agents in the antihistamines, which are structurally related to the phenothiazines, have been related to persistent involuntary movements of the face and mouth. Two females with prolonged use of antihystaminic decongestants developed oral-facial dyskinesias, which improved with haloperidol and worsened with placebo. Both patients had reduced homovanillic acid accumulation during probenecid loading, indicating functional or structural derangement of central dopamine pathways, as in patients with neuroleptic-induced dyskinesia (46). Favis reports a case of facial dyskinesia following the use of a proprietary cough syrup in recommended dose for 2 days. The condition was alleviated by IM diazepam and reoccurred when the patient took more of the medication (47). Sovner stated that the mechanism of action in antihistamine-induced dyskinesia might be an alteration of central dopaminergic pathways by blocking reuptake of dopamine by individual neurons (48).

Dystonic reactions to the halogenated phenothiazines are well documented. Sananman reported a case of dyskinesia occurring with a halogenated phenethylamine. A 43-year-old female took a single fenfluramine tablet, and within 2 hours experienced retrocollic movements of the head and neck, with tongue and throat muscle spasms which made it difficult to breathe. The reaction subsided within 90 seconds following IV diphenhydramine (49). The occurrence of dyskinesia after sympathomimetic drugs has not been widely recognized, but it is important that physicians be aware of the possibility of these side effects, because diet medications and other sympathomimetic agents are prescribed frequently.

Fann et al. reported 2 cases of bucco-facial-lingual dyskinesia occurring in patients treated with tricylic antidepressants (50). Although the tricyclic antidepressants have little effect on striatal dopamine, they possess potent anticholinergic properties similar to the neuroleptics. The appearance of dyskinesia in these patients lends support to the hypothesis that drug-induced hyperkinetic disorders are related to a diminution of CNS acetylcholine activity as well as to an increase in dopamine activity.

Two young patients treated with depot injections of flupenthixol (not currently marketed in the United States) developed choreiform movements. In one, a 40-year-old male, symptoms slowly and completely disappeared; in the other, a 28-year-old male, however, the condition failed to respond to treatment, and only when lithium was administered was there some amelioration of symptoms (51).

Palatucci reports a case of a 19-year-old psychiatric patient who developed a severe dyskinetic reaction following parenteral administration of methyl-

226   TARDIVE DYSKINESIA

phenidate. Although methylphenidate has been used successfully to reverse the acute neurotoxic side effects of phenothiazines, it caused them in this instance. The reaction persisted up to 30 hours (52).

Kirschberg described an acute extrapyramidal reaction involving dyskinetic movements of the face, arms, and legs in a 15-year-old female given two 250 mg doses of ethosuximide for petit mal seizures. Symptoms were abruptly and completely relieved by IV injection of diphenhydramine HCl (53).

Amodiaquine HCl, an effective and relatively nontoxic antimalarial drug, was implicated in 4 cases of involuntary movements. Dyskinesias included protrusion of the tongue, difficulty in speaking, excessive salivation, fasciculation of tongue and facial muscles, and intention tremor. Symptoms cleared within 3 hours in 3 patients prescribed IV benztropine mesylate; symptoms improved within 24 hours in one patient prescribed oral benzhexol (54).

Diazoxide, a nondiuretic benzothiadiazine vasodilator, is used in the long-term treatment of severe hypertension. Extrapyramidal symptoms were noted in 15% of acute and chronic hypertensive patients treated with diazoxide. Symptoms included the range of extrapyramidal reactions, such as tremulousness, restlessness, coarse rhythmical tremor, cog-wheel rigidity, fixed facies, tightness of jaw preventing opening of the mouth, and oculogyric crises. Dosage adjustment or the use of diazepam or procyclidine usually controlled symptoms (55).

Reserpine depletes brain catecholamines, and like the phenothiazines, can cause a parkinsonian syndrome. A 54-year-old male treated with reserpine for hypertension developed an oral-facial dyskinesia which persisted for 6 months (56).

TREATMENT OF TARDIVE DYSKINESIA

Drug therapy of TD has been approached along three main lines, based on the hypothesis that the condition results from a relative excess of brain dopamine. These techniques include modification of neuroleptic medication, depletion or blockade of dopamine, and cholinergic alteration (9,57,58).

Neuroleptics, dopamine-blocking agents, paradoxically can ameliorate the manifestation of the condition which they cause, and some clinicians recommend prescribing, continuing, or increasing dosage of phenothiazines in patients with TD (57,58). Turek et al. studied oral-facial dyskinesia in 56 chronic inpatients with TD during various sequences of cessation and doubling of original dose of neuroleptics alone or with antiparkinsonian agents. Results indicated a tendency for dyskinetic symptom severity to be lessened during neuroleptic treatment phases and increased during subsequent drug-free intervals. Antiparkinsonian medication failed to reduce symptom manifestation (59).

Although effective in masking symptoms, the neuroleptics are not curative, and their use in treating tardive dyskinesia is likely to aggravate the underlying pathology. The reinstatement of antipsychotic therapy should be avoided except in patients requiring neuroleptics for control of otherwise unmanageable psychotic behavior (6,9). Crane goes a step further, stating that ''patients who are very sensitive to the neurotoxic effects of neuroleptics should not receive such compounds, regardless of their mental condition'' (37).

Reserpine, which depletes dopamine by preventing intraneuronal storage, has been used effectively to treat TD, although it paradoxically can cause the syndrome (56,57). Tetrabenazine, another dopamine-depleting agent, has demonstrated effective, though short-lived, suppression of symptoms. This drug is not currently marketed in the United States, and because its effects are not lasting, it is doubtful that tetrabenazine will be prominent in the treatment of TD (9,57).

If tardive dyskinesia is due to an imbalance between the dopaminergic and cholinergic systems, drugs which would increase acetylcholine content in the striatum should restore balance and thereby control TD (60). Deanol, a putative acetylcholine precursor, has been investigated in TD with varying results. Widroe and Heisler report good results to deanol in doses of 100–500 mg daily (58). Fann et al. administered deanol to 10 patients with TD, and all 10 exhibited partial or complete relief of symptoms after 5 days (10,61). Crane, however, reported marginal improvement in only 18% of his patients treated with deanol (62).

Physostigmine, a centrally active anticholinesterase, has also shown contradictory results. All of 7 patients with TD who were prescribed the drug in one study showed significant suppression of movement at 24 hours (24). A later study by Fann et al. reports an absence of clinical changes in 10 patients whose tardive dyskinesia was treated with physostigmine (63).

Methylphenidate has been used successfully to reverse the acute neurotoxic side effects of phenothiazines (64). In patients with TD, however, it tends to aggravate symptoms. Of 17 patients with TD who prescribed methylphenidate, 6 became worse, 8 showed no change, and 3 improved (63,65).

Agents which suppress acetylcholine have been most widely used clinically to treat TD. However, the possibility that a cholinergic deficit exists in tardive dyskinesia suggests that long-term suppression of acetylcholine-dependent mechanisms may contribute to this condition. If this hypothesis is true, then a compound which elevates striatal dopamine levels would be preferable to one which suppresses the acetylcholine system in order to restore balance (66).

PREVENTION

Because of the lack of adequate substitutes for the treatment of psychoses, tardive dyskinesia has generally been accepted as an undesirable but occasionally unavoidable consequence of the benefits of prolonged drug therapy. Physicians can minimize the risk in long-term patients by titrating dose to the lowest possible levels that provide adequate control. Many patients can be satisfactorily maintained for long periods without antipsychotic drugs, and "drug holidays" are advised. These drug-free intervals help protect the patient from potential hazards of chronic administration and can allow the physician to ascertain if there is evidence of tardive dyskinesia (9,57).

The most important tool to diminish TD remains early detection of symptoms. Often early and insidious manifestations are overlooked, and the syndrome is not diagnosed until it is well established, making prognosis poorer (8,67). Patients receiving neuroleptics should be examined regularly for the appearance of early signs of emerging TD. These signs include fine vermicular movements of the tongue, circular movements of the big toe, tics in the facial region, ill-defined abnormal mouth or eye movements, mild mouthing or chewing movements, the presence of rocking or swaying movements, or the occurrence of restless limb movements in the absence of the subjective discomfort associated with akathisia (6,9). Symptoms of slight intensity, such as those listed above, are often reversible when antipsychotic medication is withdrawn. Symptoms of moderate or marked intensity are difficult to ameliorate and can become irreversible and permanent.

ACKNOWLEDGMENTS

The author gratefully acknowledges the assistance of Bruce W. Richman, M.A. and Nancy L. Berry of the Houston Veterans Administration Hospital in the preparation of this report.

REFERENCES

1. Snyder, S., Greenberg, D., Yamamura, H. Antischizophrenic drugs and brain cholinergic receptor. *Arch. Gen. Psychiatry, 21*:58–61, 1974.
2. Burch, J.G. A brief review of drug related neurologic disorders in the elderly. In *Drug Issues in Geropsychiatry*, Fann & Maddox (eds.). Baltimore: Williams and Wilkins, pp. 29–34, 1974.
3. Man, P.L. Long-term effects of haloperidol. *Dis. Nerv. Syst., 34*:113–118, 1973.
4. Haase, H.J., Janssen, P.A.J. *The Action of Neuroleptic Drugs: A Psychiatric, Neurological, and Pharmacological Investigation*. Chicago: Yearbook Medical Publishers, pp. 193–196, 1964.
5. Ayd, F.J., A survey of drug-induced extrapyramidal reactions. *JAMA, 175*(12):1054–1060, 1961.
6. American College of Neuropsychopharmacology—FDA Task Force. Neurologic syndromes associated with antipsychotic drug use. *N. Engl. J. Med., 289*(1):20–23, 1973.
7. Paulson, G.W. Tardive dyskinesia. *Annu. Rev. Med., 26*:75–81, 1975.

8. Crane, G.E. Tardive dyskinesia in patients treated with major neuroleptics: a review of the literature. *Am. J. Psychiatry Suppl.*, *124*(8):40–48, 1968.
9. Clyne, K.E., Juhl, P.P. Tardive dyskinesia. *Am. J. Hosp. Pharm.*, *33*:481–486, 1976.
10. Fann, W.E., Lake, C.R., Sullivan, J.L., Miller, R.D. Neuroleptic-induced movement disorders: pharmacology and treatment. In *Psychopharmacogenetics*, Eleftheriou, B.E. (ed.). New York: Plenum Press, pp. 169–182, 1975.
11. Fann, W.E., Lake, C.R. Treatment of drug-induced parkinsonism in the elderly patient. In *Drug Issues in Geropsychiatry*, Fann & Maddox (eds.). Baltimore: Williams and Wilkins, pp. 41–48, 1974.
12. Fann, W.E., Lake, C.R. Amantadine versus trihexyphenidyl in the treatment of neuroleptic-induced parkinsonism. *Am. J. Psychiatry*, *133*(8):940–943, 1976.
13. Klawans, H.L. The pharmacology of tardive dyskinesias. *Am. J. Psychiatry*, *130*(1):82–86, 1973.
14. Boston Collaborative Drug Surveillance Program. Drug-induced extra pyramidal symptoms. *JAMA*, *224*(6):889–891, 1973.
15. Ayd, F.J. Haloperidol: fifteen years of clinical experience. *Dis. Nerv. Syst.*, *33*:459–469, 1972.
16. Jus, A., Pineau, R., Lachance, R., Pelchat, G., Jus, K., Pipes, P., Villeneuve, P. Epidemiology of tardive dyskinesia. Part I. *Dis. Nerv. Syst.*, *37*:210–214, 1976.
17. Crane, G.E., Smeets, R.A. Tardive dyskinesia and drug therapy in geriatric patients. *Arch. Gen. Psychiatry*, *30*:341–343, 1974.
18. Kline, N.S. On the rarity of 'irreversible' oral dyskinesias following phenothiazines. *Am. J. Psychiatry Suppl.*, *124*(8):48–54, 1968.
19. Curren, J.P. Tardive dyskinesia—side effect or not? *Am. J. Psychiatry*, *130*(4):406–410, 1973.
20. Crane, G.E. Dyskinesia and neuroleptics. *Arch. Gen. Psychiatry*, *19*:700–703, 1968.
21. Greenblatt, D.L., Dominick, J.R., Stotsky, B.A., DiMascio, A. Phenothiazine-induced dyskinesia in nursing home patients. *J. Am. Geriatratic Soc.*, *16*:27–34, 1968.
22. American College of Neuropsychopharmacology—FDA Task Force. Neurological syndromes associated with antipsychotic drug use. A special editorial report. *Arch. Gen. Psychiatry*, *28*:463–467, 1973.
23. Baldessarini, R.J. Tardive dyskinesia: an evaluation of the etiologic association with neuroleptic therapy. *Can. Psychiatr. Assoc. J.*, *19*(6):551–554, 1974.
24. Fann, W.E., Lake, C.R., Gerber, C.J., McKenzie, G.M. Cholinergic suppression of tardive dyskinesia. *Psychopharmacologia*, *37*:101–107, 1974.
25. Fann, W.E., Lake, C.R. On the coexistence of parkinsonism and tardive dyskinesia. *Dis. Nerv. Syst.*, *35*:324–326, 1974.
26. Pecknold, J.C., Ananth, J.V., Ban, T.A., Lehmann, H.E. Lack of indication for use of antiparkinson medication. A follow-up study. *Dis. Nerv. Syst.*, *32*:538–542, 1971.
27. Fann, W.E., Lake, C.R., Richman, B.W. Drug-induced parkinsonism. A re-evaluation. *Dis. Nerv. Syst.*, *36*:91–93, 1975.
28. Fann, W.E., Davis, J.M., Janowsky, D.S. The prevalence of tardive dyskinesia in mental hospital patients. *Dis. Nerv. Syst.*, *33*:182–186, 1972.
29. Quitkin, F., Rifkin, A., Gochfeld, L., Klein, D.F. Tardive dyskinesia: are first signs reversible? *Am. J. Psychiatry*, *134*(1):184–187, 1977.
30. Jus, A., Pineau, R., Lachance, R., Pelchat, G., Jus, K., Pipes, P., Villeneuve, P. Epidemiology of tardive dyskinesia. Part II. *Dis. Nerv. Syst.*, *37*:257–261, 1976.
31. Hussey, H. Tardive dyskinesia. An editorial. *JAMA*, *28*(8):1030, 1974.
32. Thornton, W.E., Thornton, B.P. Tardive dyskinesia and low dosage. *Am. J. Psychiatry*, *130*(12):1401, 1973.
33. Crane, G.E. Pseudoparkinsonism and tardive dyskinesia. *Arch. Neurol.*, *27*:426–430, 1972.

34. Good, M.I. Catatonia-like symptomatology and withdrawal dyskinesias. *Am. J. Psychiatry, 133*(12):1454–1456, 1976.

35. Stimmel, G.L. Tardive dyskinesia with low-dose, short-term neuroleptic therapy. *Am. J. Hosp. Pharm., 33*:961–963, 1976.

36. Hale, M. Reversible dyskinesia caused by haloperidol. *Am. J. Psychiatry, 131*:1413, 1974.

37. Crane, G.E. Rapid reversal of tardive dyskinesia. *Am. J. Psychiatry, 130*:1159, 1973.

38. Jacobson, G., Baldessarini, R., Manschreck, T. Tardive and withdrawal dyskinesia associated with haloperidol. *Am. J. Psychiatry, 131*:910–913, 1974.

39. Moline, R. Atypical tardive dyskinesia. *Am. J. Psychiatry, 132*:534–535, 1975.

40. Marcotte, D.G. Neuroleptics and neurological reactions. *South. Med. J., 66*(3):321–324, 1973.

41. Lutz, E. Neuroleptic-induced akathisia and dystonia triggered by alcohol. *JAMA, 236*(21):2422–2423, 1976.

42. Lutz, E.G. Short-lasting akathisia during combined electro-convulsive and phenothiazine therapy. *Dis. Nerv. Syst., 29*:259–260, 1968.

43. Loudon, J.B., Waring, H. Toxic reactions to lithium and haloperidol. *Lancet, II*:1088, 1976.

44. Lake, C.R., Fann, W.E. Possible potentiation of haloperidol neurotoxicity in acute hyperthyroidism. *Br. J. Psychiatry, 123*:523–525, 1973.

45. Schaaf, M., Payne, C.A. Dystonic reactions to prochlorperazine in hypoparathyroidism. *N. Engl. J. Med., 275*(18):991–995, 1966.

46. Thach, B.T., Chase, T.N., Basma, J.F. Oral-facial dyskinesia associated with prolonged use of antihistamic decongestants. *N. Engl. J. Med., 293*(10):486–487, 1975.

47. Favis, G. Facial dyskinesia related to antihistamines? *N. Engl. J. Med., 294*(13):730, 1976.

48. Sovner, R. Dyskinesia associated with chronic antihistamines use. *N. Engl. J. Med., 294*(2):113, 1976.

49. Sananman, M.L. Dyskinesia after fenfluramine. *N. Engl. J. Med., 291*(8):422, 1974.

50. Fann, W.E., Sullivan, J.L., Richman, B.W. Dyskinesia associated with tricyclic antidepressants. *Br. J. Psychiatry, 128*:490–493, 1976.

51. Gibson, A. Choreiform movements after depot injections of flupenthixol. *Br. J. Psychiatry, 125*:111, 1974.

52. Palatucci, D.M. Iatrogenic dyskinesia—a unique reaction to parenteral methylphenidate. *J. Nerv. Men. Dis., 159*:73–76, 1974.

53. Kirschberg, G.J. Dyskinesia—an unusual reaction to ethosuximide. *Arch. Neurol., 32*:137–138, 1975.

54. Akindele, M.O., Odejide, A.O. Amodiaquine-induced involuntary movements. *Br. Med. J., 2*:214–215, 1976.

55. Neary, D., Thurston, H., Pohl, J.E.F. Development of extrapyramidal symptoms in hypertensive patients treated with diazoxide. *Br. Med. J., 3*:474–475, 1973.

56. Wolf, S.M. Reserpine: cause and treatment of oral-facial dyskinesia. *Bull. L.A. Neurol. Soc., 38*:80–84, 1973.

57. Kobayashi, R.M. Drug therapy of tardive dyskinesia. *N. Engl. J. Med., 296*:257–260, 1977.

58. Widroe, H.J., Heisler, S. Treatment of tardive dyskinesia. *Dis. Nerv. Syst., 37*:162–164, 1976.

59. Turek, I., Kurland, A., Hanlon, T., Bohm, M. Tardive dyskinesia: its relation to neuroleptic and antiparkinson drugs. *Br. J. Psychiatry, 121*:605–612, 1972.

60. DeSilva, L., Huang, C.Y. Deanol in tardive dyskinesia. *Br. Med. J., 3*:466, 1975.

61. Fann, W.E., Sullivan, J.L., Miller, R.D., McKenzie, G.M. Deanol in tardive dyskinesia: a preliminary report. *Psychopharmacologia, 42*:135–137, 1975.

62. Crane, G.E. Deanol for tardive dyskinesia. *N. Engl. J., Med., 292*:926, 1975.

63. Fann, W.E., Davis, J.M., Wilson, I.C., Lake, C.R. Attempts at pharmacological management of tardive dyskinesia. In *Psychopharmacology and Aging,* Eisodrfer and Fann (eds.). New York: Plenum Press, pp. 89–96, 1973.

64. Fann, W.E. Use of methylphenidate to counteract the acute dystonic reactions to phenothiazines. *Am. J. Psychiatry, 122*:1293–1294, 1966.

65. Fann, W.E., Davis, J.M., Wilson, I.C. Methylphenidate in tardive dyskinesia. *Am. J. Psychiatry, 130*:922–924, 1973.

66. Fann, W.E., Lake, C.R., McKenzie, G.M. Adrenergic and cholinergic factors in extrapyramidal disorders. In *Neurotransmitter Balances Regulating Behavior,* Domino, E. and Davis, J. (eds.). Ann Arbor: University Michigan Press, pp. 159–174, 1975.

67. Crane, G.E. Prevention and management of tardive dyskinesia. *Am. J. Psychiatry, 129*:466–467, 1972.

22

Methodological Approach to the Measurement of Tardive Dyskinesia: Piezoelectric Recording and Concurrent Validity Test on Five Clinical Rating Scales

CHING-PIAO CHIEN
KOOCK JUNG
and ANITA ROSS-TOWNSEND

Recently, there has been an upsurge of literature on persistent dyskinesia, reporting the effects of various drugs in changing the dyskinetic symptoms. Although various methods for measuring this syndrome have been employed, no study has yet compared the reliability and sensitivity of the instruments used by the various investigators. Before Casey and Denney's report in 1975 on the electrical recording method they developed (1), most of the evaluation methods reported were either (1) based on subjective clinical impression rating scales, with direct observation of the patient or through videotapes, or (2) on counting the frequency of involuntary movements, especially the mouth movement, per unit time. The electrical recording method, on the other hand, has made a more objective graphic evaluation of persistent dyskinesia possible. However, as most clinical facilities lack this equipment, the need for a thorough evaluation of the relative value of the various clinical rating scales continues. Concurrent validation of each clinical instrument with the electrical recording device might indicate a rational basis for establishing the superiority of one clinical instrument over the others for future clinical and research purposes.

The present study is designed to (1) determine the interrater reliability of several conventional rating scales; (2) determine the interscale correlations; and (3) determine the relative validity of these clinical rating scales by correlating the results obtained from each with those of the piezoelectric recording system.

METHODOLOGY

Rating Scales

Five rating scales presented at a National Institute of Mental Health Tardive Dyskinesia Workshop held at Ramsey Hospital, St. Paul, Minnesota, in the fall of 1974 were selected for study. These rating scales were designed and used by leading investigators in the field of persistent dyskinesia. They are listed as Scale I to V in the following order:

I. Direct Counting Method (2,3,4)

II. Oral Tardive Dyskinesia Rating Scale, by Gerlach, Thorsen, and Munkvad (5)

III. Crane Rating Scale (6)

IV. Sandoz-Wander Tardive Dyskinesia Rating Scale by Simpson (7)

V. Abnormal Involuntary Movement Scale (AIMS) from NIMH (8).*

Items not related to tardive dyskinesia were deleted from some of the above scales, and the statistical analysis was based only on the pertinent items.†
Comparison of the characteristics of each rating scale is illustrated in Table 1.

Piezoelectric Recording

This instrument consisted of a piezoelectric transducer and Grass Model 7 polygraph with preamplifier, amplifier, recorder, and rubber bulb inserted in the patient's mouth, which enabled a direct recording of bucco-linguomasticatory movements. An integrator summed the frequency and intensity of movements, permitting a direct count of the number of epochs as the measure of persistent dyskinesia by this method.

---

*Hereafter, these scales will be referred to by the Roman numerals preceding their names.

†Items included were as follows:

I. all

II. all

III. only items IA and IB (except dystonia)

IV. the first 21 items

V. items 1 to 10.

Table 1

Rating Scales for Persistent Dyskinesia

Characteristics of Scales Rating Scales	Method	Assessment of Dyskinetic Movement Frequency	Assessment of Dyskinetic Movement Intensity	Anatomical Area Observed	No. of Items
I. Direct Counting (Chien, Kazamatsuri, and Cole)	Counting the number of movements per minute	Objective	Not counted	Tongue, Lip, Jaw, Cheek	1
II. Oral Tardive Dyskinesia Rating Scale (Gerlach, Thorsen, and Munkvad)	Objective 4 point rating scale	Objective	Objective	Tongue, Jaw, Mouth	6
III. Crane's Rating Scale	Subjective 5 point rating scale	Subjective, not specified	Subjective, not specified	Tongue, Lip, Facial muscles, Extremities, Other	12+
IV. Sandoz-Wander's Rating Scale	Subjective 4 point rating scale	Subjective, specified	Subjective, specified	Eye, Eyelid, Tongue, Lip, Cheek, Jaw, Neck, Trunk, Extremities	21+
V. AIMS (NIMH)	Subjective 5 point rating scale	Subjective, not specified	Subjective, not specified	Facial Muscles, Lip, Cheek, Tongue, Jaw, Extremities, Trunk, Neck, Global judgment	9+

Subjects

Thirty-eight outpatients from a community mental-health center and a V.A. hospital were recruited for the study after they were confirmed by two clinicians to have clinical manifestation of persistent dyskinesia. Their mean age was 61.7 years; 53% were female, 84% were caucasian, 16% black; 58% carried the diagnosis of schizophrenia, 5% manic-depressive psychosis, 5% involutional paranoia, 13% depression, 16% organic brain syndrome, and 3% alcoholism; chronicity of mental illness was 22.3 years; about half had had previous ECT; 8% had had CNS infections; 29% wore dentures. They were all evaluated by five rating scales. For the piezoelectric recording, 15 of the above 38 patients were available for the study, yet only 9 patients could complete the recording successfully.

Procedure

Phase I. A staff psychiatrist and medical student trained in the use of these 5 scales rated each patient simultaneously and independently on all the scales, according to the examination procedures specified by each scale.

Phase II. A 10-minute-long piezoelectric recording was made by asking the patient to relax in his chair and to swallow as usual. Patients were assured that no electricity from the machine would enter their bodies and that no pain or harm would result from this procedure.

Statistical Analysis

In Phase I, the Pearson "r" correlation coefficient was computed to establish interrater and interscale correlations. The average score of the two raters was used for the interscale correlational analysis. In Phase II, as there were only 9 subjects' piezoelectric recordings available, the Spearman rank order correlation technique was used when piezoelectric recording scores were compared to the scores of 5 rating scales.

RESULTS

Interrater Reliability

The Pearson correlation coefficients for scales I to V described in the methodology section are r = .99, .76, .81, .85, and .87, respectively. All of these were significant at p<.01 level. The Direct Counting Method was markedly more reliable than the remaining rating scales, most of which are based on subjective impression (Table 2).

Interscale Correlations

The average correlation coefficient of each scale to the remaining 4 scales was calculated by Fisher's "z transformation" method (9). They are .35, .54, .67, .74, and .73 for scales I through V, respectively. Thus, Sandoz-Wander and AIMS appear to have the highest correlation with the others. The Direct Counting Method, due to its difference in evaluation method from the others, has the lowest correlation (.35) with the remaining scales. The r's for scales II to V were significant at p<.01, and for scale I at p<.05 (Table 3).

Table 2
Interrater Reliability
(Number of dyskinetic patients = 38)
Between Rater 1 & Rater 2

Rating Scale	Correlation Coefficient
Scale I (Direct Counting)	0.987*
Scale II (Gerlach et al.)	0.763*
Scale III (Crane)	0.814*
Scale IV (Sandoz-Wander)	0.851*
Scale V (NIMH AIMS)	0.867*

*p<0.005

Table 3
Interscale Correlation Coefficients
(N = 38, based on average scores of 2 raters)

Scale	Direct Counting	Gerlach	Crane	Sandoz-Wander	AIMS
Direct Counting	—	0.37†	0.27	0.43‡	0.37†
Gerlach	0.37†	—	0.45‡	0.63‡	0.68‡
Crane	0.27	0.45‡	—	0.87‡	0.82‡
Sandoz-Wander	0.43‡	0.63‡	0.87‡	—	0.87‡
AIMS	0.37†	0.68‡	0.82‡	0.87‡	—
Average "r"	0.35†	0.54‡	0.67‡	0.74‡	0.73‡

*p<0.05
†p<0.025
‡p<0.005

Concurrent Validity

Comparing each scale with the piezoelectric recording system resulted in the following values of Rho: .62, .67, .69, .47, and .72 for scales I to V, respectively. All except scale IV reached statistical significance at $p<.05$ (Table 4). It should be noted here that the piezoelectric recording method, although the most objective, is not free of problems. Of the 15 patients who were tested by this method, 4 were uncooperative and 2 desisted from bucco-linguomasticatory movements, resulting in only 9 usable recordings.

Table 4
Correlation of Piezoelectric Recording Scores
with 5 Rating Scales Scores
(N = 9 figures are correlation coefficients)

Rating Scales	Piezoelectric Recording
Direct Counting	0.62*
Gerlach	0.67*
Crane	0.69*
Sandoz-Wander	0.47
AIMS	0.72*

*$p<0.05$

FIGURE 1 - PIEZOELECTRIC RECORDING

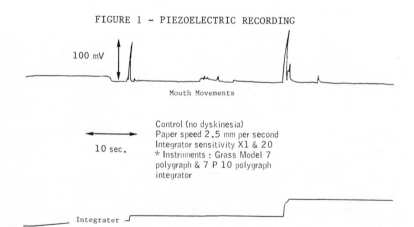

100 mV

Mouth Movements

Control (no dyskinesia)
Paper speed 2.5 mm per second
Integrator sensitivity X1 & 20
* Instruments : Grass Model 7
polygraph & 7 P 10 polygraph
integrator

10 sec.

Integrater

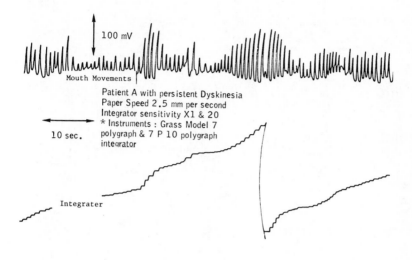

100 mV

Mouth Movements

Patient A with persistent Dyskinesia
Paper Speed 2.5 mm per second
Integrator sensitivity X1 & 20
* Instruments : Grass Model 7
polygraph & 7 P 10 polygraph
integrator

10 sec.

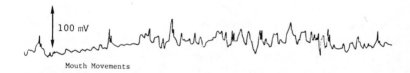

Integrater

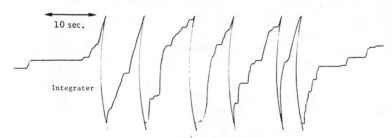

100 mV

Mouth Movements

10 sec.

Integrater

Patient C with Persistent Dyskinesia
Paper Speed 2.5 mm per second
Integrator sensitivity X 10 & 20
* Instruments : Grass Model 7
polygraph & 7 P 10 polygraph
integrator

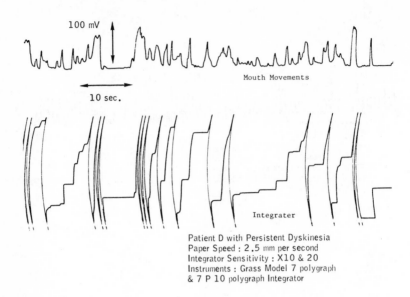

Patient D with Persistent Dyskinesia
Paper Speed : 2.5 mm per second
Integrator Sensitivity : X10 & 20
Instruments : Grass Model 7 polygraph
& 7 P 10 polygraph Integrator

DISCUSSION

The measurement of dyskinetic symptoms needs not only a reliable, sensitive, and valid tool, but also a consistent manner, time, and environment for evaluation. It is well known among clinicians that there is a great fluctuation of movements within an individual at different times and environments. The patient can stop involuntary movements through his own volition for a few seconds or minutes if he is asked to do so, although, eventually, dyskinetic movements will reappear. On the other hand, dyskinesia can be worsened when the patient is under emotional stress (10). The latter case was also clearly demonstrated in dyskinetic monkeys in a well-controlled laboratory setting (11). Therefore, in any clinical study measuring the change of tardive dyskinesia, factors other than the measurement tools should be considered as equally important as using the appropriate measurement tools. Since not every clinical facility has a polygraph machine available for piezoelectric recording, and even if so, not every patient is willing to retain the rubber bulb in his mouth for the experimental procedure, clinics have to rely heavily on the rating scales. It is obvious that two or more rating methods should be used in the same study rather than relying on one measurement method. The measurement methods in clinical observation better represent different natures of observation. In this sense AIMS, which relies on the rater's subjective clinical judgment, and the Direct Counting Method, which objectively records the frequency of involuntary movements, seem to be two practical measurements to be used conjointly in the evaluation of dyskinesia.

CONCLUSIONS

Although almost all the rating scales reach statistical significances in inter-rater reliability, in interscale comparability, and in concurrent validity, after weighing all the degrees of significance, AIMS appears to be the most recommendable clinical rating scale among the scales which rely on the rater's subjective judgment. It is also recommended to combine Direct Counting Method, which is different in nature from AIMS, in the evaluation of any dyskinesia involving bucco-linguomasticatory movements. The piezoelectric recording system, as objective as it appears, can be a useful method in the laboratory setting, but still has some practical and technical drawbacks.

REFERENCES

1. Casey, D.E., Denney, D. Deanol in the treatment of tardive dyskinesia. *Am. J. Psychiatry, 132*(8):864–867, 1975.
2. Kazamatsuri, H., Chien, C.P., Cole, J.O. Treatment of tardive dyskinesia, I. *Arch. Gen. Psychiatry, 27*:95–99 1972.
3. Kazamatsuri, H., Chien, C.P., Cole, J.O. Treatment of tardive dyskinesia, II. *Arch. Gen. Psychiatry, 27*:100–103, 1972.
4. Kazamatsuri, H., Chien, C.P., Cole, J.O. Treatment of tardive dyskinesia, III. *Arch. Gen. Psychiatry., 27*:824–827, 1972.
5. Gerlach, Thorsen, Munkvad, The movement pattern of oral tardive dyskinesia in relation to anticholinergic and antidopamine treatment. (Unpublished paper, 1975.)
6. Crane, G.E., Narango, E.R. Motor disorders induced by neuroleptics. *Arch. Gen. Psychiatry, 24*:179–184, 1971.
7. Simpson, G., Zoubok, B., Lee, J.H. An early clinical and toxicity trial of EX 11-582A in chronic schizophrenia. *Curr. Ther. Res., 19*(1):87–93, 1976.
8. National Institute of Mental Health, Psychopharmacology Research Branch. Development of a dyskinetic movement scale. *ECDEU Intercom., 4*(1):3–6, 1975.
9. McNemar, Q. *Psychological Statistics*, 2nd ed. New York: John Wiley and Sons, pp. 148–149, 1955.
10. Cole, J.O., Gardos, G. Pitfalls in the assessment of tardive dyskinesia. Abstract—VI World Congress of Psychiatry, Honolulu, Hawaii, Sept. 3, 1977.
11. Carlson, K.R. A syndrome resembling tardive dyskinesia which results from chronic methadone treatment. Presented at American College of Neuropsychopharmacology, San Juan, Puerto Rico, December 15, 1977.

Tardive Dyskinesia Scales in Current Use

ABNORMAL INVOLUNTARY MOVEMENT SCALE (AIMS)

The AIMS is a 12-item scale designed to record in detail the occurrence of dyskinetic movements. In the development of this scale, the Psychopharmacology Research Branch has had the benefit of consulting with many of the scientists who have previously devised rating scales for dyskinetic movements, and of the continuing advice of a formal consultant neurologist (Dr. Roger Duvoisin). One of the units in a PRB collaborative study (St. Paul-Ramsey Hospital) had separately undertaken the development of a rating scale and had actively carried out studies with patients showing dyskinetic movements utilizing video-recording techniques. Preliminary versions of the AIMS were used to rate video recordings of patients with dyskinetic movements, and although no formal interrater reliability studies have been conducted, there was relatively good consensus among the group doing the ratings. Because of the great need for an assessment instrument in this field, the scale is being made available to the larger scientific community through the ECDEU Battery, despite the fact that it has not been validated using psychometric procedures.

EXAMINATION PROCEDURE

Either before or after completing the Examination Procedure observe the patient unobtrusively, at rest (e.g., in waiting room).

The chair to be used in this examination should be a hard, firm one without arms.

1. Ask patient whether there is anything in his/her mouth (i.e., gum, candy, etc.) and if there is, to remove it.

2. Ask patient about the *current* condition of his/her teeth. Ask patient if he/she wears dentures. Do teeth or dentures bother patient *now*?

3. Ask patient whether he/she notices any movements in mouth, face, hands, or feet. If yes, ask to describe and to what extent they *currently* bother patient or interfere with his/her activities.

4. Have patient sit in chair with hands on knees, legs slightly apart, and feet flat on floor. (Look at entire body for movements while in this position.)

5. Ask patient to sit with hands hanging unsupported. If male, between legs, if female and wearing a dress, hanging over knees. (Observe hands and other body areas.)

6. Ask patient to open mouth. (Observe tongue at rest within mouth.) Do this twice.

7. Ask patient to protrude tongue. (Observe abnormalities of tongue movement.) Do this twice.

■ 8. Ask patient to tap thumb, with each finger, as rapidly as possible for 10–15 seconds; separately with right hand, then with left hand. (Observe facial and leg movements.)

9. Flex and extend patient's left and right arms (one at a time.) (Note any rigidity and rate on DOTES.)

10. Ask patient to stand up. (Observe in profile. Observe all body areas again, hips included.)

■ 11. Ask patient to extend both arms outstretched in front with palms down. (Observe trunk, legs, and mouth.)

■ 12. Have patient walk a few paces, turn, and walk back to chair. (Observe hands and gait.) Do this twice.

■ Activated movements

	STUDY	PATIENT	FORM	PERIOD	RATE	HOSPITAL
DEPARTMENT OF HEALTH, EDUCATION, AND WELFARE PUBLIC HEALTH SERVICE ALCOHOL, DRUG ABUSE, AND MENTAL HEALTH ADMINISTRATION NATIONAL INSTITUTE OF MENTAL HEALTH			117			
	(1-6)	(7-9)	(10-12)	(13-15)	(16-17)	(79-80)

ABNORMAL INVOLUNTARY
MOVEMENT SCALE
(AIMS)

PATIENT'S NAME

RATER

DATE

INSTRUCTIONS: Complete Examination Procedure (reverse side) before
making ratings.
MOVEMENT RATINGS: Rate highest severity observed.
Rate movements that occur upon activation one *less* than
those observed spontaneously.

Code: 0 = None
1 = Minimal, may be extreme normal
2 = Mild
3 = Moderate
4 = Severe

(Circle One)

CARD 01
(18-19)

FACIAL AND ORAL MOVEMENTS:	1.	**Muscles of Facial Expression** e.g., movements of forehead, eyebrows, periorbital area, cheeks; include frowning, blinking, smiling, grimacing	0 1 2 3 4				(20)
	2.	**Lips and Perioral Area** e.g., puckering, pouting, smacking	0 1 2 3 4				(21)
	3.	**Jaw** e.g., biting, clenching, chewing, mouth opening, lateral movement	0 1 2 3 4				(22)
	4.	**Tongue** Rate only increase in movement both in and out of mouth, NOT inability to sustain movement	0 1 2 3 4				(23)
EXTREMITY MOVEMENTS:	5.	**Upper** *(arms, wrists, hands, fingers)* Include choreic movements, (i.e., rapid, objectively purposeless, irregular, spontaneous), athetoid movements (i.e., slow, irregular, complex, serpentine) Do NOT include tremor (i.e., repetitive, regular, rhythmic)	0 1 2 3 4				(24)
	6.	**Lower** *(legs, knees, ankles, toes)* e.g., lateral knee movement, foot tapping, heel dropping, foot squirming, inversion and eversion of foot	0 1 2 3 4				(25)
TRUNK MOVEMENTS:	7.	**Neck, shoulders, hips** e.g., rocking, twisting, squirming, pelvic gyrations	0 1 2 3 4				(26)
GLOBAL JUDGMENTS:	8.	Severity of abnormal movements	None, normal 0 Minimal 1 Mild 2 Moderate 3 Severe 4				(27)
	9.	Incapacitation due to abnormal movements	None, normal 0 Minimal 1 Mild 2 Moderate 3 Severe 4				(28)
	10.	Patient's awareness of abnormal movements Rate only patient's report	No awareness 0 Aware, no distress 1 Aware, mild distress 2 Aware, moderate distress 3 Aware, severe distress 4				(29)
DENTAL STATUS:	11.	Current problems with teeth and/or dentures	No 0 Yes 1				(30)
	12.	Does patient usually wear dentures?	No 0 Yes 1				(31)

MH-9-117
11-74

Subsection 2

Smith Tardive Dyskinesia Scale

I. SUPPLEMENTARY DEFINITIONS OF ITEMS, AND INSTRUCTIONS

I. Rating severity uses the following guidelines:

0 = *Absent*. Symptom not present at all during observation period.

1 = *Slight, doubtful*. Symptom present very fleetingly during observation period, and/or so mild that it is difficult to determine whether it was just part of normal movement.

2 = *Mild*. Symptom is definitely present, although not to a severe degree. It may be present occasionally during the rating period (more than 4 times), or may have alternating small periods of being present, with periods of not being present.

3 = *Moderate*. Symptom is, at least, of moderate severity. The symptom will often be present at the majority of time of the observation period.

4 = *Severe*. Very pronounced symptoms. Symptoms are usually present throughout most of the observation period.

In making numerical judgments, rater should use his total experience in evaluating the severity of tardive dyskinesia symptoms.

In making numerical judgments, rater should consider the severity of the movement more important than its persistence over the entire time period of the observation, which should be 5–10 minutes.

In making severity ratings, rater should use the most severe intensity as the final rating. This highest severity on intensity of the symptom should be present for at least 1 minute during the observation period. If the most severe intensity of the symptom is present for less than 1 minute during the observation period, combine the most severe rating with the next severe rating occurring for more than a minute's time during the observation. (For example, if a symptom severity of 4 occurred for about 30 seconds, but a symptom severity of 2 is present for another 2 or 3 minutes of the observation period, then the final rating would be 3, marked on the TD scale. If the symptom severity of 4 is present for 1 minute, then the final rating would be 4.)

If the most severe rating is seen only after activation of the patient (e.g., after the patient had walked to and fro, following the instructions of the rater or examiner), then one should *decrease* this severity rating by 1. (For example, if a severity of 4 was seen for a minute or more after directed activation of the patient, but this level of severity was not seen earlier in the observation period, then the final scale rating would be severity rating of 3.) However, if a severity intensity of 4 was also seen before the direct activation of the patient, then the severity rating of 4 would be marked on the TD scale as the final rating for this specific symptom.

II. General Definitions

Tremor movements. Regular rhythmic movements. Tremor is most often a fine tremor, but in more severe cases can be a coarse tremor. The manifestation of tremor is identified with extrapyramidal parkinsonianlike symptoms.

Jerking movements. These are more irregular movements, usually of a coarser nature than tremors. They do not have a regular rhythmic pattern, although they may be rolling or circular. They have a more jerky quality. They are most often identified with tardive dyskinesia, although they can also be characteristic of some organic neurological syndromes.

III. Specific Definitions

1. *Fidgeting*. This is a measure of general restlessness, especially in the hands. The movements are jerky or interrupted movements in which the patient touches his body, manipulates his clothes, buttonholes, rings, etc.

7. *Salivation*. 0 = normal. 1 = excess, to the extent that pooling takes place if the mouth is open and the tongue raised. 2 = excess, occasionally causing difficulty in speaking. 3 = speaking is difficult because of the excess salivation. 4 = frank drooling.

12. *Rigid or masked face*. Rigid-looking face with little spontaneous facial expression.

13. *Grimacing*. Gesture involves the cheeks and upper face. Oral and lip-smacking movements, on the other hand, involve primarily the mouth and oral region.

14. *Pill-rolling tremor*. Alternating movements of thumb against the opposing index finger.

15. *Jerky movements of fingers and wrists*. These include jerky, interrupted movements of fingers, extension of fingers, and sometimes flexion of fingers. The fourth and fifth fingers may also be involved. These finger movements are often increased by activity, but in more severe cases (3+ to 4+) may also be prominent at rest.

19. *Neck, shoulders, head*. Movements similar to those performed in adjusting one's clothes. In more severe cases (3+,4+), tonic spasm of the head may be present; the head is thrust forward and backward.

20. *Alternating movement of knees*. Nonregualr, but some rhythmic, movements of the knees in adduction and abduction. In more severe cases, knees are moving continuously when the patient is at rest (e.g., seated).

25. *Heel walking.* Walking with main step first on heels rather than toes.

26. *Stiff or shuffling gait.* In severe cases, gait is slow and stiff. Arms are often held rigidly toward the foot. In the most severe cases, the patient has a slow, shuffling gait.

27. *Waist movements.* Movements consist of rapid forward projection of the pelvis, as if the patient must compensate for inability to keep erect posture. Body is thrown backward from waist thrown forward in severe cases.

IV. Some Supplemental Instructions

Frequent differences on some regional ratings, usually of a 1-point nature, further necessitate some standardizations of evaluation proceedings.

1. Have the patient hold his or her tongue out till told to retract, approximately 30 seconds.

2. Check to see if the patient is chewing gum or tobacco. Ask patient to remove either before evaluating mouth movement. Please make a comment under "Teeth" in the case of a patient has no teeth or does not have dentures in place.

3. Grimacing should involve the upper part of the face and cheeks, rather than only the mouth and lips.

4. Ask the patient to uncross his or her legs for evaluating knees and upper leg movements.

SMITH TARDIVE DYSKINESIA SCALE
I. GENERAL INSTRUCTIONS
SUGGESTED PROCEDURES FOR RATING PATIENT SYMPTOMS OF TARDIVE DYSKINESIA AND PSEUDOPARKINSONISM

These are suggested procedures in approaching a patient and rating him on the scales which are to be found on the following pages for symptoms of tardive dyskinesia and pseudoparkinsonism. They can be modified to fit problems in rating any particular patient where this procedure is difficult to follow because of the patient's uncooperativeness or inaccessibility.

1. Generally observe patient for total period of 5–10 minutes at each rating.

2. You can make preliminary ratings in light pencil as you observe the patient. If other behavior is seen which makes the rating higher as you continue to observe the patient, these light pencil marks can be erased and changed.

3. First, try to observe the patient from a distance, without intruding.

4. Next, go closer to the patient, and continue observations at a closer range, trying not to intrude too much.

5. Talk to the patient and observe movement of lips, mouth, face, and hands.

6. Ask the patient to open his mouth. Observe movement of tongue.
7. Ask patient to stick out his tongue. Observe tongue and see whether it is difficult for patient to hold his tongue out. Time patient for 30 seconds.
8. Have patient walk back and forth. Observe patient's gait, observe movement of hands, and observe the effects of walking on the expression of other symptoms.
9. If patient has not been observed sitting quietly at beginning, try to have patient sit quietly and observe movements.

SMITH TARDIVE DYSKINESIA SCALE
II. RATING SCALE FOR TARDIVE DYSKINESIA
AND EXTRAPYRAMIDAL SYMPTOMS

Computer Card

Column

Date: _____   1. _____

2. _____

3. _____

Study: _____   4. _____

Hospital: _____   5. _____

Patient name and/or number:

_____   6. _____

7. _____

8. _____

Rating name and/or number:

_____   9. _____

10. _____

Drugs patients are on today:

Drugs   Dose   11. _____

_____ _____ 12. _____

_____ _____ 13. _____

_____   _____   14. _____

_____   _____   15. _____

                                           16. _____

                                           17. _____

                                           18. _____

Is Diagnosis Hebephrenic Schizophrenia?

                    Yes_____ No_____   19. _____

Patient general activity and activation level:

                        0 1 2 3 4 5 6 7   20. _____

0 = Asleep
1 = Drowsy
3 = Slightly hypoactive
4 = Normal
5 = Slightly hyperactive
6 = Moderately agitated
7 = Severely agitated

                                    Age   21. _____

                                               22. _____

                                    Sex   23. _____
                                    1 = Male
                                    2 = Female

Rating scale: Unless otherwise specified,
                   0 = Not present
                   2 = Mild
                   3 = Moderate
                   4 = Severe
                   N.D. = No data or could not assess

A. GENERAL
    (TD) 1. Fidgeting   0 1+ 2+ 3+ 4+ N.D.   24. _____
             (see definitions)

B. MOUTH
    Tongue
    (PK) 2. Regular tremor   0 1+ 2+ 3+ 4+ N.D.   25. _____

(TD)   3. Jerking movements   0 1+ 2+ 3+ 4+ N.D. | 26. _____
            (side to side,
            rotating, other)

(TD)   4. Patient cannot keep   0 1+ 2+ 3+ 4+ N.D. | 27. _____
            tongue out (see
            definitions)

Salivation
(PK)   5. Extent of salivation   0 1+ 2+ 3+ 4+ N.D. | 28. _____
            (see definitions)

C.   ORAL REGION
(TD)   6. Lip smacking,   0 1+ 2+ 3+ 4+ N.D. | 29. _____
            pouting, sucking

D.   EYES
(PK)   7. Regular tremor   0 1+ 2+ 3+ 4+ N.D. | 30. _____
(TD)   8. Ticlike movements   0 1+ 2+ 3+ 4+ N.D. | 31. _____

(PK)   9. No blinking of eyes   0 1+ 2+ 3+ 4+ N.D. | 32. _____
            (see definitions)

E.   FACE
(PK) 10. Masked or rigid   0 1+ 2+ 3+ 4+ N.D. | 33. _____
            facial expression

(TD) 11. Grimacing (see   0 1+ 2+ 3+ 4+ N.D. | 34. _____
            definitions)

F.   FINGERS AND WRIST
(PK) 12. Pill-rolling tremor   0 1+ 2+ 3+ 4+ N.D. | 35. _____
            (see definitions)

(PK) 13. Regular resting   0 1+ 2+ 3+ 4+ N.D. | 36. _____
            tremor (not pill-
            rolling type)

(TD) 14. Jerky movements with 0 1+ 2+ 3+ 4+ N.D. | 37. _____
            possible extension
            and flexion (see
            definitions)

G.   ELBOWS AND ARMS
(PK) 15. Regular tremor   0 1+ 2+ 3+ 4+ N.D. | 38. _____

(TD) 16. Spastic contractions   0 1+ 2+ 3+ 4+ N.D. | 39. _____
            and jerky movements.

H.   NECK, SHOULDERS, AND HEAD
(TD) 17. Movements similar to 0 1+ 2+ 3+ 4+ N.D. | 40. _____
            those performed in

adjusting one's
clothes. Tonic spasms
that throw head back-
wards = 3+ or 4+

I. KNEES
  (TD) 18. Alternating movement 0 1+ 2+ 3+ 4+ N.D. | 41._____
              of knees. In severe
              cases patients cannot
              stop this movement.

J. LEGS AND ANKLES
  (PK) 19. Regular tremor—   0 1+ 2+ 3+ 4+ N.D. | 42._____
              leg and ankle tendon

  (TD) 20. Jerky movements   0 1+ 2+ 3+ 4+ N.D. | 43._____

K. ARM TENSION AND MOVEMENTS
  (PK) 21. Diminished arm swing 0 1+ 2+ 3+ 4+ N.D. | 44._____
              with arm rigid (not
              flaccid—see
              definitions)

L. GAIT-WALKING
  (TD) 22. Heel walking   0 1+ 2+ 3+ 4+ N.D. | 45._____
              (see definitions)

  (PK) 23. Rigid, shuffling gait 0 1+ 2+ 3+ 4+ N.D. | 46._____
              (see definitions)

M. WAIST
  (TD) 24. Rapid forward pro- 0 1+ 2+ 3+ 4+ N.D. | 47._____
              jection of pelvis
              (see definitions)

N. RESPIRATION
  (TD) 25. Involuntary move- 0 1+ 2+ 3+ 4+ N.D. | 48._____
              ments of diaphragm
              and/or grunting
              respiration.

O. MANNERISMS
  Describe any other
  special mannerisms   Teeth: 1 = Own teeth | 49._____
                     2 = False teeth
                     3 = No teeth

            Can walk: 1 = Yes | 50._____
                     2 = No
                     3 = with
                       assistance

Total scores:

(TD) Primary dyskinesia—sum of columns 27, 28, 30

51._____

52._____

(TD) Facial dyskinesia—sum of columns 27, 28, 30, 32, 35

53._____

54._____

(TD) Total body dyskinesia—sum of columns 27, 28, 30, 32, 35, 38, 40, 41, 42, 44, 46, 48, 49

55._____

56._____

(EP) Primary PK—sum of columns 34, 36, 37, 45, 47,

57._____

58._____

(EP) Total body PK—sum of columns 34, 36, 37, 39, 43, 45, 47

59._____

60._____

Subsection 3

Simpson Tardive Dyskinesia Rating Scale

I. General Instructions

Patients may be examined one at a time or in pairs. Pairs have the advantage in that the examiner can rate each patient "unawares." (The dyskinetic movements may be diminished or even absent when the patient's attention is self-focused or when the subject is aware of being rated.) Talking to one patient while rating the other produces a more accurate rating. If only one patient is present, the examiner should engage in conversation or have someone else talk to him while the examiner rates him.

Observation begins when the patient walks into the room. Observe whole body movements with particular attention to the limbs. Wrist and finger movements not readily observable at other procedures can frequently be seen when the subject is walking. Similarly, abnormalities of gait give clues to other dyskinetic phenomenon.

The patient should sit in a firm armrest chair, with his shoes and socks removed. The hands should be placed on the knees or let hung loosely, and the feet should be placed slightly apart, flat on the floor.

To examine the tongue, have the patient open his mouth wide and stick out his tongue. This should be done on at least two occasions. (A good light is essential to see the tongue movements.) Another procedure to bring out bucco-lingual movements is to ask the patient to count up to 10 or 20 in his mind or to have him tap with his hands, count his fingers or flap his hands. The tongue is observed within the buccal cavity while this procedure is being carried out. Eye tremor can be demonstrated with the eyes gently closed, and if need be, the same reinforcing procedures carried out as discussed under evaluation of the tongue. In order to rate trunk movements, the patient should be asked to stand up for at least 1 minute. He is also to be observed walking away from and towards the examiner at this time.

To elicit dyskinetic movements which are not evident at rest, the following distracting maneuvers are suggested. The patient is asked to stand with his arms straight out in front of him and his wrists bent at 90 degrees to his arms. This should be in a relaxed position. He should be told to close his eyes gently and open his mouth, keeping his tongue within the buccal cavity. This position should be held for about 30 seconds. The patient can be spoken to at this time in order to distract him and to observe tongue movements as well as finger movements—that is, slight forward and backward movements of the fingers which are choreoathetoid in nature and easily distinguishable from tremor. If no finger movements are noted, the patient can be told to close his mouth, and he can then be engaged in conversation, with his arms as described above and his eyes remaining closed. In this way, movements may be seen. In examining the feet, the patient should be in a sitting position as described above. While talking to the patient, reinforcement movements—either slapping his hand on his knees or rapidly tapping his fingers with his thumbs—can be carried out, and movement of the ankle joint and contracting and relaxing movements of the toes as well as any tapping movements can be observed. The trunk movements and other arm movements are rated while the patient is walking and standing for other tests. Whatever distractive maneuvers are used during the first examination should be used in the subsequent examination throughout any study. A minimum of 10 minutes should be spent with each patient, and approximately the same amount of time should be spent at each of the subsequent examinations.

II. SIMPSON TARDIVE DYSKINESIA RATING SCALE (FULL SCALE)

Patient_____# _____AM

Date _____Time _____PM

Setting_____Rater_____

FACE	Absent	?	Mild	Moderate	Moderately severe	Very severe
1. Blinking of eyes	1	2	3	4	5	6
2. Tremor of eyelids	1	2	3	4	5	6
3. Tremor of upper lip (Rabbit syndrome)	1	2	3	4	5	6
4. Pouting of lower lip	1	2	3	4	5	6
5. Puckering of lips	1	2	3	4	5	6
6. Sucking movements	1	2	3	4	5	6
7. Chewing movements	1	2	3	4	5	6
8. Smacking of lips	1	2	3	4	5	6
9. Bon bon sign	1	2	3	4	5	6
10. Tongue protrusion	1	2	3	4	5	6

	Absent	?	Mild	Moderate	Moderately severe	Very severe
11. Tongue tremor	1	2	3	4	5	6
12. Choreoathetoid movements of the tongue	1	2	3	4	5	6
13. Facial tics	1	2	3	4	5	6
14. Grimacing	1	2	3	4	5	6
15. Other (describe)_____	1	2	3	4	5	6
16. Other (describe)_____	1	2	3	4	5	6
NECK AND TRUNK						
17. Head nodding	1	2	3	4	5	6
18. Retrocollis	1	2	3	4	5	6
19. Spasmodic torticollis	1	2	3	4	5	6
20. Torsion movements (trunk)	1	2	3	4	5	6
21. Axial hyperkinesia	1	2	3	4	5	6
22. Rocking movement	1	2	3	4	5	6
23. Other (describe)_____	1	2	3	4	5	6
24. Other (describe)_____	1	2	3	4	5	6
EXTREMITIES (upper)						
25. Ballistic movements	1	2	3	4	5	6
26. Choreoathetoid movements—fingers	1	2	3	4	5	6
27. Choreoathetoid movements—wrists	1	2	3	4	5	6
28. Pill-rolling movements	1	2	3	4	5	6
29. Caressing or rubbing face and hair	1	2	3	4	5	6
30. Rubbing of thighs	1	2	3	4	5	6
31. Other (describe) _____	1	2	3	4	5	6
32. Other (describe) _____	1	2	3	4	5	6
(lower)						
33. Rotation and/or flexion of ankles	1	2	3	4	5	6
34. Toe movements	1	2	3	4	5	6
35. Stamping movements—standing	1	2	3	4	5	6
36. Stamping movements—sitting	1	2	3	4	5	6
37. Restless legs	1	2	3	4	5	6
38. Crossing/uncrossing legs—sitting	1	2	3	4	5	6

	Absent	?	Mild	Moderate	Moderately severe	Very severe
39. Other (describe)＿＿＿＿＿	1	2	3	4	5	6
40. Other (describe)＿＿＿＿＿	1	2	3	4	5	6
ENTIRE BODY						
41. Holokinetic movements	1	2	3	4	5	6
42. Akathisia	1	2	3	4	5	6
43. Other (describe)＿＿＿＿＿	1	2	3	4	5	6

COMMENTS

_____

_____

_____

III. SIMPSON TARDIVE DYSKINESIA RATING SCALE DEFINITIONS

FACE

1. *Blinking of Eyes*
   Repetitive and more or less continuous, or in bursts. To be distinguished from tics, which occur episodically
2. *Tremor of Eyelids*
   Isolated tremor, more frequently bilateral, but can occur unilaterally. Usually seen when eyes are closed. Fine in character
3. *Tremor of Upper Lip (Rabbit Syndrome)*
   Fine, rapid tremor confined to the upper lip
4. *Pouting of the Lower Lip*
   A thrusting out of the lower lip, as in solemnness
5. *Puckering of Lips*
   Drawstring or pursing action of the lip
6. *Smacking of Lips*
   Brisk separation of lips, which produces a sharp sound
7. *Sucking Movement*
   Self-explanatory
8. *Chewing Movement*
   Self-explanatory

9. *Bon Bon Sign*

Tongue movement within the oral cavity, which produces a bulge in the cheek, giving the impression the patient has a hard bon bon pocketed in his cheek. Occasionally, a repetitious sweeping movement of the tongue over the buccal lining, which also pushes out the mouth

10. *Tongue Protrusion*

Clonic—a rhythmic in-and-out movement of the tongue

Tonic—a continuous protrusion of the tongue

Fly catcher—a sudden shooting out of the tongue from the mouth at irregular episodes

11. *Tongue Tremor*

Fine tremor observed with the mouth open and tongue within the buccal cavity

12. *Choreoathetoid Movements of the Tongue*

A rolling, wormlike movement of the tongue muscles without displacement of the tongue from the mouth. The tongue may rotate on its longitudinal axis. Observed when the mouth is opened

13. *Facial Tics*

Brief, recurrent, stereotyped movement involving relatively small segments of the face

14. *Grimacing*

A repetitive, irregularly occurring distortion of the face. A complex movement involving large segments of facial muscles

15. & 16. *Other*

Write in items, such as unusual bucco-lingual movements, blepharospasm, repetitive sounds, etc.

NECK AND TRUNK

17. *Head Nodding*

Slower than tremor, may or may not be rhythmic. Can occur horizontally or vertically

18. *Retrocollis*

Overextension of the neck, as a result of which the head is bent backwards. Can occur with or without rigidity of the muscles of the neck and shoulder

19. *Spasmodic Torticollis*

Tonic, prolonged contracture of sternocleidomastoides on one side, resulting in a downward and lateral fixation of the chin. The head may be bent laterally

20. *Torsion Movements*

Twisting, undulant movements of the upper or lower part of the trunk (shoulder or hip girdle), resulting from mobile, spastic movements of the axial and proximal muscles. The movements are not fast, and they involve large portions of the body

21. *Axial Hyperkinesia*
   A front-to-back hip rocking movement. Resembles copulatory movements. Differs from the rocking movement in which the upper torso has to-and-fro movement
22. *Rocking Movements*
   A rhythmic to-and-fro movement of the upper torso, which occurs from a repeated bending of the spinal column in the lumbar region. Different from axial hyperkinesia, where the hips move to and fro
23. & 24. *Other*
   (Write in)

EXTREMITIES

25. *Ballistic Movements*
   Sudden, fast, large amplitude swinging movements, occurring most often in the arms and less frequently in the legs. One or both sides may be involved
26. *Choreoathetoid Movements—Choreiform Movements*
   In fingers, wrists, arms. Variable, purposeless, coarse, quick, and jerky movements, which begin suddenly and show no rhythmicity. They vary in distribution and extension
27. *Athetoid Movements*
   In fingers, wrists, arms. Continuous rhythmic, slow, writhing, wormlike movements. They almost invariably appear together with choreiform movements
28. *Finger Counting*
   Rhythmic rubbing of the thumb against the middle and index finger
29. *Caressing Face and Hair*
   Gives the impression of an absent-minded or nervous mannerism; has the appearance of being purposeful
30. *Rubbing of Thighs*
   Hands rub the outside or tops of thighs. Sporadic and nonrhythmic
31. & 32. *Other*
   (Write in)
33. *Rotation and/or Flexion of the Ankles*
   Self-explanatory
34. *Toe Movements*
   Slow, rhythmic retroflexion, usually of the big toes, although other toes can also be involved
35. *Stamping Movements (Standing)*
   Weight is shifted back and forth from one foot to the other when patient stands
36. *Stamping Movements (Sitting)*
   Flapping or tapping of the whole foot on floor when the patient is sitting, or alternate toe-and-heel tapping

37. *Restless Legs*
    Constant leg movement: jiggling of legs, of foot when leg is crossed; or
    may involve rapidly moving knees apart and together
38. *Crossing and Uncrossing Legs*
    Self-explanatory
39. *Holokinetic Movements*
    Extensive, jerky, rapid, abrupt, awkward, gross movements of large parts
    or entire body. The movement may appear to be somewhat goal-directed
    and only moderately coordinated. May begin in response to a stimulus or
    spontaneously.
40. *Akathisia*
    An inability to sit or stand still. (The verbal expression of inner restless-
    ness is not required here)
41. & 42. *Other*
    (Write in)

IV. ABBREVIATED (SIMPSON) DYSKINESIA RATING
SCALE (ADS)

Patient_____# _____Date_____Time _____AM
                                                                PM
Setting_____Study #_____Rater # _____Period _____

FACIAL AND ORAL MOVEMENTS
  1. Periocular area (blinking of eyes, tremor of eyelids) 1 2 3 4 5 6
  2. Movements of the lips (pouting, puckering, smacking) 1 2 3 4 5 6
  3. Chewing movements   1 2 3 4 5 6
  4. Bon bon sign   1 2 3 4 5 6
  5. Tongue protrusion   1 2 3 4 5 6
  6. Tremor and/or choreoathetoid movements of the tongue 1 2 3 4 5 6
  7. Other (describe)_____   1 2 3 4 5 6
NECK AND TRUNK
  8. Axial hyperkinesis (patient standing)   1 2 3 4 5 6
  9. Rocking movements   1 2 3 4 5 6
10. Torsion movements   1 2 3 4 5 6
11. Other (describe)_____   1 2 3 4 5 6
EXTREMITIES
12. Movements of fingers and wrists   1 2 3 4 5 6
13. Movements of ankles and toes   1 2 3 4 5 6

14. Stamping movements	1 2 3 4 5 6
15. Other (describe)＿＿＿＿＿＿＿	1 2 3 4 5 6
ENTIRE BODY	
16. Akathisia	1 2 3 4 5 6
17. Other (describe)＿＿＿＿＿＿＿	1 2 3 4 5 6

RATING: 1 = absent   4 = moderate

2 = ?   5 = moderately severe

3 = mild   6 = severe

V. SIMPSON TARDIVE DYSKINESIA SCALE DEFINITIONS (ABBREVIATED SCALE) (ADS)

Facial and Oral Movements

1. *Periocular area (blinking of eyes, tremor of eyelids)*
   a. *Blinking of eyes*
   Repetitive or continual involuntary shutting and opening of eyes (as distinguished from tics, which occur episodically).
   b. *Tremor of eyelids*
   Isolated fine tremor more frequently bilateral but can occur unilaterally. Usually seen when eyes are closed (not too tightly).

Rate the increase in frequency and extent of these movements. Movements should be observed separately but can be rated together or separately, as the case may be.
   1 = absent
   2 = ?
   3 = 7–10 blinks per 30 seconds
   4 = 11–13 blinks per 30 seconds
   5 = almost continuous
   6 = continuous and incapacitating
2. *Movements of the lips (pouting, puckering, smacking)*
   a. *Pouting*
   A thrusting out of the lower lip, as in solemnness.
   b. *Puckering*
   Drawstring or pursing action of the lips.
   c. *Smacking*
   Brisk separation of lips, which produces a sharp sound.
Rate the increase in frequency and extent of these movements. Movements should be observed separately but can be rated together or separately, as the case may be.

1 = absent
2 = ?
3 = occasional during observation period
4 = frequently during observation period
5 = almost continuously
6 = continuously

3. *Chewing movements*
   Self explanatory. Make sure that the patient does not have chewing gum or candy in his mouth.
Rating is based on the frequency and degree of interference with normal chewing activities.
1 = absent
2 = ?
3 = occasional chewing movements
4 = frequent chewing movements
5 = almost continuous chewing
6 = continuous chewing which interferes with normal eating and articulation

4. *Bon-bon sign*
   Tongue movement within the oral cavity, which produces a bulge in the cheek giving the impression the patient has a hard bon bon pocketed in his cheek. Occasionally a repetitive sweeping movement of the tongue over the buccal lining, which also pushes out the mouth. (Distinguish from choreoathetoid movements of the tongue)
Rating is based on the frequency and degree at which the tongue pushes against the cheek within the oral cavity.
1 = absent
2 = ?
3 = occasionally
4 = obvious most of the time
5 = almost continuous
6 = continual sweeping movements involving whole cheeks and buccal cavity

5. *Tongue protrusion*
   a. *Clonic*
      A rhythmic in and out movement of the tongue
   b. *Tonic*
      A continuous protrusion of the tongue
   c. *Fly catcher*
      A sudden shooting out of the tongue from the mouth at irregular episodes
Rating is based on the frequency, degree, and duration of tongue protrusion in and out of the mouth cavity.
1 = absent

2 = ?

3 = occasional protrusion of tongue

4 = frequent protrusion

5 = almost continuous protrusion of the tongue

6 = pronounced protrusion with swollen tongue as if it has
no room in the mouth

6. *Tremor and/or choreoathetoid movements of the tongue*

a. *Tremor*

Fine rapid to slow tremor observed with the mouth open and tongue within the buccal cavity.

b. *Choreoathetoid movements of the tongue*

Rolling, wormlike movement of the tongue muscles without displacement of the tongue from the mouth. The tongue may rotate on its longitudinal axis. Observed when the mouth is open.

Both movements should be observed separately but could be rated together, as the case may be. (Distinguish from bon-bon sign, which is continual irregular movements within the oral cavity with the mouth closed.)

Rating is based on the intensity and frequency of the tongue movements.

1 = absent

2 = ?

3 = brief and occasional wormlike tongue movements

4 = tongue moves several times in all directions on
its longitudinal axis

5 = almost continuous rolling

6 = continuous and incessant twisting, folding and rolling
all over the oral cavity so that the underside of the
tongue is exposed

7. *Other*

Write in items such as the Rabbit Syndrome, a fine, very rapid tremor of the upper lip (5 per second), tics, or grimacing.

Neck and Trunk

8. *Axial hyperkinesis (patient standing)*

A front-to-back hip-rocking movement. Resembles copulatory movements, and differs from the rocking movement, where it is the upper torso which has to-and-fro movement.

Rating is based on the frequency and range of the movements of the pelvis when standing.

1 = absent

2 = ?

3 = seen occasionally

4 = seen most frequently
5 = almost continuous long range movements of the pelvis
6 = continuous swinging of the pelvis

9. *Rocking movements*
Continuous or episodic, rhythmic to-and-fro or side-to-side movement of the upper torso, which occurs from a repeated bending of the spinal column in the lumbar region while sitting (as distinguished from axial hyperkinesia, where the hips move to and fro while standing).
1 = absent
2 = ?
3 = occasional to-and-fro movements
4 = episodic movements with small range
5 = almost continuous to-and-fro movements with small range
6 = continuous to-and-fro movements with large range

10. *Torsion movements*
Twisting undulant movements of the upper or lower part of the trunk (shoulder or hip girdle). The movements are not fast, and they involve large portions of the body.
Rating is based on frequency and intensity.
1 = absent
2 = ?
3 = occasional
4 = episodic
5 = almost continuous—small range
6 = continuous twisting of large portions of the body

11. *Other*
Write in items such as head nodding, retrocollis, and torticollis

Extremities

12. *Movements of fingers and wrists*
Irregular, purposeless, coarse, jerky (nonrhythmic and rhythmic) movements (resembling guitar playing), which begin suddenly and may last for brief period or may be continuous. They may involve a few fingers or the whole hand and wrist. Wrist movements are more rhythmic and are occasionally jerky and wormlike. Both invariably appear together.
Rating is based on frequency and intensity.
1 = absent
2 = ?
3 = seen occasionally in a few fingers—low in intensity
4 = seen most of the time during observation involving the whole hand with marked intensity
5 = continuous wormlike movements involving all the fingers of whole hand

   6 = continuous, wormlike, irregular movements of the
       whole hand and wrist
13. *Movements of ankles and toes*
    Involves rotation and flexion of ankles. Slow range, irregular, coarse,
    involuntary movement of toes, episodic or continuous.
Rating is based on intensity and frequency.
   1 = absent
   2 = ?
   3 = seen occasionally
   4 = seen most of the time during observation, ankle
       rotating and flexing
   5 = almost continuously
   6 = seen continuously with marked intensity
14. *Stamping movements*
    Flapping or tapping of whole foot on the floor, either in sitting or standing.
Rating is based on intensity and frequency.
   1 = absent
   2 = ?
   3 = seen only few times
   4 = seen most of the time
   5 = almost continuously
   6 = seen continuously
15. *Other*
    Write in items such as pill rolling-like movements (these are not classical
    pill-rolling movements, but involve repetitive movement of the thumb
    across several fingers), carressing or rubbing of face and/or hair.

Entire Body

16. *Akathisia*
    Involuntary restlessness (may be continuous or may be observed as out-
    bursts of activity), with inability to sit or stand still. (Verbal expression of
    inner restlessness is not required here.)
Rating is based on the frequency and intensity of restlessness.
   1 = absent
   2 = ?
   3 = infrequent jiggling
   4 = pacing, jiggling most of the time
   5 = pacing up and down; continuous jiggling
   6 = unable to sit and stand still
17. *Other*
    Write in items such as holokinetic movements, i.e. extensive, abrupt,
    gross movements of large parts or entire body.

Gerlach Tardive Dyskinesia and Parkinsonism Rating Scale

The tardive dyskinesia is scored twice during each evaluation: (1) while unoccupied and undisturbed (passive), and (2) while performing certain voluntary movements, e.g., drawing a spiral or doing hand movements (active). The oral tardive dyskinesia syndrome is recorded separately according to the following items:

a. *Hypermotility* (frequency), estimated from 0 to 6
b. *Amplitude*

Mouth opening	*Tongue protrusion*
0–½ cm 1	within mouth ... 1
½–1 cm 2	to the lips 2
1–1½ cm 3	0–1 cm 3
1½–2 cm 4	½–1 cm 4
2–2½ cm 5	1–1½ cm 5
2½–3 cm 6	1½ > cm 6

c. *Duration of each separate tongue protrusion/mouth opening*

1 second 0
1–5 seconds 1
6–10 seconds 2
> 10 seconds .. 3

24

The Prevalence of Tardive Dyskinesia

GEORGE CRANE
and ROBERT C. SMITH

This chapter reviews the prevalence of tardive dyskinesia (TD) in several major survey studies conducted since 1964. Table 1 summarizes the results of these studies.

As can be seen in Table 1, the prevalence of tardive dyskinesia varies from about 0.5% to 56% in the different studies. This discrepancy is probably due, in a large part, to a number of factors which varied in the different studies. These include:

1. *The definition of the tardive dyskinesia syndrome.* A very broad definition can inflate the rate of prevalence of tardive dyskinesia by including other motor disorders which have some similarities. On the other hand, a narrow definition—for example, defining TD in terms of one or two oral-buccal signs—would exclude many patients, especially younger patients or early cases in which jerky movements of the extremities more often predominate. Another factor which can influence prevalence rates is whether the "positive" cases of TD include only those patients with moderate or severe TD symptoms or also count patients with mild or questionable symptoms.

2. *Method of obtaining information for assessment.* This factor can also have a large influence on prevalence rates. In some studies, information was obtained by questionnaire surveys of the staff, while in others, direct observations of the patient was used. Some of the observational studies used clinically trained raters or very experienced clinicians, while others are based on ratings or impressions of a large number of physicians, nurses, technicians in different hospitals with various degrees of knowledge and training. More recent studies have used quantitative rating scales and/or consensus among several trained raters or experienced clinicians.

Table 1
Some Prevalence Studies of Tardive Dyskinesia

Author(s)	(Ref)	Year	Special Conditions	Neuroleptic Treated Patients (a)		Non-Neuroleptic Treated Patients (b)	
				Number	% TD	Number	% TD
Pryce & Edwards	(1)	1966	(s)	27	70.4	15 (c)	13.3
Demars	(2)	1966	(o)	371	7	117	13.7
Degkwitz	(3,5)	1967		1209	22	912	1.5
						1500 (g)	1
Crane & Paulson	(6)	1967		182	14		
Hoff & Hoffman	(7)	1967		10,000	0.5		
Turunen & Achte	(8)	1967	(o)	400	6		
Siede & Müller	(9)	1967	(g)	404	11		
Crane	(10)	1968		305	24		
				379	28		
Eckmann	(11)	1968		804	3		
Heinrich et al.	(12)	1968		554	17	201	3
						110 (g)	2
Paulson	(13)	1968		500	10		
Greenblatt et al.	(14)	1968	(g)	52	39		
Villineuve et al.	(15)	1969	(o)	3280	2		
Edwards	(16)	1970	(o)	184	19		
Dynes	(17)	1970	(o)	1200	8		
Hippius & Lange	(18)	1970		531	32	137	14
Crane	(19)	1970		127	27		
Lehman et al.	(20)	1970	(o)	350	6.5		
Poxburg	(21)	1970	(g)	120	2		
Kennedy et al.	(22)	1971		63	40		
Brandon et al.	(23)	1971		625	24	285	19
Fann et al.	(24)	1972		204	36		
Crane	(25	1973		926	17	46	2
						150	0
Crane & Smeets	(26)	1974	(g)	31	42	8	0
Jus et al.	(27)	1975		330	56 (?)	2	0 (?)
Bell & Smith	(28)	1978		1329	26		

			Patients with TD Not Divided by Whether They Received Neuroleptics	
			Number	% TD
Hunter et al.	(29)	1964	450	2.9
Faurbye et al.	(30)	1964	417	26.1
Dincmen	(31)	1966	1700	3.4

Table 1 (Key)

Number = number of patients. % TD = percent of patients with tardive dyskinesia.

(a) Patients who were classified by original researchers as receiving neuroleptics (or who were classified by us as receiving more than occasional neuroleptics on basis of authors' original description or tables)

(b) Patients who received no neuroleptics or occasional neuroleptics

(c) Because of very small numbers of patients who received "0" neuroleptics, patients who received 0–6 months of neuroleptics were combined in this specific sample, and compared with patients with 7–29 months of neuroleptics.

(g) Exclusively geriatric sample

(o) Only oral dyskinesia scored (not dyskinesia in other body parts)

(s) Author indicates that only moderately severe or severe cases were counted as positive dyskinesia

(?) Whether the two neuroleptic-free patients had TD is not absolutely certain from authors' original report.

---

3. *Characteristics of the patients.* Age of patient has clearly been shown to be associated with the prevalence of tardive dyskinesia, and sex of patient has been implicated in some studies. Large differences in these characteristics of the patients in different samples may therefore give different apparent prevalence rates of tardive dyskinesia.

4. *Medication treatment of the patient.* The type of drugs the patients have received and the length of treatment may be an important variable influencing the rate of prevalence of tardive dyskinesia in a specific sample or population.

One or more of these factors may have contributed to the marked variation of tardive dyskinesia in some of the studies listed in Table 1. For example, some studies reporting a low incidence of tardive dyskinesia include only cases of oral dyskinesia (for example, those of Dynes and of Lehmann et al. [17, 20]), or only more severe cases of their number of positive cases. The very low incidence in Hoff and Hoffman's study (8) may be due to poor reporting and observation techniques, since their data were based on the reports of many different observers at fourteen different institutions. The high percentage of tardive dyskinesia reported in some of the studies may be due to such factors as (a) a sample composed exclusively of geriatric patients (such as in Greenblatt, et al. [15] and Crane and Smeets's [27] studies); (b) samples composed of special populations in which most patients have received large doses of neuroleptic drugs; and (c) samples which include a considerable number of patients with motor disorders unrelated to drug-induced dyskinesia. A few of the factors which may influence the apparent prevalence rates of TD are discussed in greater detail in the sections below.

NEUROLEPTIC HISTORY OF THE PATIENTS

Since most of the patients who have a high incidence of tardive dyskinesia are chronic schizophrenics or other chronically hospitalized patients, the question has been raised whether neuroleptic drugs are definitely responsible for tardive dyskinesia or whether the chronic disease itself or long-term institutionalization, with its concomitant emotional and physical effects, may be responsible for the development of tardive dyskinesia. The epidemiological evidence, however, specifically associating treatment with neuroleptics as the important etiological factor in TD, is strong. Several studies have compared tardive dyskinesia in chronic patients regularly treated with neuroleptics with TD in patients who have received none or very occasional treatment of neuroleptics. In all but one of the studies listed in Table 1—in which sufficient information was provided to divide the patient population into two subsamples of patients, those who had received neuroleptics and those who had not—there is a higher rate of tardive dyskinesia in patients who received neuroleptics. A few studies showed appreciable rates (10–20%) of tardive dyskinesia in patients who have not received neuroleptics, but these studies may have some important methodological deficiencies. For example, the Brandon et al. (24) study found a 19% prevalence rate of tardive dyskinesia in patients not taking neuroleptics, compared with the 24% rate for patients on neuroleptics. In this study, the drug-treated population at risk was defined as patients who had three or more months of pharmacotherapy, and the researchers also may have counted a fair number of questionable cases in their enumeration of TD. Most researchers agree that tardive dyskinesia is much less likely to develop without at least two or three years of treatment with neuroleptics; therefore, the neuroleptic-treated population may have been diluted by many low-risk subjects. In some of their results, these authors subdivided their total sample by severity of dyskinesia, and about 60% of their positive TD cases had mild or doubtful dyskinesia of the mouth. Doubtful dyskinesia of the mouth is difficult to assess accurately in patients with organic brain disorders or older mental patients. The authors did not divide their patients with only mild or doubtful TD into the two treatment groups—i.e., those patients on neuroleptics versus those not treated with neuroleptics—but it is likely that many of the patients rated as dyskinetic in the nonneuroleptic group may not have had definite signs of tardive dyskinesia. All of the fourteen patients in their study who were rated as severe dyskinesia cases had a history of treatment with neuroleptics. Overall, most of the prevalence studies have reported dyskinesia occurring only in patients treated with neuroleptics, or 8 to 20 times more frequently in patients treated with neuroleptics as compared to a 0% to 3% prevalence rate of drug-free chronic patients.

Another factor contributing to the reported differences in the prevalence of TD has to do with when a study was carried out. Patients who were evaluated in 1975 had, in general, a longer exposure to drugs than those studied in 1970. Duvoisin (32) reported a very high prevalence of TD in an outpatient population in 1977. Ten years ago it seemed to be limited to chronic hospital populations.

Most of the prevalence studies have been done in the United States or Western Europe. One might still argue that chronic psychiatric patients who receive drug therapy in the United States, in the United Kingdom, or in Western Europe are selected groups of patients, since it is now customary for such patients to receive chemotherapy at some time during their hospitalization. On the other hand, up until the middle 1960's drugs were seldom prescribed to chronic patients in Turkish hospitals. Therefore, in the 1960's I examined 150 male patients in the chronic wards of a Turkish hospital, most of whom were schizophrenic patients. Of those patients who have never or only very occasionally received drugs, none manifested symptoms of tardive dyskinesia. This sample of Turkish patients was then matched for age, sex, and diagnosis with patients in a U.S. hospital who were heavily treated with neuroleptics and other medication. The difference between the two samples was highly significant with the U.S. patients having a much higher frequency of tardive dyskinesia.

CURRENT DRUG TREATMENT

High doses of neuroleptic medication suppress the abnormal movements of TD, either partially or totally, at least for several weeks or months. This masking phenomenon was first described by Hunter *et al.* (33), Degkwitz *et al.* (3–5) and others in the early 1960's, and has been confirmed by subsequent studies (see, for example, Crane and Naranjo [34]). And in up to 40% of initially asymptomatic patients, TD first manifests itself, or existing symptoms become better defined, as a result of drug withdrawal. The interval between discontinuation of neuroleptic medication and emergence of TD varies from one day to several weeks. In the study of geriatric patients by Crane and Smeets (26), tardive dyskinesia was most pronounced at the end of the second drug-free week, with no further increase during the following 10 weeks. It is therefore possible that in a population of patients who were evaluated while they were on standard high doses of neuroleptics, a lower rate of TD could be found than in a population recently withdrawn from neuroleptics. However, a recent study by Smith (28), which used a sample of patients, most of whom had received considerable amounts of neuroleptics, recorded no difference in the rate of TD in patients who were not receiving neuroleptics on the day they were rated, compared with those who were still on neuroleptics on the day of rating.

AGE AND SEX

A good deal of the variation in the prevalence of tardive dyskinesia in different studies may be due to age differences in the different samples. Many studies have shown that prevalence of TD is associated with age, and that the syndrome rarely occurs in patients under 30. The greatest prevalence is found in patients over 50 or 60 (see Table 2).

Because of this fact, samples composed exclusively of geriatric patients or those with a high percentage of patients who were over 50 would be expected to show a much higher prevalence rate of tardive dyskinesia than samples with a more even age distribution which included a larger number of younger age patients. Some of the very large samples, such as those in the studies of Hoff and Hoffman (7) and Villeneuve (15), probably included a much larger percentage of younger patients, and this may have contributed to the much lower prevalence rate recorded in these studies. One approach to correct for age effects in computing population prevalence rates is to compare the age distribution of the sample studied with the age distribution of the patients in the total population at risk, and then adjust prevalence rates accordingly. The study by Smith (28) surveyed tardive dyskinesia in Illinois state hospitals, using a stratified sampling procedure so as to have a sample which had approximately 50% of the patients above the age of 50 and 50% below the age of 50. The prevalence of definite TD in this sample was about 26%. However, the age-adjusted prevalence rate, which was calculated on the actual age

Table 2
Age and Tardive Dyskinesia in
Several Survey Studies

Author(s)	(Ref)	Percent of Patients with Tardive Dyskinesia			
		Age of Patient			
		< 40	40-50	51-60	61+
Brandon et al.	(23)	1.9	9.4	16.6	32.2
Fann et al.	(24)	22.2	26.5	34.0	45.0
Bell & Smith	(28)	7.0	25	27	33
Crane	(25)	4.7[a]	9.7[a]	13.2[a]	32.7[a]
Jus et al.	(27)	40.2[b]		60.0[b]	

Each number represents percent of patients at given age group in study who were counted as positive cases of tardive dyskinesia by original researchers. Some researchers included in their enumeration of cases those with doubtful or minimal signs while others counted patients with definite signs or moderate dyskinesia. In some studies the authors presented age data divided into different age categories. In Crane study (a) age ranges were < 44, 44–54, 55–65, 65+ years old. In Jus et al. study (b) age ranges were 20–49 and 50–69 years of age.

distribution of all patients in the Illinois state mental hospitals, was half this rate, about 12%.

Although TD occurs much less frequently in younger patients below 30 or 40, clinical reports (35) have indicated that the syndrome can clearly occur in younger patients after a few years or sometimes after only a few months of neuroleptic therapy. Especially in these younger patients, the period of observation after removal of drugs is important, because in younger patients the symptoms of TD are more likely to be very much diminished or to disappear after a drug-free period. In other cases, TD symptoms in these patients may diminish after an initial increase in TD symptoms shortly after drug withdrawal.

According to several studies and reviews, tardive dyskinesia is more common in females than in males. However, five of thirteen large-scale survey studies have not shown a significant difference between the sexes. On the average, institutionalized females are 5 to 6 years older than males, reflecting a similar trend in general population, and therefore the report of higher prevalence of tardive dyskinesia in females may be a function of age rather than of sex. In one study by Bell and Smith (28), which had a fairly wide age range, the authors controlled for both age and sex of patient; there was a small (3.6%) but statistically significant higher rate of tardive dyskinesia in female patients, and there was no statistical interaction between age and sex in their effect on TD. Even if it becomes more definitely established that the prevalence of tardive dyskinesia is significantly greater in females than males, a very small sex difference between male and female prevalence rates may not have too much practical significance for drug treatment in older patients, since both older male and female patients have a fairly high prevalence rate of TD.

SYNDROME SEVERITY AND PREVALENCE RATES

Most reviews of TD survey studies have presented the rates of TD as a "present" or "absent" determination. Many of the original studies on which these reviews are based also rated the syndrome as present or absent or used a very gross method of estimating severity. The fairly high prevalence rates of TD reported in some studies can arise from counting as "positive" cases a considerable number of patients who have only mild or doubtful TD signs. What constitutes minimum symptoms for definite diagnosis of TD has not been defined. TD signs can also vary from day to day. Therefore, patients with minimal or doubtful symptoms of TD, even if some of them do represent "true" cases of definite TD in their early or mild stages, may be the most difficult to accurately assess. Some of the differences in prevalence rates noted in Table 1 are probably due to differences in the degree of motor symptoms the researchers took as their cut-off points for enumeration and positive cases of TD.

The prevalence of TD, broken down by severity of the disorder from a few studies, is summarized in Table 3. If we add or subtract the doubtful or slight symptom categories, the TD prevalence rate can change from 56 to 23 in some of the studies.

OTHER ABNORMAL MOVEMENT DISORDERS SIMILAR TO TARDIVE DYSKINESIA

The confusion of other motor abnormalities or side effects with TD may also influence prevalence rates. The extent to which this confusion with other syndromes influenced rates in some of the early survey reports of prevalence of TD cannot be fully evaluated. The picture of TD, however, is fairly clear, and as a general rule, the diagnosis should present little difficulty to the experienced clinician or trained rater in spite of the many variations and combinations of symptoms.

Abnormal movements, however, including the oral-buccal syndrome of TD, have been known to occur in a variety of physical conditions, and therefore in doubtful cases the rater may need additional information provided by clinical history, family history, and a more thorough neurological evaluation to distinguish these syndromes from TD. For example, two papers from France (36,37) reported cases manifesting symptoms similar to those of drug-induced TD in patients who were not currently treated with neuroleptics. On more careful clinical history, however, these patients were found to have either

Table 3

Severity of Tardive Dyskinesia Signs and Prevalence Rates

Author(s)	(Ref.)	Percent of Identified Tardive Dyskinesia Cases Which Have Given Degree of Severity of Dyskinesia Symptoms				Total Prevalence (Percent)	
		Doubtful	Slight Minimal or Mild	Moderate or Definite	Moderately Severe or Severe	All Cases	All Cases Minus Doubtful & Slight Categories
Crane	(25)	28.6		42.9	28.6	25	17.9
Jus et al.	(27)		59.1		40.9[a]	56	22.9
Bell & Smith	(28)		35	35	30	40	26
Brandon et al.	(23)	8.9	48.8	35.5	6.6	23.4	9.9

[a]Moderate and severe categories combined in authors original report.

suffered from massive neurological diseases or to have been treated with neuroleptics for reasons other than schizophrenia at some time in the past. Adventitions movements of the mouth and postural disorders have been described in senile or atherosclerotic patients who have not received neuroleptics (38,39). Poorly fitting dentures are occasionally accompanied by oral movements resembling TD (40). The dyskinesia of amphetamine intoxication, thyrotoxicosis, and anoxia at least superficially resemble some of the movements seen in TD patients who have been treated with neuroleptics. The dyskinetic motor abnormality which develops in some of the patients with Parkinson's disease who are treated with L-dopa may be indistinguishable from dyskinesia due to neuroleptics. In such cases, however, the etiology can be established without difficulty, and the disorder may be corrected by proper medical measures. The question is periodically asked as to whether abnormalities in hebephrenic or catatonic schizophrenics are drug-induced or manifestions of their psychiatric disorders. In general, the stereotypic movements of chronic schizophrenics are semivoluntary and often serve a purpose, even though their meaning is obscure. Posture in extension with flexion of the head or chest are characteristic catatonic features which may resemble some of the posture seen in TD. Similarly, the presence of rocking and swaying movements in mental defectives or in chronic psychotics may be either a manifestation of their primary disease or the result of long-term neuroleptic administration.

Thus, problems of differential diagnosis of TD do exist in some cases, but many unnecessary and inconclusive discussions as to whether the motor disorders of a patient is drug-induced TD can be avoided by an appropriate neurological examination and clinical neurological history of every candidate for neuroleptic therapy before we begin drug administration. More difficult is the differential diagnosis between TD secondary to these drugs and dyskinesia occurring naturally, because both conditions have many clinical conditions in common. Furthermore, a disease like Huntington's chorea may be misdiagnosed and treated with routine neuroleptic therapy for many years before the emergence of the motor components of the disorders (41). Similar motor abnormalities of sporadic encephalitis and other diseases of the central nervous system may be preceded by mental symptoms and are often treated with neuroleptics. Therefore, the emergence of dyskinesia in such conditions could erroneously be attributed to drug therapy. We believe, however, that in most routine samples of patients seen in psychiatric settings, in which the evaluation of TD is made by experienced clinicians directly observing TD or by a trained rater using the TD scales, the percentage of "false positive" cases rated erroneously as drug-induced TD is quite small. It would be further reduced if routine clinical history and neurological laboratory tests were investigated for any patient whose TD symptoms are somewhat unusual or whenever neurological diseases are suspected.

REFERENCES

1. Pryce, I.J., Edwards, H. Persistent oral dyskinesia in female mental hospital patients. *Br. J. Psychiatry*, *112*:983–987, 1966.

2. Demars, J.C.A. Neuromuscular effects of long-term phenothiazine medication, ECT and leucotomy. *J. Nerv. Ment. Dis.*, *143*:73–79, 1966.

3. Degkwitz, R. Uber die Ursachen der persistierenden extrapyramidalen Hyperkinesen nach langfristiger Anwendung von Neuroleptika. *Activitas Nerv. System.*, *9*:389–399, 1967.

4. Degkwitz, R., Wenzel, W., Binsack, K.F., Herkert, H, Luxenburger, O. Zum Probleme der terminalen extrapyramidalen Hyperkinesen an Hand von 1600 langfristig mit Neuroleptica Behandelten. *Arzneim. Forsch.*, *16*:276–278, 1966.

5. Degkwitz, R., Binsack, K.F., Herkert, H., Luxenburger, O., Wenzel, W. Zum Probleme der persistierend Hyperkinesen nach langfristiger Anwendung von Neuroleptika. *Nervenarzt*, *38*:170–174, 1967.

6. Crane, G.E., Paulson, G. Involuntary movements in a sample of chronic mental patients and their relation to the treatment with neuroleptics. *Int. J. Neuropsychiatry, 3*:286–291, 1967.

7. Hoff, H., Hoffman, G. Das persistierende extrapyramidale Syndrom bei Neuroleptika Therapie. *Wien. Med. Wochenschr.*, *117*:14–17, 1967.

8. Turunen, S., Achte, K.A. The bucco-lingual-masticatory syndrome as side effect of neuroleptic therapy. *Psychiatr., Quart.*, *41*:268–280, 1967.

9. Siede, H., Müller, H.F. Choreoform dyskinesia as side effect of phenothiazine medication in geriatric patients. *J. Am. Geriatrics Soc.*, *15*:517–522, 1967.

10. Crane, G.E. Tardive dyskinesia in schizophrenic patients treated with psychotropic drugs. *Aggressologie*, *9*:209–218, 1968.

11. Eckmann, F. Zur Problematik von Dauerschanden nach neuroleptischer Langzeitbehandelung. *Ther. Ggw.*, *107*:316–323, 1968.

12. Heinrich, K., Wegener, I., Bener, H.J. Spate extrapyramydale Hyperkinesen be neuroleptischer Langzeit-Therapie. *Pharmakopsychiatr., Neuropsychopharmakol.*, *1*:169–195, 1968.

13. Paulson, G.W. Permanent or complex dyskinesias in the aged. *Geriatrics, 23*:105–110, 1968.

14. Greenblatt, D.L., Stotsky, B.A., DiMascio, A. Phenothiazine-induced dyskinesia in nursing home patients. *J. Amer. Geriatrics Soc.*, *16*:27–34, 1968.

15. Villineuve, A., Lavalee, J.C., Limieus, L.H. Dyskinesia tardive post-neuroleptique. *Laval Med.*, *40*:832–827, 1969.

16. Edwards, H. The significance of brain damage in persistent oral dyskinesia. *Br. J. Psychiatry, 116*:271–275, 1970.

17. Dynes, J.B. Oral dyskinesia, occurrence and treatment. *Dis. Nerv. Syst., 31*:854–859, 1970.

18. Hippius, H., Lang, J. Zur Problematik der spaten extrapyramydalen Hyperkinesen nach langfristiger neuroleptischer Therapie. *Arzneim. Forsch.*, *20*:888–890, 1970.

19. Crane, G.E. High doses of trifluoperazine and tardive dyskinesia. *Arch. Neurol.*, *33*:176–180, 1970.

20. Lehman, H.L., Ban, T.A., Saxena, B.M. A survey of extrapyramidal manifestations in the inpatient population of a psychiatric hospital. *Laval Med., 41*:909–916, 1970.

21. Poxburg, P.A. Treatment of phenothiazine induced oral dyskinesia. *Br. J. Psychiatry, 116*:277–280, 1970.

22. Kennedy, P.F., Hershon, I.H., McGuire, R.J. Extrapyramidal disorders after prolonged phenothiazine therapy. *Br. J. Psychiatry, 118*:509–518, 1971.

23. Brandon, S., McClelland, H.A., Protheroe, C. A study of facial dyskinesia in a mental hospital population. *Br. J. Psychiatry, 118*:171–184, 1971.

24. Fann, W.E., Davis, J.M., Janowsky, D.S. The prevalence of tardive dyskinesia in mental hospital patients. *Dis. Nerv. Syst., 33*:182–186, 1972.

25. Crane, G.E. Persistent dyskinesia. *Br. J. Psychiatry, 122*:395–405, 1973.

26. Crane, G.E., Smeets, R.A. Tardive dyskinesia and drug therapy in geriatric patients. *Arch. Gen. Psychiatry, 30*:341–343, 1974.

27. Jus, A., Pineau, R., Lachance, G., Pelchat, K., Jus, K., Pires, P., Villeneuve, R. Epidemiology of tardive dyskinesia. Part I. *Dis. Nerv. Syst., 37*:210–214, 1976.

28. Bell, R.C.H., Smith, R.C. Tardive dyskinesia: characterization and prevalence in a statewide system. *J. Clin. Psychiatry, 39*:39–47, 1978.

29. Hunter, R., Earl, C.J., Janz, D. A syndrome of abnormal movements and dementia in leucotomized patients treated with phenothiazines. *J. Neuro. Neurochirur. Psychiatry, 27*:219–223, 1964.

30. Faurbye, A., Rasch, P.J., Petersen, P.B., Brandborg, G., Pakkenberg, H. Neurological symptoms in pharmacotherapy of psychosis. *Acta Psychiatr., Scand., 40*:10–27, 1964.

31. Dincmen, K. Chronic psychotic choreo-athetosis. *Dis. Nerv. Syst., 27*:399–402, 1966.

32. Annis, G., Leopold, M., Duvoisin, R., Schwartz, A.H. A survey of tardive dyskinesia in psychiatric out-patients. *Am. J. Psychiatry, 134*:1367–1370, 1977.

33. Hunter, R., Earl, C.J., Thornicroft, S. An apparently irreversible syndrome of abnormal movements following phenothiazine medication. *Proc. Roy. Soc. Med., 57*:758–762, 1964.

34. Crane, G.E., Naranjo, E.R. Motor disorders induced by neuroleptics: a proposed new classification. *Arch. Gen. Psychiatry, 24*:179–184, 1971.

35. Tarsy, D., Granacher, R., Braloneer, M. Tardive dyskinesia in young adults. *Am J. Psychiatry, 134*:1032–1034, 1977.

36. Delay, J., Deniker, P., Dalle, B., Colonna, L. Syndrome choreique idiopathique rappelant la semiologie dimpregnation chronique parles neuroleptiques. *Ann. Medico-psychol., 125*:784–788, 1967.

37. Graux, P., Arnott, G., Pettit, H., Piquet, B. Dyskinesies bucco-linguals reversibles des personnes agees. Societe Fransaise de Neurologie, Seance, May 8, 1969.

38. Appenzeller, O., Biehl, J.P. Mouthing in the elderly. *Neurology, 17*:290.

39. Altrocchi, P.H. Spontaneous oral facial dyskinesia. *Arch. Neurol., 26*:506–511, 1972.

40. Sutcher, H.D., Underwood, R.B., Beatty, R., Sugar, D. Orofacial dyskinesia. *JAMA, 216*:1459–1463.

41. Crane, G.E. Tardive dyskinesia and Huntington's chorea: drug-induced and hereditary dyskinesias. In *Advances in Neurology*, vol. 1, Barbeau, A., Chases, T.N., Paulson, G.W. (eds.). New York: Raven Press, pp. 115–122.

25

Neuroleptic Drugs and Other Factors Predisposing to Tardive Dyskinesia

GEORGE E. CRANE

INTRODUCTION

Although epidemiological evidence clearly implicates neuroleptic drugs in the etiology of tardive dyskinesia (TD), the relationship of types of neuroleptics, dose of neuroleptics, or other treatment, medical conditions, or characteristics of the patient to the risks for developing tardive dyskinesia have not been well defined. Two previous studies (1,2) show that very high doses of chlorpromazine and trifluperazine (administered in two experimental projects) predisposed patients to TD. This chapter will review two studies based on patients who received more routine treatment with neuroleptics.

STUDY 1

Methods

Subjects in this first study were 669 patients selected from the chronically hospitalized population of Spring Grove State Hospital. They were selected from a larger population of 900 patients, who were surveyed for tardive dyskinesia by the author and his associates in 1970; 231 patients were excluded because of poor cooperation or inadequacy of available medical records. Some characteristics of the patient population and their drug treatment is summarized in Table 1. Records of the patients' drug history were obtained from their medical charts, and any indications of neurological disorders were obtained from medical histories, laboratory tests, and clinical evaluations. All neuroleptic medication was converted to chlorpromazine equivalents (CPZ-E).

A number of the variables used in this study are defined below:

1. *Maximum dose of neuroleptics*. This is based on the highest doses prescribed for at least 6 months at any one time during the course of treatment. In those cases in which the highest dose was administered for less than 6 months, it was averaged with the next highest dose.

2. *Duration of treatment*. This is the number of years of drug therapy. If this could not be determined in a specific patient because of frequent or prolonged absences from the hospital or an inadequate medical record, the patient was excluded from the study.

3. *Continuity of treatment*. This is the percentage of years of neuroleptic drug exposure from the initiation of neuroleptic treatment up to 1970, when the drug-history survey was conducted (i.e., number of years on neuroleptics; 1970 was year first treated with neuroleptics).

4. *Antiparkinsonian medication*. This refers to the antiparkinsonian drugs administered at the time of the drug-history survey.

5. *Central nervous system (CNS) disorder*. This includes organic brain diseases diagnosed at the time of admission or in the course of hospitalization. It also includes specific conditions, such as convulsive disorders, postleucotomy status, or active or inactive CNS syphilis. (Patients with other neurological diseases which manifest themselves in extrapyramidal disorders—Huntington's chorea, viral encephalitis, or clear idiopathic parkinsonism—are not included in the sample.)

Symptoms of TD and parkinsonism were recorded separately and were rated on a scale ranging from a minimum of 0 to a maximum of 6 for each disorder.

Table 1
Characteristics of Chronic Patients in Drug History Study

1. Median age	53 years
2. Sex	Male 287, female 382
3. Median maximum dose	430 mg
4. Median duration treatment	6.5 years
5. Continuous treatment	> 90%, 217; <90%, 452
6. Median current dose	240 mg
7. Antiparkinsonian medication	Yes 165, no 504
8. CNS disorder	Yes 112, no 557
9. Median total years hospitalized	16
10. Median years continuous hospitalization	12

All examinations were carried out without knowledge of drug history or neurological diseases of the patient.

Results

The prevalence of TD and parkinsonian symptoms in this sample, which is summarized in Table 2, is comparable to that of other studies of samples reporting a fairly high percentage of tardive dyskinesia. There were, however, relatively few (2.4%) cases which were rated as very severe. Parkinsonian symptoms are less prevalent than those of TD in this sample. Since the sample included a considerable number of elderly patients, some of the parkinsonian symptoms may be due to age.

Table 3 shows the results of a correlation analysis investigating the relationship of several drug-history, epidemiological, and disease variables to TD

Table 2
Prevalence of Tardive Dyskinesia and Parkinsonism

Severity Rating of Symptoms	Tardive Dyskinesia		Parkinsonism	
	Number	%	Number	%
Minimal (1, 2)	213	32	159	24
Moderate (3, 4)	71	11	65	10
Severe (5, 6)	16	2.4	17	2.5

Table 3
Coefficient of Correlation (r) between Tardive Dyskinesia and Drug History

	Zero Order Correlation	Partial Correlation with TD Controlling for						
dis.	Tard. dysk.	Age	Mx dose	Dur. tr.	Cont. tr.	Curr. ds	Antpk.	CNS dis.
1. Age	0.2496	—	0.2636	0.2515	0.2746	0.2441	0.2609	0.2521
2. Max. dose	0.0720	0.1902	—	NS	NS	0.1561	NS	NS
3. Dur. treat.	0.1409	0.1423	0.1214	—	NS	0.1734	0.1277	0.1402
4. Cont. treat.	0.0500	NS	NS	NS	—	NS	NS	NS
5. Curr. dose	-0.0627	NS	-0.1521	-0.1200	NS	—	NS	NS
6. Antipark.	0.1200	0.1453	NS	NS	NS	0.1356	—	0.1200
7. CNS dis.	-0.0155	NS	NS	NS	NS	NS	NS	—

Note: r with absolute value > 0.12 is statistically significant at $p < .01$

scores in this sample of patients. Older age was significantly related to higher TD scores, and this finding is consistent with the results of many other epidemiological surveys of this disorder. Contrary to some speculations, preexisting CNS disease was not related to the development in TD. This is seen both in nonsignificant zero order correlation as well as in the partial correlations which controlled for some other possible confounding variables.

Several drug treatment variables were related to TD, as is evident in either zero order or partial correlations with TD scores. The maximum dose of neuroleptics a patient had received was positively related to his TD score, whereas his current neuroleptic dose was negatively related to TD score. Although there was no statistically significant correlation between maximum dose and TD score in the zero order correlation, there was a significant positive correlation of maximum neuroleptic dose and TD score when either the variables of age or current dose were controlled for. The patient's current dose had a slight (nonsignificant) negative relationship to this TD score in the zero order correlation, and this relationship became more significantly negative when either maximum dose or duration of treatment was controlled for in partial correlations. The number of years a patient had been treated with neuroleptics (duration of treatment variable) was positively and significantly related to his TD score as evident both in zero order correlation and most of the partial correlations. However, the percent of time the patient was on neuroleptics during his total duration of treatment (continuity of treatment variable) was not significantly related to TD score in either the zero order or partial correlations. Antiparkinsonian medication the patient was on at the time of evaluation for TD was positively related to his TD score, and this relationship became slightly stronger when age or current dose of neuroleptics was controlled for in partial correlations.

Data on the effects of length of hospitalization on TD were not reported in Table 3, because the correlation between the duration of hospitalization and duration of treatment was so high that the separation of these two effects was impossible. Consequently a smaller subsample (287 patients) admitted to the hospital prior to 1955 (the year when wide-scale use of neuroleptics began at Spring Grove) was also analyzed. In this subsample there was no significant relationship between years of hospitalization and duration of treatment. The coefficient of correlation between TD score and hospitalization in this subsample was + .05. This suggests that institutionalization in a mental hospital itself does not produce neurological side effects manifested as TD, at least in a very chronic patient population.

In view of the importance of age as a contributor to tardive dyskinesia, the variable maximum doses and durations of treatment were also analyzed separately in a sample of 311 patients 55 years of age or older. (See Figs. 1 and 2.) In this subsample all the correlations between either maximum dose or duration of treatment and TD score were significantly positive. The prevalence of TD

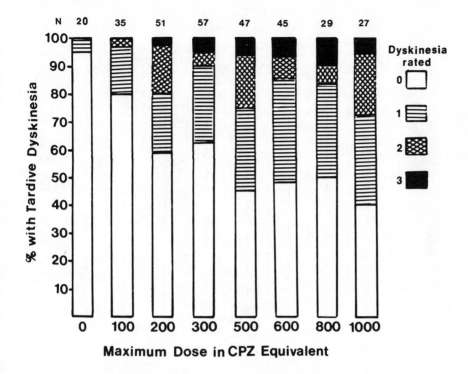

Figure 1.   Maximum dose of neuroleptics and tardive dyskinesia in patients over the age of
55. See text for definition of maximum dose and tardive dyskinesia ratings.

increased sharply in subjects who received in excess of 200 mg of chlorpromazine equivalent for 6 months or longer. In patients receiving 500 mg/day
CPZ-E for 6 months or longer, total TD prevalence was about 50% to 55%, but
did not seem to increase any further with higher doses of neuroleptics, although slightly more moderate and severe cases were found at the highest
neuroleptic dose level. Similarly, the prevalence of TD became quite substantial in patients receiving 2 years of neuroleptic therapy, and it continued to
increase in a montonic fashion with increasing duration of treatment up to 8
years of duration of treatment. In this subsample, patients who were treated for
short periods of time also received rather small doses of neuroleptics.

STUDY 2

The second study was conducted between 1970 and 1972 at Spring Grove
State Hospital. It focused on geriatric psychiatric patients above the age of 60
whose illness required hospitalization.

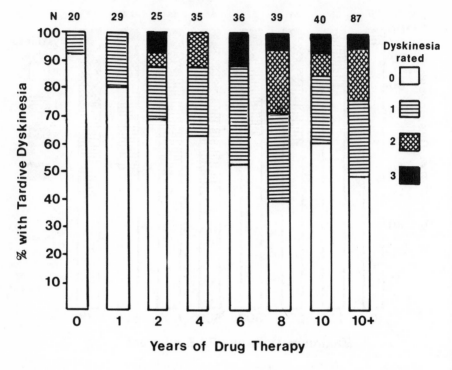

Figure 2.   Duration of neuroleptic therapy and tardive dyskinesia in patients over the age of 55. See text for definitions of variables.

Method

All patients admitted to the Geriatric Services of Spring Grove State Hospital beginning in January 1970 were included in the study, providing they met the following criteria: (1) They had no previous treatment with neuroleptic drugs or admissions to mental hospitals, except for short confinement in hospitals which had well-documented drug histories, so that we could be certain that there was no substantial prior neuroleptic exposure; (2) they were not bedridden; and (3) they were being treated with one or more neuroleptic drugs at the time of admission to the study. A number of patients who had never received neuroleptic drugs were also included to provide a continuum drug exposure from zero to a maximum during the 28-month study duration.

The 39 patients who qualified for the study had the following characteristics: sex—24 male, 15 female; age—median 74 years; range—63–89 years; length of hospitalization—median 14 months; range—1–29 months.

Drug history data was recorded for the length of time the patient was treated with neuroleptics. Drug variables were similar to those described in Study 1 with the following considerations: (a) The time span was much shorter since no patients had received neuroleptics prior to entering the study; and (b) maximum dose was the dose prescribed at any given time during the course of neuroleptic therapy, and there was *no* requirement that this dose had to be maintained for at least 6 months.

The rating of TD was based exclusively on motor abnormalities observed in the oral region with a six-point scale: 0, absent; 1, questionable; 2, minimal; 3, moderate; 4, moderately severe; 5, severe; and 6, extremely severe. (However, the last two ratings were not used, since no patient exhibited dyskinesia of a severe nature.) Oral dyskinesia rather than total body dyskinesia was rated, because motor disorders in other parts of the body could not be assessed with any degree of objectivity in this population. After the first TD rating, all patients were taken off medications and then were reexamined after 2 and 12 weeks of cessation of neuroleptics.

Results

Moderate dyskinesia was observed at one or more ratings in 12 of the patients, while another 15 patients exhibited only questionable or minimal manifestations of TD (scores 1 or 2) at one or more ratings. The fact that 4 of the patients who had questionable or minimal ratings had no history of drug treatment with neuroleptics indicates that a low grade of motor abnormality in the oral region may not be drug-induced in a geriatric population of this type.

Ten of the 19 patients who had received a total amount of neuroleptics above the median of 16.2 gms CPZ equivalent manifested TD of at least moderate proportions, while only 2 of the remaining 20 were so affected (Fishers exact test, $p = .005$). In a similar analysis carried out on the 31 patients who had received neuroleptics, the difference in the prevalence of TD between these patients who had received higher versus patients on lower amounts of neuroleptics (divided at the median dose) was also significant (Fishers exact test, $p = 0.05$). When patients were subdivided on other variables—maximum dose (median of 75 mg), or duration of treatment (median 11 months)—Fishers exact test analysis of the samples divided at the median showed similar results: patients with drug history above the median on these variables had significantly more cases of TD. Correlation of analysis gave similar results. The total amount of neuroleptics (grams CPZ equivalents) a patient had received was significantly correlated with the severity of his dyskinesia at the initial evaluation ($r = .31$, $p < .05$), and at 2 weeks ($r = .46$, $p < .01$). Maximum dose was also correlated with dyskinesia score at 2 weeks.

Table 4
Relationship between Total Amount of Neuroleptics and Occurrence of Tardive Dyskinesia in Geriatric Patients (All Patients)

		Tardive Dyskinesia Present*	Absent*
Total neuroleptics†	> 16 gms	10	9
	< 16 gms	2	18

*Present = score of at least 3 on one of three ratings. Absent = all TD scores 0–2.
†Total Neuroleptics since admission to hospitals in gms CPZ equivalents. Statistical significance: Fisher's exact test, p = .005.

Table 5
Relationship between Tardive Dyskinesia and Maximal Daily Dose of Neuroleptics in Geriatric Patients Treated with Neuroleptics

		Tardive Dyskinesia Present*	Absent*
Maximal dose† Neuroleptic	> 75 mg	10	8
	≤ 75 mg	2	11

*See legend to Table 4.
†Maximal dose on neuroleptics (CPZ equivalents) on any day of treatment. Statistical significance: Fisher's exact test, p = .027.

DISCUSSION

It should be realized that data obtained from these types of largely retrospective studies of drug history must be interpreted with some caution, because the administration of drugs, their dosage, and use of antiparkinsonian agents were not random procedures. However, it is important to note that both studies showed TD significantly related to drug-history variables, especially maximum dose of neuroleptics. The use of high doses of neuroleptics and the concomitant use of antiparkinsonian medication contributes to TD primarily in older patients, a finding which is in agreement with the results from a previous study (1). This correlation of drug-history variables with TD appeared stronger in the older geriatric population (Study 2). In these geriatric patients, the total amount of neuroleptics a patient had received was also significantly correlated with TD. However, in the geriatric patients the neuroleptic doses were considerably lower; only 3 of the patients in Study 2 had a maximum dose of 200 mg CPZ equivalents per day, whereas in the subsample of patients over 55 from Study 1 the majority of patients had a maximum dose of CPZ equivalents over 200 mg. In the larger Study 1 subsample of patients over 55 years of age, the prevalence of TD rose sharply in patients with maximum doses over 200 mg CPZ equivalents per day, whereas in the somewhat older geriatric sample of Study 2, 10 of the 12 patients with at least moderate dyskinesia had maximum doses of below 200 mg CPZ equivalents per day. This suggests that in older geriatric patients (i.e., over 60), the maximum dose threshold for significant risk of TD may be considerably lower than in a somewhat younger sample of elderly patients.

Duration of treatment with neuroleptics, especially more than 2 years of treatment with neuroleptics, is related to the development of TD. The duration of treatment variable may not provide satisfactory information as to the length of drug exposure necessary for the development of TD, because the symptoms detected at the time of the surveys may have been present for an unknown length of time prior to this date. The appearance of the TD syndrome, however, increases sharply after the second year of neuroleptic therapy.

Our studies show that organic brain disease (at least as a medical diagnosis rather than as a rate or a degree of intellectual impairment) was not related to TD score, and therefore they suggest that this may not be an important risk factor. This result is in agreement with some previous studies. However, the patient's age is unquestionably an important risk factor for TD, and it interacts with the toxicity of neuroleptic drugs.

It is important to bear in mind, however, that the age and drug-history variables explain only a relatively small part of the variation in TD scores. Although the partial correlations between the independent variables— maximum dose of neuroleptics, total amount of neuroleptics, or duration of treatment—and the dependent variable, TD, were statistically significant, they were fairly small, generally .20 or less in the larger study. Each of the drug-history factors would "explain" (based on the value of r^2) less than 5% or 10% of the variability in TD ratings. Even the highest correlation ($r = .46$) between total amount of neuroleptics and TD score found at the second TD rating in the older geriatric sample (Study 2) would only explain about 20% of the variation in TD scores. Other factors, undefined in these studies, relating to the individuals' vulnerability to neurotoxicity of neuroleptics must therefore also play a major role. Otherwise, it would be difficult to explain why certain subjects in their 30's and 40's do develop rather severe dyskinesia after an intake of neuroleptic medication which is small to moderate, while a sizable percentage of elderly subjects do not show signs of TD despite fairly extensive exposure to neuroleptic drugs. Since these individual vulnerability factors have not been identified, however, the physician should be cautious in the administration of neuroleptic drugs, especially high doses, for all patients.

REFERENCES

1. Crane, G.E. Tardive dyskinesia in schizophrenic patients treated with psychotropic drugs. *Aggressologie*, *9*:209–218, 1968.
2. Crane, G.E. High doses of trifluoperazine and tardive dyskinesia. *Arch. Neurol.*, *33*:176–180, 1970.

26

Drug Variables in the Etiology of Tardive Dyskinesia: Application of Discriminant Function Analysis

GEORGE GARDOS
JONATHAN O. COLE
and RICHARD A. LA BRIE

INTRODUCTION

Clinical descriptions of schizophrenia have tended to emphasize charac-teristic movement abnormalities, such as stereotypies and mannerisms (1). During the late 1950's a syndrome was described, characterized by sponta-neous involuntary movements of the face, mouth, tongue, and the extremities (2), which has come to be known as persistent or tardive dys-kinesia. This syndrome is generally believed to be associated with the pro-longed administration of neuroleptics. However, since this issue is still de-bated (3), it is necessary to summarize the evidence implicating neuroleptics in the etiology of tardive dyskinesia.

1. There is a temporal association between neuroleptic treatment and the onset of tardive dyskinesia. Tardive dyskinesia has only been reported since the introduction of neuroleptics and published prevalence rates have tended to increase over the years paralleling the increase in the number of patients who have been on drugs for many years. For instance, Villeneuve *et al.* (4) found that 2.2% of drug-treated hospitalized patients showed tardive dyskinesia.

Approximately eight years later a group of investigators using the same rating scale in a similar population obtained a prevalence rate of 56% (5). Whatever other factors may have played a role in this astonishing increase in prevalence rate, one may safely conclude that there has been a significant increase in the number of tardive dyskinesia cases during the last ten years.

There are also numerous case reports documenting the appearance of tardive dyskinesia following neuroleptic therapy supporting the association between neuroleptic therapy and the onset of dyskinesia.

2. Studies comparing neuroleptic-treated with nondrug-treated patient groups show significantly more tardive dyskinesia among drug-treated patients (6,7,8). While one can always question the comparability of drug and nondrug groups, it is reasonable to accept these data as strong indirect evidence implicating neuroleptics.

3. The demonstration that withdrawal or dose reduction of dopamine-blocking drugs (9,10,11) or the administration of L-dopa (12) is often followed by increased dyskinesia supports the notion that dopaminergic mechanisms are involved and thus tends to confirm indirectly the connection between prolonged neuroleptic therapy and tardive dyskinesia.

The implication of neuroleptics in the etiology of tardive dyskinesia warrants the investigation of the relative contribution of drug variables such as type of drug, dosage, length of treatment, and the interaction of drug and nondrug variables. As to the type of neuroleptics which may cause tardive dyskinesia, the most accurate statement that can be made is that any neuroleptic drug has the capacity to induce tardive dyskinesia. Since it has been suggested that patients who develop pseudoparkinsonism (13) are more likely to be later afflicted with tardive dyskinesia, piperazine phenothiazines such as perphenazine (Trilafon) have been assumed to be more likely to lead to tardive dyskinesia than drugs such as thioridazine (Mellaril), which has a lower propensity for causing pseudoparkinsonism. The evidence in favor of this hypothesis, however, is not convincing. Amount and duration of neuroleptic medication have been found by some studies to be associated with tardive dyskinesia, but these findings are by no means unanimous.

The role of long-acting phenothiazines in the pathogenesis of tardive dyskinesia is undetermined. It can be argued that since maintenance therapy with injectible neuroleptics such as fluphenazine decanoate (Prolixin Decanoate) tends to introduce lower mg amounts of the drug into the body than corresponding oral dosage, depot fluphenazine therapy would be less likely to induce tardive dyskinesia. Conversely, one might argue that depot fluphenazine releases the drug less evenly than oral dosage, leading to fluctuating concentrations in the blood and in the brain and thereby sensitizing dopamine receptors more readily. Unfortunately, systematic comparisons between oral and depot therapy as they relate to dyskinesia are not available as yet.

The status of research regarding non-drug variables is rather confusing. There is fairly good evidence suggesting older age and female sex are contributing factors, but the evidence implicating variables such as EST or brain damage is less clear cut.

The problem in isolating etiological factors contributing to the development of tardive dyskinesia is basically threefold. First, there are too many demographic and treatment variables to consider in each patient. It is an exceptional patient who has not had several different neuroleptics and perhaps EST as well. Second, the assessment methods employed leave a great deal to be desired in terms of sensitivity, reliability, and validity. Third, the univariate statistical approach which has been utilized in almost all of the studies so far cannot deal adequately with highly correlated variables, such as age, dose, duration of treatment, and chronicity.

The study sample consisted of 50 chronic psychotic state hospital inpatients. Data on demographic variables and on those drug and non-drug treatment variables thought to be important in the causation of tardive dyskinesia were obtained by examination of the medical records going back 10–20 years or more in many cases. Neuroleptics were classified as low-potency and high-potency types to test whether the latter showed higher correlations with dyskinesia.

Tardive dyskinesia was assessed by a rating scale developed by G.M. Simpson at Rockland State Hospital (14). It consists of 33 items denoting commonly observed abnormal movements in patients with tardive dyskinesia rated on 2- or 4-point scales. Using the scale, we have achieved interrater reliability of .92 for total score (sum of 33 items) (15). On the basis of the total score, patients were assigned to ''dyskinesia group'' (score of 40 or more, N = 23) and ''no dyskinesia group'' (score of 39 or less, N = 27). While the cutoff score is somewhat arbitrary, it was chosen on the basis of a frequency distribution of scores in 100 patients. The Simpson total scores showed a correlation of .78 with global ratings of dyskinesia obtained simultaneously.

In order to determine which variables discriminated best between the dyskinesia and no dyskinesia groups, a stepwise discriminant function analysis was carried out. In this statistical procedure discriminators are entered to the equation in successive steps. The variable to be entered at each step has the largest unique contribution to discrimination.

RESULTS

Tables 1 and 2 summarize the data obtained from the medical record. The patient sample was predominantly male chronic schizophrenics who have received large quantities of neuroleptics of several kinds over a long period of time. Total amount was evenly divided between low- and high-potency drugs.

DISCUSSION

According to the discriminant function equation, three drug variables—the number of months on low-potency neuroleptics, time since initial neuroleptic therapy began, and total amount of depot fluphenazine received—and two other variables—abnormal EEG and previous EST—significantly predicted

Table 1
Demographic and Non-Drug Treatment Variables

Sex	39 men	
	11 women	
Age	23-65 $\bar{x}$ = 47.5 ± 13.0	
Previous EST		# patients
	Yes	22
	No	28
Abnormal neurological	Definite	20
findings	Questionable	5
	None	25
EEG	Abnormal	10
	Questionable	4
	Normal	36
Total dosage of	None	6
antiparkinson drugs	Low	21
	Moderate	18
	Heavy	5

Table 2
Drug Variables

	Range	Mean ± S.D.
Total amount of neuroleptics (in gram CPZ eq.)	28–4595	1769 ± 1367
Length of neuroleptic therapy (in years)	2–21	14.3 ± 4.8
Maximum dose for at least one month (in mg CPZ eq.)	90–4750	1430 ± 1048
Total amount of depot fluphenazine (in gram CPZ eq.)	0–500	60.0 ± 98.2

	Low potency	High potency
Types of Drugs	Chlorpromazine	Piperazines
	Thioridazine	Thiothixene
	Mesoridazine	Haloperidol
	Chlorprothixene	Molindone
Total amount	0–3162	0–6244
(in gram CPZ eq.)	$\bar{x}$ = 839 ± 809	$\bar{x}$ = 836 ± 997
Duration of treatment	0–152	0–171
(in months)	$\bar{x}$ = 62.1 ± 41.9	$\bar{x}$ = 52.1 ± 44.3

Table 3
Discriminant Function Analysis

	Significance	D.F. coefficient	Dyskinesia group vs. no dyskinesia group
Duration of low-potency neuroleptic treatment	.001	.20	$t = 3.01\, p < .005$
Previous EST	.001	.10	$t = 1.65\, p < .11$
Length of neuroleptic therapy	.002	.12	$t = 2.77\, p < .01$
Total amount of depot fluphenazine	.003	.13	$t = 2.15\, p < .05$
EEG	.004	.12	$t = 1.74\, p < .09$

membership in the dyskinesia group. In view of the modest sample size, only tentative conclusions can be offered. The data do not support the notion that piperazines and other high-potency neuroleptics are more strongly associated with tardive dyskinesia than low-potency neuroleptics. The emergence of low-potency neuroleptic duration as a strong discriminator was unexpected and is not readily explicable. The amount of depot fluphenazine also contributed significantly to discrimination. There is no unequivocal clinical interpretation which can be given, since most fluphenazine patients also received other neuroleptics at different times. However, the fact that depot fluphenazine treatment was a significant discriminator is compatible with the hypothesis that injectible neuroleptics are more, rather than less, likely to lead to tardive dyskinesia than comparable oral therapy. The emergence of previous EST and abnormal EEG in the equation tends to support research which has implicated these variables in the etiology of tardive dyskinesia. Contrary to some research, however, in our study sex, age, diagnosis, antiparkinson use, and high potency neuroleptics did not contribute significantly to the discrimination.

The stepwise discriminant function procedure appears to be suitable for the study of etiological factors. Our five discriminators correctly classified 74% of cases. However, remembering that pure guessing would achieve 50% correct assignment, it is obvious that our equation is not particularly powerful. Increasing the sample size, obtaining complete drug-history information and maximizing the validity, reliability, and sensitivity of the method used for assessing tardive dyskinesia would undoubtedly result in better discrimination in future studies.

ACKNOWLEDGMENTS

This investigation was supported by NIH Research Grant MH 27505 from the National Institute of Mental Health.

REFERENCES

1. Marsden, C.D., Tarsy, D., Baldessarini, R.J. Spontaneous and drug-induced movement disorders in psychotic patients. In *Psychiatric Aspects of Neurological Disease*. Benson, D.F., Blumer, D. (eds.). New York: Grune and Stratton, pp. 219–266, 1975.
2. Sigwald, J., Bouttier, D., Courvoisier, S. Les accidents neurologiques des medications neuroleptiques. *Rev. Neurol.*, *100*:553–595, 1959.
3. Turek, I.S. Drug-induced dyskinesia: reality or myth? *Dis. Nerv. Syst.*, *36*:397–399, 1975.
4. Villeneuve, A., Lavalle, J.C., Lemieux, L.H. Dyskinesie tardive postneuroleptique. *Laval Med.*, *40*:832–837, 1969.
5. Jus, A., Pineau, R., Lachance, R., Pelchat, G., Jus, K., Pires, P., Villeneuve, R. Epidemiology of tardive dyskinesia. Part I. *Dis. Nerv. Syst.*, *37*:210–214, 1976.
6. Faurbye, A., Rasch, P.J., Bender, H.J., Peterson, P., Brandborg, G., Pakkenberg, H. Neurological symptoms in pharmacotherapy of psychosis. *Acta Psychiatr. Scand.*, *40*:10–27, 1964.
7. Heinrich, K., Wegener, I., Bender, H.J. Spate Extrapyramidale Hyperkinesen bei neuroleptischer Langzeittherapie. *Pharmakopsychiatr. Neuropsychopharmakol.*, *1*:169–195, 1968.
8. Crane, G.E. Dyskinesia and neuroleptics. *Arch. Gen. Psychiatry, 19*:700–703, 1968.
9. Pryce, I.G., Edwards, H. Persistent oral dyskinesia in female mental hospital patients. *Br. J. Psychiatry, 112*:983–987, 1966.
10. Degkwitz, R., Wenzel, W. Persistent extrapyramidal side effects after long-term application of neuroleptics. In *Neuropsychopharmacology* (International Congress Series #129). Brill, H. (ed.). New York: Excerpta Medica, pp. 608–615, 1967.
11. Gardos, G., Cole, J.O. Maintenance antipsychotic therapy: is the cure worse than the disease? *Am. J. Psychiatry, 133*:32–36, 1976.
12. Hippius, H., Logemann, G. Zur Wirkung von Dioxyphenylalanin (L-dopa) auf extrapyramidalmotorische Hyperkinesen nach langfristiger neuroleptischer Therapie. *Arzneim. Forsch.*, *20*:894–895, 1970.
13. Crane, G.E. Persistent dyskinesia. *Br. J. Psychiatry, 122*:395–405, 1973.
14. Simpson, G.M., Zoubok, B., Lee, H.J. An early clinical and toxicity trial of Ex 11–532A in chronic schizophrenia. *Curr. Ther. Res., 19*:87–93, 1976.
15. Gardos, G., Sokol, M., Cole, J.O., Sniffin, C. Eye color and tardive dyskinesia. *Psychopharmacol. Bull., 22*:(2), 7–9, 1976.

27

Past History of Drug and Somatic Treatments in Tardive Dyskinesia

CHING-PIAO CHIEN
ANITA ROSS-TOWNSEND
and MAUREEN DONNELLY

Although involuntary choreoathetoid movements similar to tardive dyskinesia may occur in 1 to 3 percent of the population that has never received neuroleptics (1,2), the prevalence of tardive dyskinesia among the neuroleptic-treated patients ranges from 0.5% to as high as 56% in the literature (3,4). While the diversity of prevalence may be attributable to the different degrees of severity of symptoms used for inclusion criteria, as well as to sex, age and setting of the population, it is fairly consistent that neuroleptics are considered to be the major causative agents for this syndrome (1,4–9). With the advent of new knowledge regarding the neuropharmacological mechanism of neuroleptics at the synaptic site, it is postulated that after a prolonged period of blockade of dopamine receptors by neuroleptics, disuse supersensitivity of dopamine receptors in the nigrostriatal system may occur as the pathophysiology of tardive dyskinesia (10–15). Based on this hypothesis, clinicians were cautioned that (1) anticholinergic antiparkinsonian agents could worsen tardive dyskinesia due to their potentiation of dopaminergic activity as the result of inhibition of cholinergic activity (16); (2) dopamine-depleting agents, such as reserpine or tetrabenazine, may lead to dyskinesia after a prolonged period of depleting dopamine at the presynaptic neuron, leading to disuse supersensitivity at the postsynaptic dopamine receptors (17,18); (3) patients with previous history of possible CNS damage—due to either CNS infection, convulsion and head trauma, excessive electroconvulsive treatment, insulin shock treatment, or lobotomy—were vulnerable to tardive dyskinesia (19–21). It was suggested that preexisting subclinical pathology of the nigrostriatal system might cause impaired presynaptic reuptake and inactivation of dopamine, leading to dopaminergic hyperactivity (22,23).

Reflecting the public concerns on tardive dyskinesia, Massachusetts and New York have recently planned state-wide education programs to familiarize mental health workers with this syndrome (24,25). Precautionary measures, such as drug holidays and minimum therapeutic dosage, among others, are emphasized. While part of these precautions frequently noted in the recent literature has been validated by epidemiological and clinical data analyses, some of them, such as the preventive effect of drug holidays, are based purely on logical speculation. More data based on retrospective and prospective studies are needed. The present study was designed to explore the following hypotheses, with the hope that the more information will be available for generalization and confirmation as to the causative factors of tardive dyskinesia and for the future prevention of this alarming syndrome:

1. The total lifetime dosage of dopamine-blocking neuroleptics is higher in dyskinetic patients than in nondyskinetic patients.

2. The total lifetime dosage of dopamine-depleting agents, such as reserpine, is higher in dyskinetic patients than in nondyskinetic patients.

3. The total lifetime dosage of anticholinergic antiparkinsonian agents is higher in dyskinetic patients than in nondyskinetic patients.

4. Tardive dyskinesia is not dose-related to catecholamine- or indolamine-potentiating agents, such as tricyclic antidepressants or methylphenidate.

5. Past history of CNS events is more frequent in dyskinetic patients than in non-dyskinetic patients.

6. Dyskinetic patients have had longer duration on neuroleptics, and shorter and less frequent drug-free periods, than nondyskinetic counterparts.

7. Although depot fluphenazine has been identified to be highly used in dyskinetic groups (8,9), the total oral neuroleptic dosage prior to depot-fluphenazine treatment is higher in dyskinetic patients than in nondyskinetic patients.

8. Dyskinetic patients were exposed more frequently to and received a greater amount of high-potency neuroleptics than did the nondyskinetic patients.

METHOD

All clinicians in the Albany Medical College—Capital District Psychiatric Center—Veterans Administration consortium were asked to nominate patients who exhibited abnormal involuntary movements. These patients were screened by two psychiatrists for tardive dyskinesia (TD), which resulted in a total of 31 patients ascertained for the definite presence of TD on the Abnormal Involuntary Movement Scale (i.e., mild, moderate, or severe on Item 8).

Because these patients were drawn from several heterogeneously different treatment units and each treatment unit was believed to be a possible important source of variance, control subjects were also chosen from the same unit where the dyskinetic patients came from to match the number and demographic characteristics of tardive dyskinesia patients. The various subgroups matched for age, sex, chronicity, diagnosis, and race were combined to constitute the control group consisting of 31 patients.

The results of this matching process and a demographic description of the TD and non-TD samples appear in Table 1. It should be noted that the two groups are not significantly different at the 5% level of confidence in any respect.

Procedure

A medical student was assigned to perform chart reviews of each TD and non-TD subject, collecting all pertinent information on past drug history and selected neurological and somatic treatment variables. A total lifetime drug intake for each patient was computed within each drug category. For neuroleptic drugs, total lifetime drug intake was calculated by converting each neuroleptic drug into chlorpromazine milligram equivalents, with the exception of depot fluphenazine, for which no generally accepted conversion formula exists. Hollister's conversion chart was employed for this purpose (26). Reserpine was separated from all dopamine-blocking neuroleptics and was calculated independently as a dopamine-depleting agent. For the analysis of differences among the two groups in high-potency neuroleptic drugs used, any neuroleptic with chlorpromazine dosage equivalency below 50 was classified as a high-potency neuroleptic. All antidepressant drugs were converted into imipramine equivalents.

RESULTS

As can be seen in Table 2, which compares the TD and non-TD groups on total lifetime drug intake, the TD group received a significantly higher amount of neuroleptics (p<.025), depot fluphenazine (p<.01), and reserpine (p<.05), which was used in some cases as an early antipsychotic drug. The TD group also showed a significantly higher lifetime dosage for the antiparkinsonian agents; biperidin (p<.05), trihexyphenidyl HCl (p<.05), and a trend in the same direction for benztropine mesylate (p<.10). No differences were noted for either tricyclics or methylphenidate. Thus, the tardive dyskinesia group received significantly more dopamine-blocking, depleting, and anticholinergic drugs than the non-TD group.

Table 1
Demographic Characteristics of Tardive Dyskinesia (N = 31)
and Matched Non-Tardive Dyskinesia

Variable	Tardive Dyskinesia Group		Control*	
Age	M = 57.68	SD = 12.03	M = 52.29	SD = 12.11
Chronicity	M = 20.69	SD = 11.44	M = 18.15	SD = 12.60
Sex	N	%	N	%
Male	17	55	17	55
Female	14	45	14	45
Race	N	%	N	%
White	25	81	25	81
Black	6	19	6	19
Diagnosis	N	%	N	%
Schizophrenic	20	65	20	65
Affective disorder	4	13	4	13
Organic brain syndrome	5	16	4	13
Alcoholism	1	3	2	6
Other psychoses	1	3	1	3

*Tardive dyskinesia and control groups showed no statistically significant difference at p<.05 by t-test and Chi-square test performed for demographic variables.

Table 2
Comparison of Tardive Dyskinesia and Control Groups on Total Lifetime Drug Intake

Drug	Tardive Dyskinesia Group (N = 31)		Control Group (N = 31)		t	p*
	Mean (mg)	SD	Mean (mg)	SD		
Neuroleptics (in mg CPZ eq.)	630,951	734,639	315,722	426,326	2.05	<.025
Depot fluphenazine	1,605	3,305	98	417	2.52	<.01
Reserpine	285	856	19	90	1.72	<.05
Biperidin (Akineton)	540	1,720	1	6	1.75	<.05
Trihexyphenidyl HCl (Artane)	3,272	8,921	469	1,233	1.73	<.05
Benztropine mesylate (Cogentin)	925	2,349	237	676	1.57	<.10
Antidepressants	25,382	55,568	19,654	35,175	.48	ns
Methylphenidate (Ritalin)	15,183	65,852	6,745	27,063	.66	ns

*one-tailed test

Were these mean differences due to differences in the number of individuals taking these drugs or to the higher dosages prescribed for individual TD patients? Table 3 shows the number of individuals within each group receiving each drug, and compares the two groups by means of X^2 and Fisher's exact probability test (used only for neuroleptic drugs). The results indicate that the TD groups had a significantly larger number of individuals assigned to depot fluphenazine, biperiden, and trihexyphenidyl HCl, but that the two groups were statistically similar with respect to the number of patients receiving reserpine, methylphenidate, the antidepressants, and benztropine mesylate.

The next analysis focused on lifetime dosages only for patients assigned to each drug. The means, standard deviations, and t-values were recomputed, excluding patients not assigned to these drugs, to determine if group differences noted in Table 2 were attributable to higher dosages prescribed for those TD patients assigned to that drug. The results of these comparisons are noted in Table 4, which shows that the TD patients had larger lifetime amounts of oral neuroleptics ($p < .06$) and depot-fluphenazine ($p < .04$). Trends in the same direction were noted for reserpine and biperidin. Thus, for the oral neuroleptics, although there were no differences between TD and non-TD groups with respect to the number of patients assigned to the drug, the TD patients clearly received significantly higher dosages than did those in the non-TD group. For depot fluphenazine, the TD group definitely had more individuals receiving that drug and significantly higher dosages taken as compared with the non-TD group (see Table 4).

The data permitted some analyses which could shed light on the current dogma regarding the efficacy of drug holidays in preventing TD, through the

Table 3
Comparisons of Number of Individuals from
Tardive Dyskinesia and Control Groups Receiving Various Drugs

Drug	Number of Patients Who Received Drug			
	Tardive Dyskinesia Group	Control	X^2	p^*
Neuroleptics	31	28	— †	< .12
Depot fluphenazine	16	7	5.60	< .02
Reserpine	4	2	0.74	NS
Biperidin (Akineton)	8	1	6.37	< .02
Trihexyphenidyl HCl (Artane)	17	9	4.24	< .02
Benztropine mesylate (Cogentin)	15	9	2.45	NS
Antidepressants	17	16	.06	NS
Methylphenidate (Ritalin)	7	7	0	NS

*one-tailed test
†Fisher's exact test

examination of the prescribing patterns for neuroleptics. More specifically, the two groups were compared for (1) duration of neuroleptic usage; (2) total length of drug-free periods once neuroleptic therapy had begun; (3) number of drug-free periods exceeding one week; (4) number of drug-free periods exceeding one month; and (5) average daily dosage, to test the hypotheses that the TD group would have a longer duration on drugs, higher average daily dosages, and shorter and less frequent drug-free periods. Table 5 shows that there were no differences between the groups on these variables except for a trend ($p < .10$) suggesting longer duration of neuroleptic usage in the TD group.

It was also possible to examine the data with respect to two other controversial etiological issues: (1) Is depot fluphenazine artificially implicated in the etiology of TD because patients who are assigned to this drug often fail to respond to the gamut of oral neuroleptics and therefore might have previously received larger lifetime doses of oral neuroleptics? (2) Did the TD group receive different types of neuroleptic drugs (i.e., more high-potency drugs as compared to low-potency neuroleptics) than the non-TD group? Theoretically, if TD is more likely to develop in those patients with a history of extrapyramidal symptoms, then we would expect that the TD patients should have received more high-potency neuroleptics.

Results of the intergroup comparisons for neuroleptic drug therapy summarized in Table 5 indicate a trend in the expected direction ($p < .10$) suggesting that TD patients who received depot fluphenazine had a higher prior level of oral neuroleptic medication prior to the first dose of depot medication than did non-TD patients. The TD group also tended to receive more dosage of low-potency ($p < .10$) as well as high-potency neuroleptics ($p < 0.05$), excluding depot fluphenazine. These two findings would be expected on the basis of previous findings that the TD group had a higher mean for all neuroleptics (Table 2). To control for the greater amount of neuroleptics received by the TD group, a ratio of high-potency–low-potency neuroleptics (in CPZ equivalents) was computed for each patient, and the groups were compared for mean differences with respect to this ratio. Table 5 shows that the two groups were not statistically significantly different, even at the lax 10% level of confidence. Chi-square test was then applied to examine the number of patients in two groups receiving and not receiving high-potency neuroleptics; again, no statistical significance was found between the two groups. There was no statistically significant difference between TD and control groups when the number of patients receiving low-potency neuroleptics in the two groups was examined.

Previous reports have also investigated the role of neurological factors in TD. In the present study, each case record was reviewed for the presence of (1) head trauma, (2) CNS infection, (3) seizures, (4) lobotomy, (5) ECT, and (6) insulin shock therapy. Comparison between the TD and non-TD groups

Table 4
Dosage Comparisons of TD and Non-TD Patients Receiving Various Drugs

Drug	Tardive Dyskinesia Group Mean (mg)	SD	N	Non-TD Group Mean (mg)	SD	N	Mann Whitney U Test p*
Neuroleptics (in mg CPZ eq.)	630,951	743,639	31	347,620	434,986	28	<.06
Depot fluphenazine	3,109	4,106	16	435	838	7	<.04
Reserpine	2,136	1,345	4	294	289	2	<.07
Biperidin (Akineton)	1,969	3,051	8	32	0	1	<.10
Trihexyphenidyl HCl (Artane)	5,965	11,496	17	1,614	1,902	9	=.16
Benztropine mesylate (Cogentin)	1,912	3,131	15	706	1,144	9	ns
Antidepressants	46,285	69,005	17	38,074	41,553	16	ns
Methylphenidate (Ritalin)	67,238	132,662	7	29,875	53,441	7	ns

*one-tailed test

Table 5
Intergroup Comparisons on Neuroleptic Drug Therapy Variables

	Tardive Dyskinesia Group Mean	SD	Non-TD Group Mean	SD	t	df	p
Duration of Neuroleptic Usage (days)	3,592	2,435	2,629	2,460	1.55	60	<.10
Length of Drug-Free Period (days)	1,411	1,504	1,318	1,593	.22	54	ns
Number of Drug-Free Periods > 1 Week	2.81	2.72	2.38	2.86	.58	54	ns
Number of Drug-Free Periods > 1 Month	2.30	2.13	2.17	2.80	.19	54	ns
Average Daily Dose Neuroleptics (mg)	237	298	150	248	1.25	60	ns
Total Oral Neuroleptic Prior to Depot Fluphenazine (gm)	284	704	95	252	1.39	59	<.10
Total Low-Potency Neuroleptic (in gm CPZ eq.)	419	689	210	315	1.54	60	<.10
Total High-Potency Neuroleptic (in gm CPZ eq.)	212	314	106	170	1.91	60	<.05
Ratio High-Potency/Low-Potency Neuroleptic	7.04*	14.73	22.12*	62.33	1.06	40	ns

*Only subjects who received both types of neuroleptics were included in this analysis: N = 22 TD and 20 non-TD.

showed that no differences were revealed by Fisher's exact probability test in the number of cases positive for any of these variables.

For statistical purposes, three scores for each patient on these CNS variables were made. The first was a total CNS score which ranged theoretically from 0 to 6, and which simply represented the number of items on which the patient's history was positive. A second score, called the endogenous triad, represented a sum of the first three items (trauma, infection, and seizure). The last score, or the "iatrogenic" triad, representing the sum of the last three items consisting of lobotomy, ECT, and IST, represented manipulations of the CNS through prescribed somatic treatment. The TD and non-TD groups were then compared for mean differences in total CNS score, endogenous triad, and iatrogenic triad. There were no statistically significant differences between groups on any of these variables (see Table 6).

DISCUSSION

In a retrospective study based on the past history solely from the medical record, the investigators often encountered difficulty in collecting the accurate data of medication and somatic treatments history. Even if the record was perfect, a question would still remain as to the compliance of patients to the prescribed drugs. Few studies with research questions like this study's were carried out using medical records as data resources. In the pioneering study by Greenblatt *et al.* of dyskinesia in nursing home patients, the authors were able to conclude a definite relationship between dyskinesia and phenothiazine medication, although cumulative drug dosage and length of treatment with drugs were not studied in greater depth in relation to dyskinesia (1). Similarly, in studies by Gardos *et al.* (8) and by Chouinard *et al.* (9), using elegant stepwise multiple discriminant function analysis, the authors were able to single out several factors significantly related to dyskinesia, although their findings were not consistently identical.

Table 6

Comparison of CNS Factors in TD and Non-TD Patients

CNS Factors	Tardive Dyskinesia Group		Non-TD Group				
	Mean	SD	Mean	SD	t	df	p
Total CNS Factors	.97	.84	.87	.81	.50	60	NS
Endogenous Triad	.32	.60	.23	.43	.53	60	NS
Iatrogenic Triad	.65	.61	.65	.80	.0	60	NS

In our study, due to the relatively low mobility of our patients in this semirural region, most of the records showed little interruption of continuity and revealed a reasonably usable track of records. Despite this advantage, our data on accumulated lifetime dosage, duration of medicine, and drug-free period may represent overestimation or underestimation due to the special nature of methodology used. However, the chance of such shortcomings should be equally distributed between the two groups. The relative weight of each variable as formulated in the eight hypotheses, therefore, is considered to be informative.

Our data have confirmed all research hypotheses except Hypothesis 5 and part of Hypotheses 6 and 8. CNS events, either as a whole or divided into the endogenous triad and iatrogenic triad, were not significantly different for dyskinetic and nondyskinetic groups. Our findings were somewhat similar to those of Greenblatt et al. (1), who found no relationship of dyskinesia to chronic brain syndrome in nursing home patients. The findings of Chouinard et al. that no correlations exist between dyskinesia and brain damage, ECT, and IST are consistent with ours. However, in view of the finding of Gardos et al. (8) that abnormal EEG and ECT were significantly correlated with tardive dyskinesia, and the earlier literature indicating a positive relationship between dyskinesia and CNS events (19,21), more studies are needed to reconcile these inconsistent findings.

The value of drug holidays for the prevention of TD was, unfortunately, not unequivocally confirmed by our data. The number of drug-free periods, although as few as three in about ten years' duration of drug treatment, was about the same in both groups. We would expect such a meager drug-free period in the TD group, but it is difficult to explain why the control group did not manifest dyskinesia with so few drug-free periods. Our other finding, that dyskinetic patients had significantly longer periods of neuroleptic treatment than the nondyskinetic patients, may, however, support indirectly the value of drug holidays. More vigorous effort should be put forth in this area in future research.

As to whether tardive dyskinesia has more correlation with high-potency neuroleptics than low-potency neuroleptics, our finding, similar to that of Gardos et al. (8), could not support the common clinical notion that high-potency neuroleptics are more inductive to dyskinesia. Crane suggested that tardive dyskinesia could be expected predominantly in patients previously exhibiting significant drug-induced parkinsonism (27). High potency drugs which are well known for their high incidence of extrapyramidal side effects would then be expected to produce more tardive dyskinesia. This hypothesis is not substantiated by our findings. Due to the relative scarcity of studies exploring this question, more studies are obviously needed to clarify this academically interesting issue.

Finally, regarding the role of depot fluphenazine in tardive dyskinesia, our findings as well as those of Gardos *et al.* (8) and Chouinard *et al.* (9) consistently show its significance in the dyskinesia group. However, our data also show that there is a higher total amount of oral neuroleptics taken by the dyskinetic group than by the nondyskinetic group prior to the first injection of depot fluphenazine. Higher total dosage of antiparkinsonian agents was also seen in dyskinetic patients, suggesting that more usage of depot fluphenazine was concomitant with more antiparkinsonian drugs. Viewing all these factors, the role of depot fluphenazine in tardive dyskinesia, at least in our study, is synergetic with other factors and cannot be singled out as an independent causative agent.

CONCLUSION

Thirty-two dyskinetic patients were compared to an equal number of matched nondyskinetic patients for their past history of psychotropic medication and CNS events, including intrinsic and extrinsic factors of possible brain assault. Eight hypotheses were tested and the following were confirmed:

1. The total lifetime dosage of dopamine-blocking neuroleptics is higher in dyskinetic patients than in nondyskinetic patients.

2. The total lifetime dosage of dopamine-depleting agents, such as reserpine, is higher in dyskinetic patients than in nondyskinetic patients.

3. The total lifetime of anticholinergic antiparkinsonian agents is higher in dyskinetic patients than in nondyskinetic patients.

4. Catecholamine or indolamine-potentiating agents, such as tricyclic antidepressants and methylphenidate, were not dose-related to tardive dyskinesia.

5. CNS events, including head trauma, CNS infection, convulsion, ECT, IST, and lobotomy, are not related to tardive dyskinesia as significant factors.

6. Dyskinetic patients have had longer duration on neuroleptics, but the number of drug-free periods they have is equal to that of nondyskinetic patients. The drug holiday as a prevention for tardive dyskinesia is only partially and indirectly confirmed. More studies are needed in the future for unequivocal confirmation.

7. Although depot fluphenazine has been identified to be highly used in the dyskinetic group, the total oral neuroleptic dosage prior to depot fluphenazine treatment is higher in dyskinetic patients than in nondyskinetic patients. The role of depot fluphenazine in tardive dyskinesia is synergetic with higher previous oral neuroleptic dosage and higher dosage of antiparkinsonian agent in dyskinetic group.

8. High-potency neuroleptics are not found to be preferentially related to tardive dyskinesia as compared to low-potency neuroleptics.

REFERENCES

1. Greenblatt, D.L., Dominick, J.R., Stotsky, B.A., DiMascio, A. Phenothiazine-induced dyskinesia in nursing-home patients. *J. Am. Geriatr. Soc., 16*(1):27–34, 1968.
2. Mettler, F.A., Crandell, A. Neurologic disorders in psychiatric institutions. *J. Nerv. Ment. Dis., 128*:148–159, 1959.
3. Kazamatsuri, H., Chien, C.P., Cole, J.O. Therapeutic approaches to tardive dyskinesia—a review of the literature. *Arch. Gen. Psychiatry, 27,* 1972.
4. Asnis, G.M., Leopold, M.A., Duvoisin, R.C., Schwartz, A.H. A survey of tardive dyskinesia in psychiatric outpatients. *Am. J. Psychiatry, 134*(12):1367–1370, 1977.
5. Crane, G.E. Persistent dyskinesia. *Br. J. Psychiatry, 122*:395, 1973.
6. Crane, G.E. Clinical psychopharmacology in its 20th year. *Science, 181*:124, 1973.
7. Baldessarini, R.J. Tardive dyskinesia: an evaluation of the etiologic association with neuroleptic therapy. *Can. Psychiatr. Assoc. J., 19*:551, 1974.
8. Gardos, G., Cole, J.O., LaBrie, R.A. Drug variables in the etiology of tardive dyskinesia application of discriminant function analysis. In *Progress in Neuropsychopharmacology,* vol. 1. Oxford: Pergamon Press, pp. 147–154, 1977.
9. Chouinard, G., Annable, L., Chouinard, A.R. Factors related to tardive dyskinesia. Presented at American Psychiatric Association Annual Meeting, Toronto, Canada, May 3, 1977.
10. Carlsson, A. Biochemical implications of dopa-induced actions on the central nervous system with particular relevance to abnormal movements. In *L-Dopa and Parkinsonism,* Barbeau, A., McDowell, F.H. (eds.) Philadelphia: Davis, pp. 205–213, 1970.
11. Klawans, H.L., Jr. *The Pharmacology of Extrapyramidal Movement Disorders.* Basel: S. Karger, pp. 7–47, 74–80, 1973.
12. Klawans, H.L., Jr. The pharmacology of tardive dyskinesia. *Am. J. Psychiatry, 130*:82, 1973.
13. Tarsy, D., Baldessarini, R.J. Pharmacologically-induced behavioral supersensitivity to apomorphine. *Nature (New Biol.), 245*:262, 1973.
14. Tarsy, D., Baldessarini, R.J. Behavioral supersensitivity to apomorphine following chronic treatment with drugs which interfere with the synaptic function of catecholamines. *Neuropharmacology, 13*:927, 1974.
15. Tarsy, D., Baldessarini, R.J. The pathophysiologic basis of tardive dyskinesia. *Biol. Psychiatry, 12*(3):431–449, 1977.
16. Kiloh, L.G., Smith, S.J., Williams, S.E. Antiparkinson drugs as causal agents in tardive dyskinesia. *Med. J. Aust., 2*:591, 1973.
17. Degwitz, R. Extrapyramidal motor disorders following long-term treatment with neuroleptic drugs. In *Psychotropic Drugs and Dysfunction of the Basal Ganglia,* Crane, G.E., Gardner, R. (eds.). U.S. Public Health Service Publication No. 1938, Washington, D.C., pp. 12–13, 1969.
18. Wolf, S.M. Reserpine: cause and treatment of oral-facial dyskinesia. *Bull. Los Angeles Neurol. Soc., 38*:80–84, 1973.
19. Kline, N.S. On the rarity of "irreversible" oral dyskinesias following phenothiazines. *Am. J. Psychiatry, 124*(8):48–54, supp., 1968.
20. Hunter, R., Earl, C.J., Janz, D. A syndrome of abnormal movements and dementia in leucotomized patients treated with phenothiazines. *J. Neurol. Neurosurg. Psychiatry, 27*:219–223, 1964.
21. Hunter, R., Earl, C.J., Thornicroft, S. An apparently irreversible syndrome of abnormal movements following phenothiazine medication. *Proc. R. Soc. Med., 57*:758–762, 1964.
22. Korczyn, A.D. Pathophysiology of drug-induced dyskinesias. *Neuropharmacology, 11*:601, 1972.

23. Christensen, E., Moller, J.E., Faurbye, A. Neuropathological investigation of 28 brains from patients with dyskinesia. *Acta Psychiatr. Scand., 46*:14, 1970.
24. Preventing drug-induced dyskinesia. *Medical World News*, 76–77, February 6, 1978.
25. Tardive dyskinesia. Memo. 78–1, Division of Mental Health, State of New York, Dept. of Mental Hygiene, Jan. 3, 1978.
26. Hollister, L.E. *Clinical Use of Psychotherapeutic Drugs.* Springfield, Ill.: Charles C. Thomas, p. 33, 1973.
27. Crane, G.E. Pseudoparkinsonism and tardive dyskinesia. *Arch. Neurol., 27*:426, 1972.

28

History of Neuroleptic Drugs and Tardive Dyskinesia

ROBERT C. SMITH
MICHAEL STRIZICH
and **DAVID KLASS**

INTRODUCTION

A good deal of epidemiological evidence (reviewed in Chapter 24) now clearly relates neuroleptic drugs to the pathogenesis of tardive dyskinesia (TD), and research in animal models (reviewed in the first part of this book) also clearly supports the idea that chronic treatment with neuroleptic drugs produces increases in the sensitivity of dopamine receptors and can produce symptoms in animals which are similar to some of those seen in patients with tardive dyskinesia. A question of considerable importance that remains unanswered is whether any of the neuroleptic drugs or treatment regimens have a greater risk of inducing tardive dyskinesia in schizophrenic patients who are maintained on antipsychotic medication. This paper, which attempts to investigate this question, presents preliminary findings from a study of drug history and tardive dyskinesia in chronically hospitalized mental patients.

METHOD

One hundred and three patients, 50 years of age or older, at Manteno Mental Health Center were selected for the drug-history study (from a larger survey study of TD), using stratified random sampling procedures based on the patients' dyskinesia and parkinsonian scores for their initial ratings. The drug-history patient sample was stratified so that it would include patients with varying degrees of severity of TD and parkinsonian symptoms, but contain a larger number of patients in the more severe TD categories. Most patients were rated for TD on at least two or three separate occasions with the Smith Tardive Dyskinesia Scale (pp. 247–254). Since the facial dyskinesia subscale (derived from several of the individual items) gave stronger correlations with most of the drug-history variables than the total dyskinesia subscale, most of the analysis will be presented in the terms of mean facial dyskinesia scores. The amount of neuroleptic drugs a patient had received over his or her entire period of hospitalization in the state system was quantified from the medication records and doctors' orders. Because of changes in recording procedures in the late 1960's, drug-history records from 1968 onward proved to be more accurate; therefore, mostly post-1967 drug-history data will be used in this preliminary report. The amount of neuroleptics was measured both in grams and in the chlorpromazine equivalents (CPZ–E), using the conversion ratios of Davis (1).

RESULTS

The total amount of neuroleptics that a patient had received was not positively related to his tardive dyskinesia score. Indeed, the opposite relationship appeared to be true: the patient's TD score was negatively correlated with his total amount of neuroleptics, whether this was calculated in grams or CPZ equivalents (see Table 1). Patients who had received larger amounts of total neuroleptics also had a lower percentage of severe TD ratings (see Fig. 1). TD score also correlated negatively ($r = -.16$, $p < .05$) with the amount of neuroleptics the patient was receiving on the days of his TD ratings. Since it has been shown that higher doses of neuroleptics can at least temporarily reduce or mask TD symptoms, it is possible that the negative correlation between facial dyskinesia and the total amount of neuroleptics the patient had received over several years might be a "spurious" result, simply reflecting the fact that these patients were continued on high doses of neuroleptic drugs during the period of TD ratings. Although the correlation between total amount of neuroleptics a patient had received over many years and the amount of neuroleptics he was receiving on the day of TD ratings was moderate ($r = .43$ to $.52$, $p < .001$), there was still a significant negative partial correlation ($r = -.17$, $p < .05$) between the total amount of neuroleptics and facial TD scores when the dose of neuroleptics on the day of rating was controlled for.

A few of the measures reflecting the concentration of neuroleptic dosage the patient had received were, however, positively related to the patient's tardive dyskinesia score. When total amount of neuroleptics was controlled for, the variable of maximum dose of neuroleptics (max. CPZ-E) the patient had received, as well as another measure of "concentration" of neuroleptic dosage (CON), were both positively related to facial TD score. (Partial correlations with facial TD were: max. CPZ-E, $r = +.17$, $p < .05$; CON, $r = +.12$ for

Table 1
Relationship Between Tardive Dyskinesia and Drug History

Drug-History Variable	Zero Order Correlation	Partial Correlation Controlling for Total Neuroleptics
1. Total Amount of Neuroleptics (CPZ eq.) Received over Course of Hospitalization	−.26‡	—
2. Maximum Amount of Neuroleptics in a Single Year (CPZ eq.)	−.21‡	+.17*
3. Amount Thioridazine (CPZ eq.)	−.22‡	−.14†
4. Amount Thioridazine (gms)	−.22**	−.13†
5. Proportion of Neuroleptics Given as Fluphenazine (gms)ᵃ	+.29‡	+.28‡
6. Proportion of Neuroleptics Given as Intramuscular Fluphenazineᵇ	+.70**	—ᶜ

Each number is Pearson Correlation Coefficient (r) of the variable on the left side of the table with mean facial tardive dyskinesia score, or partial correlation of the same variable with mean facial tardive dyskinesia controlling for the total neuroleptics the patient had received over years of treatment. N = 99–103 patients for variables 1 to 5, and n = 12 patients for variable 6 (i.e., only 12 patients had received any appreciable amount of intramuscular fluphenazine). Statistical significance of r value: † p < .10; *p < .05; **p < .01; ‡ p < .005. The^a is grams fluphenazine/grams total neuroleptics patient received. The^b is mg CPZ equivalents intramuscular fluphenazine/grams CPZ equivalents total neuroleptics received. The^c is CPZ equivalents of total neuroleptics is controlled for in original variables 6.

1967 + drug data, and r = +.16 for total drug data, p < .10 and p < .05 respectively.)

Only one drug, fluphenazine, consistently had a small to moderately significant positive correlation with TD score (see Table 1). The proportion of fluphenazine that a patient had received as part of his neuroleptic treatment correlated positively and significantly with his tardive dyskinesia score. This association was much higher for depot (intramuscular) fluphenazine than for the oral fluphenazine. In a small number of patients (n = 12) who received any appreciable amount of intramuscular fluphenazine enanthate, the correlation between facial dyskinesia and the proportion of neuroleptic medication given as fluphenazine was fairly high (r = .70, p ≈ .01). The 5 patients in this group who had definite facial dyskinesia had received about twice as high a proportion of fluphenazine in their neuroleptic treatment (mean ± s.e.m. mg CPZ-E fluphenazine/gms CPZ-E total neuroleptics = 258 ± 47) than patients with no signs or with borderline signs of facial dyskinesia (mean fluphenazine 109 ±

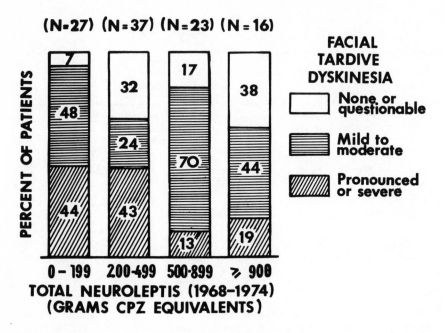

Figure 1.   Percent of patients administered differing amounts of total neuroleptics, who had given severities of facial tardive-dyskinesia symptom scores.

27), and this difference was statistically significant (t = 2.52, df = 9, p < .05). The total amount of thioridazine a patient had received tended to have a consistently small negative association with dyskinesia score, although only some of these correlations were statistically significant. No other single drug had a consistent positive or negative association with TD score. Most of the zero order or partial correlations for any other single neuroleptic versus facial TD score ranged from −.10 to +.10, and these correlations also varied considerably depending on which other variable was being controlled for in the partial correlation.

DISCUSSION

Our finding, that the total amount of neuroleptics a patient has received is *negatively* rather than *positively* related to his TD score, runs counter to some intuitions which might be drawn from the extensive epidemiological and experimental evidence which definitely gives neuroleptics a causative role in the etiology of TD. However, when we reviewed the available literature, we found only one or two prior studies (2,3) which suggested that patients who had received higher total amounts of neuroleptics had a higher prevalence or more severe manifestations of TD. In both of these studies, most of the patients, including those at the high end of the total neuroleptic distribution, had received relatively small to moderate total amounts of neuroleptics (e.g., 1.5–112.5 gms CPZ-E in the Crane study [3]). In contrast, in a study by Crane which reported no relationship between the total amounts of neuroleptics a patient had received and TD (4), many of the patients had received much higher total quantities of neuroleptics (up to 2500 gms CPZ-E). In the current sample, most of our chronic patients had received more than 200 gms CPZ-E, and many had received over 500 gms CPZ-E during their many years of neuroleptic treatment. The 37 patients who received the lowest total amounts of neuroleptics (<200 gms CPZ-E) clearly had the most severe cases of TD. Therefore, the results of the current study, as well as of one of the studies by George Crane (4), argue that for schizophrenic patients who have been given a lot of neuroleptics for many years, the total quantity of neuroleptics they have received is not the main drug variable related to the risks or severity of TD.

In patients with these types of drug histories, the dosage of neuroleptics appears to be a slightly more important variable in regard to TD. The small but significant partial correlation, showing that the maximum dose of neuroleptics a patient received in a given year was positively associated with his TD score ($r = +.17$), is very similar both in direction and in magnitude to findings reported earlier by George Crane (5) that maximum dose of neuroleptics was positively associated with TD score ($r = +.19$). The Crane drug-history study had a sample of 600 patients, many of whom were chronic schizophrenics. Other studies by Crane (4,6) conducted in samples in which some patients were specially treated with high doses of neuroleptics, also showed higher rates of TD in the high-dose patients. These results suggest that, in many patients, the pattern of concentration of neuroleptic administration over time may be more important than the total amount of neuroleptics in contributing to the risks of TD.

Our interesting finding—that one drug, fluphenazine, and particularly depot fluphenazine, was the only neuroleptic drug which had fairly consistent positive correlations with TD scores—should be viewed with the caution appropriate to preliminary results because of the following: (1) Most patients were treated with several neuroleptics, and no patient received only fluphenazine. (2) Although we tried to control for some confounding factors (i.e., through partial correlations), it is still possible that a factor that we did not control for might account for the significant positive correlations with fluphenazine. (3) Some patients who had not received substantial amounts of fluphenazine also had definite TD. (4) In a single sample, in which many correlations are computed, it is statistically possible to find a few significant correlations on a chance basis. (5) Our results on intramuscular fluphenazine, where we found the strongest relationship between fluphenazine and TD, are based on a small subsample.

On the other hand, it is important to note that at least four other independent studies of the relationship between the patient's drug-history or, specifically, depot fluphenazine and TD (See Cahpters 26, 27, 29 and 7) have also shown a significant association of TD with intramuscular fluphenazine. However, since the use of depot fluphenazine treatment has definite clinical advantages in the management of chronic schizophrenics in the community, we feel that it is important that these results, which are based largely on retrospective studies, should be confirmed in better controlled prospective studies before this useful mode of neuroleptic treatment is summarily abandoned.

If depot fluphenazine is more conclusively proven to be associated with particularly higher risks of tardive dyskinesia, this may provide leads about the pharmacological or structural properties of neuroleptics which may make them particularly toxic in regard to this disorder. Some preliminary reports on blood levels of patients receiving depot fluphenazine indicate that plasma levels are fairly low, especially towards the end of each 2- to 3-week depot injection cycle. This would suggest that plasma levels of neuroleptics may not be a major factor related to the development of TD. However, fluphenazine is extensively taken up into fat stores in the body and is very slowly released. It may, therefore, be present in pharmacologically toxic concentrations in some of the highly lipid CNS tissues for a much longer time than many other neuroleptics. Experimental pharmacological and histological studies in animals after chronic depot fluphenazine administration may help clarify whether any specific properties of this drug can be related to the pathophysiological mechanisms involved in the development of TD.

REFERENCES

1. Davis, J.M. Dose-equivalence of anti-psychotic drugs. *J. Psychiatr. Res.*, *11*:65–69, 1977.
2. Pryce, I.G., Edwards, H. Persistent oral dyskinesia in female mental hospital patients. *Brit. J. Psychiatry*, *112*:983–987, 1966.
3. Crane, G.E., Smeets, R.A. Tardive dyskinesia and drug therapy in geriatric patients. *Arch. Gen. Psychiatry*, *30*:341–343, 1974.
4. Crane, G.E. Tardive dyskinesia in schizophrenic patients treated with psychotropic drugs. *Aggressologie*, *9*:209–218, 1968.
5. Crane, G.E. Factors pre-disposing to drug-induced neurological side effects. In *Ad. in Biochem. Psychopharm.*, vol. 9. New York: Raven Press, pp. 269–279, 1974.
6. Crane, G.E. High doses of trifluoperazine and tardive dyskinesia. *Arch. Neurol.*, *33*:176–180, 1970.
7. Chouinard, G., Chouinard, A.R. Factors related to tardive dyskinesia. Scientific proceedings, 130th Annual Meeting, American Psychiatric Association, Washington, D.C., p. 52, 1977.

29

Depot Fluphenazine and Tardive Dyskinesia in an Outpatient Population

ALAN C. GIBSON

THE INCIDENCE OF TARDIVE DYSKINESIA WITH DEPOT FLUPHENAZINE TREATMENT

A large majority of papers reporting tardive dyskinesia relate to survey studies done on chronic schizophrenics maintained for relatively long periods of time in mental institutions. However, the increasing use of depot phenothiazine injections has meant that a large number of relatively asymptomatic or less symptomatic schizophrenics can be maintained in the community. In the study reported in this paper, done in an English seaside town with a population of over 200,000 (which is my catchment area), only 70 schizophrenics remain in long-term psychiatric hospitals. The remainder of these psychotic patients are visited in their homes by nurses who work entirely in the community. We began this maintenance treatment with depot phenothiazines in 1966 and have increased its use since then; only a small percentage of patients have refused the maintenance depot injection (about 4% per year).

Of 450 patients maintained in the community with nurse home visits, 246 were receiving depot fluphenazine at the beginning of 1974 when we began a prospective study to investigate the incidence and progression of tardive dyskinesia (TD) that might be associated with depot fluphenazine. These patients have been examined by me for tardive dyskinesia and psychiatric symptoms at least at yearly intervals and often more frequently. By the beginning of 1977 the number of patients in the original sample still remaining in the study had fallen from 240 to 217, and 49 (22%) of these 217 patients had developed tardive dyskinesia. The prevalence of tardive dyskinesia in this sample of patients in the prospective study increased over the 3 years since the beginning of the study: at the beginning in 1974 it was 7%; by 1975, 14%; by 1976, 19%; and by 1977, 22%. The majority of individuals with tardive dyskinesia symptoms showed the primary BLM syndrome of relatively mild degree. Those patients with BLM facial symptoms of TD had severity of symptoms as follows: 73% of the TD cases showed only infrequent movement of the lower face and tongue; 17% of the cases showed constant movement of the face and tongue; 10% of the cases showed significant protrusion of the tongue in addition to any tongue or facial movements. Some of the 49 patients with TD symptoms also developed choreiform movements of the extremities, and one patient had dyskinetic movements of the shoulders and trunk also.

There was little difference in age or sex characteristics in the patients who developed TD on depot fluphenazine injections and those who did not. The mean age of patients who developed TD was 57 years, which was slightly older than the mean age (51 years) of all patients receiving depot fluphenazine. However, all of the patients that developed TD were over the age of 40, and 35 patients (71%) were in the 50–70 year-old age group. The sex of the patient was not related to the development of TD; the ratio of males to females in the entire sample was 5 to 2, and there was a very similar sex ratio in those patients who developed symptoms of TD.

We are not certain whether the previous medication history of the patients who developed TD was any different than those who did not develop TD symptoms, but the clinical data that we do have suggests there was no large difference in the amount or type of medication the two subgroups had previously received. All the patients maintained on depot fluphenazine had previously received oral neuroleptic treatment before being placed on the depot medication sometime after 1966. The average number of years of oral medication of the total sample was (mean ± s.d.) 11 ± 10.8 years, and the subgroup of the patients who developed TD on depot fluphenazine had an average of 11.6 ± 11.2 years of oral medication. Although accurate records of the total amount and specific drugs given each patient over the entire course of his treatment with neuroleptics were not available or were too difficult to collate, all the patients had been treated by the same group of psychiatrists and staff. Therefore, it is likely that the patients who developed TD had fairly similar drug histories of oral neuroleptics compared to those who did not develop TD symptoms.

Our clinical evidence does indicate, however, that the development of TD was related to the number of years the patients had been maintained on intramuscular fluphenazine injections. Figure 1 shows that the longer a patient had been maintained on intramuscular fluphenazine injections, the greater the risk of developing TD. Whereas only 5% of the patients who had been receiving depot fluphenazine for about a year had developed some signs of TD, almost 40% of patients who had been maintained on depot fluphenazine for 11 years had signs of TD.

Since the dosage of the depot fluphenazine was fairly similar for most patients over the course of their years of treatment (25 mg every 3 weeks), it is difficult to make an analysis of whether the dosage of depot fluphenazine was related to development of TD. A few patients who were on larger doses of depot fluphenazine (up to 75 mg every 2 weeks) took somewhat longer to show evidence of TD, but after six years three of these higher dose patients showed clear signs of TD.

To summarize the findings at the beginning of the prospective studies, 7% of the patients showed TD, and by the end of an additional 3 years of treatment with depot fluphenazine 22% of the patients showed signs of TD; this is about a threefold increase in prevalence.

ATTEMPTS AT MANAGEMENT, TREATMENT, AND PREVENTION OF TD

Between 1974 and 1975 no attempt was made to treat TD as it arose, nor was any reduction in patients' medication made, since it was felt at the time that the risks of producing psychiatric relapse in a schizophrenic outpatient population were too great to try this latter strategy. However, as noted above, the incidence and severity of TD in these patients continued to increase. In the

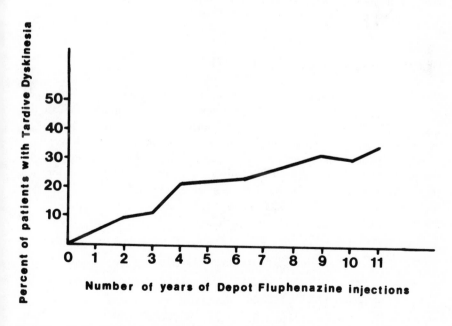

Figure 1.   Years of treatment with depot fluphenazine and the development of tardive dyskinesia.

course of the first year not only did more cases of TD occur, but four of the existing cases developed more severe mouth movements and two of these also developed choreiform movements of the extremities. Therefore, over the next three years several treatment strategies were tried out on a clinical basis. These involved (1) addition of medication thought to benefit specifically symptoms of TD; (2) reduction of dosage, drug holidays, and/or extended periods of drug-free management; or (3) switching the patient from fluphenazine to other oral or intramuscular neuroleptics.

Addition of Treatment Drugs for Dyskinesia

Over a three-year period groups of six patients at a time had potential therapeutic agents for tardive dyskinesia added to their existing neuroleptic medication. These included the drugs amantadine, deanol, lithium, clonazepam, and bromocriptine. None of these medications had a substantial clinical effect on the patients' TD. Ten patients were included in a larger trial in a sodium valproate study (7), and this drug also appeared to have no substantial amenorative effect on TD symptoms in the dose we used (600 mg/day). Another drug, tetrabenazine, was effective in reducing TD symptoms for a number of months in some patients, but we found that no patient could tolerate this medication for longer than six months because of the concomitant depression that it produced.

Changes in Dosage or Cessation of Medication

A reduction in depot fluphenazine dosage was attempted at some time in 31 of the patients who had developed TD symptoms. We attempted to reduce the fluphenazine dosage to 12.5 mg of the depot fluphenazine monthly. However, we were able to achieve this goal of maintenance therapy on a much lower dose of depot fluphenazine in only nine of the candidates. In these nine patients symptoms of TD were substantially reduced or disappeared after maintenance therapy on the considerably lower fluphenazine dose, although in three cases the symptoms of TD first exacerbated before they declined or disappeared. Three years later seven of these nine patients are still relatively psychiatrically asymptomatic, but in two of these cases the TD symptoms have reappeared even at the lower dose.

In 1977, an additional 100 patients who had not developed TD and had previously been maintained on fluphenazine at the standard dose of 25 mg per 3 weeks, were selected for a dose reduction trial. Up to the time of writing it has been possible to reduce dosage in 61 of these 100 patients without deterioration in psychiatric functioning; 43 are being maintained on a dose of 12.5

mg/month and the other 18 are able to be maintained on a dose of 18.75 mg/month of depot fluphenazine.

Drug holidays for periods of 8 to 9 weeks, when depot fluphenazine injections were temporarily stopped, was also attempted in an effort to see whether this would reduce the risk of manifestation of tardive dyskinesia. Eighteen patients receiving depot fluphenazine, 10 in a dose of 12.5 mg/month and 8 in a dose of 25 mg/3 weeks, most of whom had not developed active signs of TD, were suspended from their regular fluphenazine injections for a drug holiday of 8 to 9 weeks. Three of these 18 patients were unable to complete the drug holiday protocol because they developed increasing withdrawal and secretiveness, and one patient had to be readmitted to the hospital because of frank ideas of reference and disturbing hallucinations. These three patients reconstituted psychiatrically when depot fluphenazine was restored. The other 15 patients did not experience an exacerbation of their psychoses during the drug holiday, and half of them said they felt better without the depot fluphenazine injections. In three patients buccal-lingual TD symptoms first developed or became more prominent during the drug holiday. The uncovering of previously masked TD in these patients was regarded as a welcome sign and lead to a change in our clinical management of these patients; they will not be restarted on fluphenazine until their TD symptoms disappear unless an exacerbation of their psychiatric symptoms into a frank psychosis may necessitate restarting neuroleptic medication.

Change of Neuroleptic Medication

Since depot fluphenazine seemed to be associated with a large increase in TD, some patients have been switched to other oral or intramuscular medication in order to clinically evaluate whether a change to other neuroleptics would reduce or eliminate TD symptoms and whether the patients could be psychiatrically maintained on these other neuroleptic regimens.

Nineteen patients with tardive dyskinesia were thought to have sufficient insight and reliability to warrant a return to maintenance oral medication. The drug selected for most patients was pimozide because of the good results with this drug in TD reported by Fog and Pakkenberg (1) when they treated cases of dyskinesia with a combination of pimozide and tetrabenazine. Pharmacological evidence based on animal experiments reported by Costall and Naylor (2) has also shown that pimozide was particularly effective in reducing gnawing, hyperactivity, and other dyskinetic movements induced by intracerebral injections of dopamine.

The initial clinical results with pimozide were almost too striking to be believed. In 16 out of 17 patients, TD symptoms were either abolished or so greatly reduced in severity that they would only be apparent to someone who had known that the patient had previously had these symptoms. The dose of pimozide that we used was usually 4 mg/day though this dose had to be increased to 8 mg/day in 4 patients in order to control their psychosis. This initial excellent result with pimozide has, unfortunately, not been completely maintained. After a period ranging from 2 to 3 years from the time pimozide was begun, the dyskinetic symptoms have begun creeping back in 10 of the 16 patients who had shown substantial initial improvements. The recurring symptoms were most apparent as rapid, though very slight, buccal-lingual masticatory movements. Towards the end of 1977 the remaining 6 pimozide patients who showed no return of TD symptoms were taken off of all neuroleptic medication for one month. By the end of this one-month period only one of these 6 patients who had shown no evidence of TD when on pimozide continued to show no evidence of BLM TD syndrome after drug withdrawal; the other 5 had redeveloped some evidence of TD symptoms. Restarting pimozide in these drug-free patients abolished again the TD movements. It is important to note that the TD symptoms which reoccurred in the pimozide patients were quite mild compared to the symptoms of TD most patients had on depot fluphenazine. The time it took for symptoms of TD to reoccur on pimozide was greater than the time it took for recurrence of TD symptoms with haloperidol, as described by Kazamazuri et al. (3). The Kazamazuri et al. study reported that TD symptoms were initially suppressed in psychotic patients with a dose of 8 mg/haloperidol per day, but the majority of these patients had a reemergence of symptoms during the first 12 weeks of chronic haloperidol medication. It generally took 2 to 3 years for TD symptoms to reemerge in pimozide-treated patients, and the symptoms from pimozide were fairly mild.

We have similar results in a few cases switched to oral thioridazine. Two patients elected to switch to oral thioridazine rather than oral pimozide from depot fluphenazine. Both patients had a substantial reduction or disappearance of TD symptoms. The dyskinetic symptoms returned, however, after 18 months of oral thioridazine medication.

In 15 patients, depot fluphenazine had been replaced by depot fluspiriline. Ten of these 15 patients initially showed the same dramatic improvement in reduction or elimination of TD symptoms as occurred with the patients switched from fluphenazine to oral pimozide. It is interesting to note that fluspiriline closely resembles pimozide in its chemical structure. Since we only began the fluspiriline medication about a year and a half ago we have no information, at the current time, as to whether TD symptoms will reemerge on depot fluspiriline. However, in the light of the relapse in TD symptoms after 2 to 3 years with oral pimozide, we believe that one should not be overconfident that patients treated with depot fluspiriline will not have a similar course. The 5 patients who showed no reduction in TD symptoms when switched to depot fluspiriline were among the patients who had TD symptoms at the start of our prospective study in 1974; these may have been longer term resistant TD cases, although we do not know exactly how long their TD symptoms existed prior to 1974.

DISCUSSION

Our results, which show a 22% rate of TD in outpatients maintained on depot fluphenazine, and the rise in the prevalence of TD from 7% to 22% over only a 3-year period of chronic maintenance treatment on this depot regimen, indicates clinically significant risk of tardive dyskinesia may accompany this very useful mode of treatment, which has allowed many schizophrenics to be maintained in the community. One other recent clinical report by Marriett (4) described a somewhat lower rate of TD with depot fluphenazine, i.e., about 5% in the patients he observed. However, the rate of TD can be heavily influenced by the definition and the severity of cutoff points for diagnosing a positive case of TD. Marriett may have counted only unmistakable or more severe cases of TD, whereas this study included patients with both relatively mild as well as more severe symptoms in the enumeration of positive TD cases. Seventy-three percent of the patients with TD in our study had relatively mild symptoms, although we had observed these patients over several years and felt more certain of the presence of the disorder, even in the mild cases. If one were to exclude all of these more mild cases, however, then the prevalence rate in our sample would drop from 22% to 6%. On the other hand, if we had been more lenient in our criteria, we might have come up when an even higher prevalence rate than the 22% we report. For example, we excluded patients who could not keep their feet still, since we felt it would be difficult to differentiate TD from akathisia in these cases.

It is certainly possible that other factors which we could not completely control might be responsible in part for this high rate of TD associated with depot fluphenazine. For example, once a patient was put on fluphenazine, he may have been getting more medication than he received from a similar amount of oral drug, because any problems with patient compliance in drug taking or medication ingestion were avoided with the intramuscular regimen. Patients who developed TD were also a few years older than total sample, and patients also aged 3 years during the course of the study between 1974 and 1977; older age has been associated with a greater incidence of TD. It is important to remember, however, that we were dealing with fairly small age differences between the groups in our study—2 to 5 years on the average—and small differences in age have not been associated with great disparities with the rate of TD in the previous TD literature.

Assuming that depot fluphenazine is more likely to be a causative factor in the higher incidence of TD as compared to oral dosing, is there any reason why this might be so? One possible explanation based on pharmacokinetic considerations comes from the work of Curry. Curry (5) reported low chlor-promazine plasma levels following oral administration in certain patients, and demonstrated that this may be due to reduced absorption of the drug in the gut wall or greater first-pass metabolism. Adamson *et al*. (6), examining 97 chronic inpatient schizophrenics, showed 39 to have low plasma levels of unmetabolized chlorpromazine. If poorer gut-wall absorption or greater first-pass metabolism of orally ingested neuroleptics is a characteristic of many chronic schizophrenic patients, then these patients would have lower levels of neuroleptic drugs in their blood and brain when they received oral antipsychotic medication. If higher drug levels were related to greater toxicity and risks of developing tardive dyskinesia, then patients on oral medication might have their own protection mechanism against this effect of prolonged neuroleptic medication. This protection would be bypassed by giving injectable depot phenothiazines. This speculation must be considered as a tentative suggestion which must be confirmed by further research.

Some of the treatment regimens we tried that involved adjustments in dosage or changes in neuroleptic medication did seem to substantially reduce or temporarily abolish the symptoms of tardive dyskinesia in many of the identified cases in this prospective study. Switching to oral pimozide eliminated symptoms of tardive dyskinesia in most patients for a period of 2 to 3 years, but continued maintenance on pimozide led to a reemergence of TD symptoms after this time. Intramuscular fluspiriline, which is similar to pimozide in structure but which can also be given in depot form, had a similar ameliorative effect on TD symptoms oral pimozide; therefore, it may be a safer drug than fluphenazine for patients who require depot medication. However, one disadvantage of fluspiriline is that it must be given on a weekly basis, whereas depot fluphenazine can be given every 2 to 4 weeks. Consequently, fluspiriline may be somewhat less useful in outpatient or community situations in which the patient cannot come to the clinic or be given injections on a weekly basis. Also, it is my clinical impression that fluspiriline appears to be a somewhat less effective antipsychotic than fluphenazine, although this difference has not been established in controlled studies. Oral pimozide treatment did not appear to have "cured" most of the patients of their TD, even in those few cases in which the patient did not redevelop TD symptoms after 2 or 3 years of oral pimozide treatment. In 5 of 6 patients who never manifested TD symptoms on pimozide, mild TD symptoms were "unmasked" when the oral pimozide maintenance therapy was stopped. The TD symptoms which developed on pimozide were, nevertheless considerably milder than those seen with the same patients when they were on fluphenazine. Furthermore, to my knowledge the clinical literature does not report cases of TD associated with pimozide,although this drug has not been used as extensively for a long period of time as several other neuroleptics. Even without a change in medication, the simple strategy of reducing fluphenazine dosage also reduced or eliminated the clinical manifestations of TD symptoms in 7 of 9 patients. Therefore, this also may be a useful strategy to try in patients who have to be maintained on depot medication. Overall, one or more of these changes in the patients' pharmacotherapy regimens arrested or reversed the symptoms in 35 (71%) of the 49 identified TD cases in this prospective study. It should be remembered, however, that these therapeutic trials were uncontrolled open clinical studies and did not have a double-blind design or placebo control. Furthermore,this high percentage of very favorable results of treatment may be due, in part, to the fact that in most of our patients, TD symptoms were caught relatively soon after they were first manifested. The changes in pharmacotherapy regimens were generally initated within 6 months to 2 years after symptoms were discovered. In a patient population in which most patients had had dyskinetic symptoms which had persisted for many years, or in which many patients had severe TD symptoms, results of these treatment regimens may not produce the high rate of success that we found in our sample.

Although not formally part of our prospective study, another clinical observation warrants mention because of its relevance to the risk of TD and maintenance depot therapy of schizophrenic patients. In my view, depot flupenthixol is not an attractive alternative to depot fluphenazine. In 157 patients maintained on depot flupenthixol reviewed by the author, the rate of TD was about 24%; this is similar to that seen with fluphenazine. However, the dyskinesias seen in patients on flupenthixol in the identified TD cases were generally more severe and the occurrence of accessory choreiform movements was much more frequent.

The clinical significance of the risk of developing TD with depot fluphenazine must not be overstated, and should be balanced with the substantial benefits of this form of treatment. Routine use of depot preparations has allowed the majority of schizophrenic patients in our area to be treated in their homes and has substantially reduced the need for long-term hospitalization and the rate of relapse which may occur when the patients do not take an oral neuroleptic. The depot preparations may therefore be the most important practical advance in the treatment of chronic schizophrenia since the introduction of chlorpromazine in the 1950's. The development of symptoms of mild TD, of which many patients are unaware of in any case, is a small price to pay if a lifetime in the hospital can be avoided. Moreover, in none of the cases with mild TD that we identified in our prospective study did the dyskinesia become substantially worse over the 3-year period if the TD was identified early and changes in pharmacotherapy that I described above were instituted. Nevertheless, it seems that every clinician has the obligation to discover the lowest dose of neuroleptic on which his patients can be maintained without increases in psychiatric symptoms, and also to investigate the length of drug holidays his patient can tolerate. In appropriate patients a cessation of medication for an extended period of time may also be tried if the social and psychological consequences of relapse are not severe. There remains considerable work to be done to establish guidelines for the best practical neuroleptic regimens which will minimize the risks of TD.

REFERENCES

1. Fog, R., Pakkenberg, H. Combined nitoman-pimozide treatment of Huntington's chorea and other hyperkinetic syndromes. *Acta. Neurol. Scand., 46*:249–251, 1970.
2. Costall, B., Naylor, R.J. Behavioral characterisation of neuroleptic properties. Read at Symposium in Dopamine at Royal Society of Medicine, London, Oct. 21, 1977.
3. Kazamazuri, H., Ching-piao, C., Cole, J.O. Long-term treatment of tardive dyskinesia with haloperidol and tetrabenazine. *Amer. J. Psychiatry, 130*:479–482, 1973.
4. Marriett, P.F. Letter: potentiation of tardive dyskinesia: possible drug interaction. *Br. Med. J., 2*:139, 1975.
5. Curry, S.H., Davis, J.M., Janowsky, D.S., Marshall, H.H.L. Factors affecting chlorpromazine plasma levels in psychiatric patients. *Arch. Gen Psychiatry, 22*:209–214, 1970.
6. Adamson, L., Curry, S.H., Bridges, P.K., Firestone, A.F., Lavin, N.I., Lewis, D.M., Watson, R.D., Xavier, C.M., Anderson, J.A. Fluphenazine decanoate trial in chronic inpatient schizophrenics failing to absorb oral chlorpromazine. *Dis. Nerv. Syst., 34*:181–191, 1973.
7. Gibson, A.C. Sodium valproate and tardive dyskinesia. *Br. J. Psychiatry, 133*:82, 1978.

30

Dystonic and Dyskinetic Reactions Induced by H₁ Antihistaminic Medication

ROBERT E. SMITH
and EDWARD F. DOMINO

Although histamine and *tele*-N-methylhistamine are found in the striatum, relatively little is known concerning their function in the extrapyramidal motor system. Antihistaminics which penetrate the blood-brain barrier are primarily H₁ antagonists. In addition, some show anticholinergic and dopamine potentiating properties. Hence, it is of interest to point out that several reports have suggested a relationship between the administration of antihistaminic medication and the appearance of acute dystonias (1–3) or the production of oral-facial dyskinesias (4,5). A survey of the literature reveals many citations in which H₁ antihistamines were utilized in the treatment of extrapyramidal side effects; two additional case reports were found in which the clinical description strongly suggests the occurrence of dystonic symptoms following acute high doses of diphenhydramine (6,7), and there is one case report (8) of reversible oral dyskinesia following chronic use of mebhydrolin, a tetrahydro-γ-carboline derivative with H₁ antagonist properties. The number of case reports in the literature is small, yet it is important to review these cases and to attempt to understand the possible mechanism underlying these reactions. The acute dystonias will be discussed separately from the dyskinesias seen following chronic administration.

ACUTE DYSTONIAS

This extrapyramidal side effect is defined as a fixed, or relatively fixed, attitude in association with some other extrapyramidal disorder of movement.

325

Clinical signs are, characteristically, distortion of the lips and tongue, trismus, torticollis, tortipelvis, or athetoid posturing of the extremities. These signs and symptoms occur alone or in various combinations.

Clinical Features of H_1 Antihistamine-Induced Dystonia

The five case reports (1–3,6,7) published describe the appearance of dystonic signs following the acute administration of H_1 antihistamines. No reports were found that describe solely fixed positions or attitudes during or after long-term treatment. Thus, the literature reflects an extremely small frequency of occurrence for this reaction. In the 12 months following the publications of the series of reports in the United States during late 1976 and early 1977, the manufacturer of diphenhydramine received only one report from physicians related to the production of either dystonias or dyskinesias by H_1 antihistamines. This suggests that increased clinician awareness has not resulted in a dramatic increase in the rare frequency indicated by the literature.

The patient population in which the acute dystonias were observed is characterized in Table 1. Only children and young adults are represented. There is no evidence of sexual predisposition. The concurrent disease states may reflect an association between allergic disorders involving histamine release and the occurrence of the dystonic reaction.

The H_1 antihistamines purportedly causing the adverse reaction and the clinical presentation are given in Table 2. The early onset of signs and symptoms following initiation of the drug is notable. One patient had an immediate control of symptoms lasting for several hours from diazepam, but the reaction reoccurred; another patient had no response to the same agent. One patient was sedated with a barbiturate, but symptoms persisted. Treat-

Table 1
Characterization of Patients Showing Acute Dystonic Reactions to H_1 Antagonists

	Case 1	Case 2	Case 3	Case 4	Case 5
Age	3 yr–11 mo	19 yr	19 yr	3 yr–6 mo	1 yr–6 mo
Sex	Male	Female	Female	Male	Female
Reason for prescribing antihistamine	Urticaria & Periorbital Edema	"Cold"	Allergic Reaction	Hay Fever	Accidental Ingestion Parent With Hay Fever
Reference	(1)	(2)	(3)	(6)	(7)

Table 2
H₁ Antagonist and Clinical Features of Induced Acute Dystonic Reactions

	Case 1	Case 2	Case 3	Case 4	Case 5
Drug	Diphenhydramine	Doxylamine, Ephedrine, Dextromethorphan, Acetaminophen, & Alcohol	Diphenhydramine	Diphenhydramine	Diphenhydramine
Duration of drug administration	17 hr	2 days	Unknown	3 days	6 hr
Time from last dose until onset of symptoms	2 hr	Unknown	Unknown	20 min	6 hr
Symptoms					
Torticollis	+	+	+		
Facial grimacing	+			+	+
Tongue protrusion		+		+	
Dysarthria	+	+	+		
Trismus					
Purposeless or athetoid movements	+			+	+
Delirium/mental confusion	+			+	+
Duration of symptoms	18 hr	Intermittent > 6 hr	6 hr	4 hr	14 hr
Reference	(1)	(2)	(3)	(6)	(7)

ment was variable. In most cases the symptoms were allowed to run their course, with treatment being only close clinical monitoring.

The acute dystonias caused by neuroleptic antipsychotic drugs have an identical clinical presentation to those reported to be induced by H_1 antihistamines (9). They occur soon after treatment is instituted and are characterized by trismus, facial grimacing, tongue protrusion, distortion of the lips, dysarthria, torticollis, or retrocollis, and purposeless or athetoid movements of the extremities. Incidence rates are higher in children and young adults. Children demonstrate a greater frequency for involvement of the extremities (10). Thus, we have H_1 antihistamines with proven efficacy in treating acute dystonic reactions due to neuroleptics that also produce an identical clinical picture of acute dystonia in subjects not receiving neuroleptic medication.

Etiology

The biochemical changes and mechanisms within the central nervous system that lead to the production of dystonic phenomena are not known. This statement applies equally well to dystonias seen following neuroleptic use and to those which occur as a part of a specific neuropathological disorder, i.e., dystonia musculorum deformans. One theory (9) on the neuropharmacology of neuroleptic-induced dystonias is based upon the similarities between these movement disorders and L-dopa-induced dyskinesia. It is suggested that a rebound increase in nigral inhibition of the basal ganglia produces the acute dystonias and purposeless movements. However, the L-dopa-induced reactions occur during chronic administration of the drug and are not seen at the onset of treatment. The fact that acute doses of other dopamine agonists are not characterized by dystonic adverse effects also speaks against this explanation. It has also been reported that methylphenidate is an effective treatment for acute dystonias (11).

Observations of the time course for dystonic reactions following neuroleptics has produced a second proposed mechanism to explain dystonias (12). This study suggests that acute disruption of the dopaminergic-cholinergic balance toward cholinergic dominance underlies the mechanism which produces acute dystonias. The time course suggests that as the plasma level of the drug falls, the anticholinergic properties dissipate before the antidopamine properties producing cholinergic dominance appear and before the appearance of dystonic symptoms. Neuroleptics which are essentially pure dopamine antagonists would thus be expected to be associated with a greater incidence of acute dystonias. This indeed is the situation.

Histamine has been shown to activate cholinergic neurons in the striatum (15). If cholinergic dominance plays a role in producing dystonias, patients with allergic disorders involving histamine may be at risk for an idiosyncratic reaction to antihistamines and for the appearance of dystonias. A drug with both anticholinergic and H_1 antihistaminic properties, such as diphenhydramine, may be associated with a temporary overshooting by compensatory mechanisms following cholinergic blockade. The small incidence figures for this reaction suggest that other factors must be involved in a predisposition to respond to antihistamines with dystonia. A genetic factor may be involved analogous to the susceptibility of first-degree relatives of patients with torsion dystonia to the production of dystonias following low doses of neuroleptics (16).

Late-Occurring Dyskinesias

Late-occurring dyskinesia or tardive dyskinesia is characteristically associated with the chronic administration of antipsychotic drugs (phenothiazines, butyrophenones, etc.), and is a hyperkinetic movement disorder. A variety of diverse involuntary movements are seen, including oral-facial dyskinesia, chorea, athetosis, dystonia, hemiballismus, tics, and other abnormal postures (9). Our literature survey produced only two references (4,5) in which three case reports were described of patients developing late-occurring dyskinesia following prolonged use of H_1 antihistamines. Table 3 characterizes the patient population in which the late-occurring dyskinesias were seen. All patients were 55 years of age or older at the time the case reports appeared in the literature. This suggests that an aging central nervous system was a contributing factor, since the chronic utilization of H_1 antihistamines is also frequently seen in younger patients. Both sexes were represented in the three case reports. The clinical summaries indicate chronic allergic rhinitis as the underlying condition requiring chronic administration of the antihistamines. This may simply reflect the clinical situation when this class of drugs is used for prolonged periods of times. However, the "allergic substrate" may be a requirement for the appearance of the movement disorder. Only more

Table 3
Characterization of Patients Showing Late-Occurring
Dyskinesias to H_1 Antagonists

	Case 1	Case 2	Case 3
Age	55	65	57
Sex	Male	Male	Female
Underlying medical condition	Recurrent rhinitis	Allergic rhinitis	Allergic rhinitis
Reference	(4)	(4)	(5)

extensive study of the problem will assist in determining which conclusion will hold true.

The H_1 antihistamine purportedly causing the adverse effect and the clinical presentation is given in Table 4. All patients were administered a combination of an antihistaminic and a sympathomimetic for either the total duration of drug exposure or the majority of the time. However, the one subject who was placed on only an H_1 antihistamine following 17 years on a combination product did not develop his movement disorder until three years after the institution of only this antihistamine.

The initial clinical presentation for all subjects was characterized by the occurrence of blepharospasm as the first evidence of a movement disorder. With time, other facial dyskinesias appeared. Case 2 was unique in that a 3-per-second tremor of the mandible and soft palate was noted. Tremor is not considered to be a typical movement disorder associated with the tardive dyskinesia and seen following the chronic use of neuroleptics. In other aspects the clinical presentations are consistent with the reported signs and symptoms seen with tardive dyskinesia.

All subjects were withdrawn from their H_1 antihistaminic preparations and either improvement or no change in their clinical states was observed. Thus,

Table 4

H_1 Antagonist and Clinical Features of
Late-Occurring Dyskinesias

	Case 1	Case 2	Case 3
Drug	Brompheniramine Phenylephrine Phenylpropanolamine	Chlorpheniramine Phenylpropanolamine Isopropamide	Chlorpheniramine
Total duration of drug administration	10 yr	5 yr	27 yr
Time from initiation of drug therapy to onset of symptoms	5 yr	3 yr	20 yr
Signs and symptoms			
Facial dyskinesia	+	+	+
Blepharospasm	+	+	+
Oral involvement	+	+	+
Extremities involvement	+		
Neck involvement	+	+	
Dysphagia	+		−
Dysarthria	+	+	−
Response to discontinuation of antihistamine	No change	Improved	Improved
Reference	(4)	(4)	(5)

H_1 antihistaminic-associated dyskinesias could be characterized by persistence of signs and symptoms following drug withdrawal, but not an exacerbation of the movement disorder. All symptoms were subsequently controlled by the administration of haloperidol.

Phenomenological Comparisons of Late-Occurring H_1 Antihistamine-Induced Dyskinesias with Other Hyperkinetic States

The onset of symptoms with H_1 antihistamines is unique in that all three cases reported that blepharospasm occurred first and predated other signs and symptoms by several months to two years. Dyskinetic movements of this nature have been classified as complex dyskinesias, oculo-facial type (17). They may be present as bizarre movements of the surrounding facial muscles, blinking, or a vertical rotation of the eyes less sustained than in the typical oculogyric crisis. This clinical picture is reported to be induced by neuroleptics, but a study of tardive dyskinesia in chronic schizophrenic patients reported only a rare occurrence for this type of complex dyskinesia (17). Thus, blepharospasm is not commonly seen in tardive dyskinesia induced by neuroleptics, suggesting that H_1 antihistamine-induced dyskinesia may differ phenomenologically.

Tardive dyskinesia and L-dopa-induced hyperkinesia have been demonstrated to differ from one another on phenomenological criteria (18). The movement disorders induced by L-dopa differ on the frequency of periorbital, neck, and extremities symptoms (almost solely seen in L-dopa subjects). In contrast, tardive dyskinesia is localized almost exclusively to the oral region. The blepharospasm and neck involvement seen in the H_1 antihistamine-induced cases suggests a closer analogy to L-dopa-induced dyskinesia than to tardive dyskinesia. Since L-dopa dyskinesias are not seen in normal subjects (19), H_1 antihistamines may require an abnormal CNS to produce a dyskinetic syndrome.

CONCLUSION

Recent reports have indicated that H_1 antihistamines are associated with the appearance of acute dystonias and late-occurring dyskinesias. A literature survey discovered only a few more case reports, thus suggesting that both reactions occur only rarely. It is hoped that greater clinical awareness will add further information on the frequency and clinical presentations of these unusual adverse effects. In those patients that present with an acute dystonic reaction, H_1 antihistamines should be ruled out as possible contributing factors before they are routinely given as therapy. Patients who present with a late-

occurring dyskinesia should be screened for chronic H₁ antihistamine use, and
if present, the drugs should be withdrawn and the patients closely followed.
Further studies are required to more completely understand the pathogenesis of
these reactions.

REFERENCES

1. Lavenstein, B.L., Cantor, F.K. Acute dystonia: an unusual reaction to diphenhydramine. *JAMA*, *236*:291, 1976.
2. Favis, G.R. Facial dyskinesia related to antihistamine? *N. Eng. J. Med.*, *294*:730, 1976.
3. Brait, K.A., Zagerman, A.J. Dyskinesia after antihistamine use. *N. Eng. J. Med.*, *296*:111, 1977.
4. Thach, B.T., Chase, T.N., Bosma, J.F. Oral-facial dyskinesia associated with prolonged use of antihistaminic decongestants. *N. Eng. J. Med.*, *293*:486–487, 1975.
5. Davis, W.A. Dyskinesia associated with chronic antihistamine use. *N. Eng. J. Med.*, *293*:486–487, 1975.
6. Weil, H.R. Unusual side effect from Benadryl. *JAMA*, *133*:393, 1947.
7. Chitwood, W.R., Moore, C.D. The toxicity of antihistaminic drugs: a case report and discussion. *Virginia Med. Month.*, *78*:132–135, 1951.
8. Wörz, R. Späte extrapyramidale hyperkineseh während langzeitiger einnahme von mebhydrolin. *Dtsch. Med. Wschr.*, *98*:1071–1074, 1973.
9. Marsden, C.F., Tarsy, D., Baldessarini, R.J. In *Psychiatric Aspects of Neurologic Disease*. Benson, D.F., Blumer, D. (eds.). New York: Grune and Stratton, pp. 219–265, 1975.
10. Ayd, F.J. A survey of drug-induced extrapyramidal reactions. *JAMA*, *175*:102–108, 1961.
11. Davis, J.M., Cole, J.O. Antipsychotic agents. In *Comprehensive Textbook of Psychiatry*. Freedman, A.F., Kaplan, H. (eds.). Baltimore: Williams and Wilkins, pp. 1921–1941, 1975.
12. Garver, D.L., Davis, J.M., Dekirmenjian, H. *et al.* Dystonic reactions following neuroleptics: time course and proposed mechanisms. *Psychopharmacol.*, *47*:199–201, 1976.
13. McLennan, H., York, D.H. The action of dopamine on neurons of the caudate nucleus. *J. Physiol.*, *189*:393, 1967.
14. Deniker, P. Experimental neurological syndromes and the new drug therapies in psychiatry. *Compr. Psychiatry*, *1*:92–102, 1960.
15. Nowak, J.Z., Maślinski, C. Cholinergic link in the histamine-mediated increase in homovanillic acid in the rat striatum. *Agents and Actions*, *7*:27–30, 1977.
16. Eldridge, R. The torsion dystonias: literature review and genetic and clinical studies. *Neurology* (Minneap), *20*:1–78, 1970.
17. Crane, G.E., Naranjo, E.R. Motor disorders induced by neuroleptics. *Arch. Gen. Psychiatry*, *24*:179–184, 1971.
18. Gerlach, J. Relationship between tardive dyskinesia, L-dopa-induced hyperkinesia and parkinsonism. *Psychopharmacol.*, *51*:259–263, 1977.
19. Klawans, H.L., Paulson, G.W., Ringel, S.P., *et al.* Use of L-dopa in the detection of presynaptomatic Huntington's chorea. *N. Eng. J. Med.*, *286*:1332–1334, 1972.

31

Effects of Apomorphine and Amphetamine on Tardive Dyskinesia

ROBERT C. SMITH
CAROL TAMMINGA
and JOHN DAVIS

INTRODUCTION

Some of the hypotheses about the pathophysiological basis of tardive dyskinesia (TD) in man have been based on behavioral and biochemical studies of the effects of chronic neuroleptic drugs in animals, which have provided evidence for supersensitivity of postsynaptic dopamine receptors after termination of treatment with chronic neuroleptics (see Chapters 2–12 of this volume). The behavioral evidence for supersensitivity in animals comes from studies using the strategy of provocative tests with dopamine agonists, which have shown an increased effect of these drugs on stereotyped behavior, turning behavior, and/or locomotor activity in rats and mice withdrawn from chronic neuroleptics. Apomorphine, a direct-acting dopamine agonist, and amphetamine, an indirect-acting dopamine agonist, have been the drugs most frequently utilized in these animal studies.

Is the postsynaptic supersensitivity theory relevant to the human clinical syndrome of tardive dyskinesia? Some indirect evidence from psychopharmacological studies in patients with tardive dyskinesia is consistent with the postsynaptic supersensitivity hypotheses. When neuroleptic drugs such as haloperidol that block postsynaptic dopamine receptors (1) are administered to patients with symptoms of tardive dyskinesia, the symptoms are at least temporarily reduced (2). Other drugs such as reserpine that deplete biogenic amine stores in the presynaptic neurons also reduce symptoms of tardive dyskinesia (3). Chronic administration of L-dopa increases dopamine in pre-synaptic neurons, and some studies have also shown that it increases symptoms of tardive dyskinesia (4). However, both L-dopa and reserpine act primarily through their effect on the presynaptic neuron; therefore, their behavioral effects are not directly relevant to tests of a postsynaptic supersensitivity hypothesis of tardive dyskinesia.

In the study reported in this chapter, we used the same two drugs—apo-morphine and d-amphetamine—that have been used in the behavioral tests in the animal model, and we conducted analogous provocative tests in patients with tardive dyskinesia who had been withdrawn from neuroleptic drugs. We measured the behavioral effects of these drugs on the movement-disorder scores in patients with tardive dyskinesia. If the dopamine-agonist tests in animals chronically given neuroleptic drugs, which have been used to demon-strate supersensitivity, can also be applied to analogous tests in patients with the clinical syndrome of TD, then a postsynaptic supersensitivity hypothesis would predict that both apomorphine and d-amphetamine should increase symptoms of tardive dyskinesia in man.

METHODS

Patients with tardive dyskinesia were hospitalized on the research ward of the Illinois State Psychiatric Institute. Most of the patients were chronic schizophrenic patients (RDC chronic schizophrenia or chronic schizo-affective schizophrenia), between the ages of 25 and 73, who had been on neuroleptic medication for at least several years, and most had moderate to severe symptoms of tardive dyskinesia. The characteristics of some of these patients are summarized in Table 1 of Chapter 38, which reports other aspects of our study with these patients.

Tardive dyskinesia symptoms were evaluated with the Smith Tardive Dys-kinesia Scale, an observational scale in which many body parts are separately evaluated for dyskinetic and extrapyramidal symptoms (see copy of scale on p. 249). The primary measures used in these statistical analyses were 2 summary scores derived from sums of the scores of specified body parts: (1) oral-buccal-lingual dyskinesia (BL-TD), and (2) total tardive dyskinesia symptoms (the sum of all dyskinesia items) (total TD).

Tardive dyskinesia ratings were done by the principal investigators and nursing staff on the research ward who had achieved a fairly high degree of intrarater reliability (r = .80–.95 on summary scores). Tardive dyskinesia ratings were done routinely several times a week directly on the ward (observa-tion ratings) and also at specific times after acute drug administration. Fre-quent videotapes (TV) of the patients' movements were also made, and these were scored together at a later date. The observational ratings were usually a consensus of two trained raters.

We used double-blind placebo-controlled procedures to evaluate behavioral effects of apomorphine and amphetamine. All the patients in this study had been taken off their neuroleptic drugs and other psychotropic medications at least one week before testing, and most of the patients had been off drugs for periods of 3 to 6 weeks.

In procedures used to evaluate the behavioral effects of apomorphine, each of the patients received several doses of apomorphine (ranging from 0.75 to 6.0 mg) or saline placebo by subcutaneous injection at about 9 A.M. The patients did not eat breakfast on the morning of drug administration. Some patients did not complete the full series of all apomorphine doses, because they developed side effects of clinically significant nausea and/or vomiting at one of the lower doses, and further testing days were halted when these side effects occurred. Drug and saline days were interspersed with a saline day scheduled after every 1 or 2 active drug days. Observational ratings of tardive dyskinesia were done 20 to 30 minutes after administration of apomorphine, and a TV tape was done between 40 and 60 minutes after administration of apomorphine.

In the evaluation of the effects of amphetamine, either oral or intravenous (i.v.), procedures were used. In the oral protocol, the patients received an elixir of 20 mg of d-amphetamine sulfate, 1-amphetamine sulfate, or placebo solution on 2 different days, and observational and TV tape TD ratings were done at several points between 30 and 120 minutes after administration of the medication. Because preliminary testing in a few patients did not reveal marked effects or the oral amphetamine, we then switched to an i.v. amphetamine protocol. In the i.v. amphetamine protocol, 15 to 25 mg of d-amphetamine sulfate of saline placebo was administered intravenously through a scalp vein over a 10 to 15 minute time period. The blood pressure and psychological response of the patients were used to help determine the rate of administration and whether the drug should be stopped before the full 25 mg dose had been administered. One patient who had shown minimal physiological and behavioral responses with lower doses also received trials with two higher doses of i.v. amphetamine. Observational ratings of tardive dyskinesia were made before medication, at 5 or 10 minute intervals for a 45 minute period after the administration of medication, and again at 1½ to 2 hours after medication administration.

Because of our clinical observations in some of the early patients in the series, of the effects of amphetamine in apomorphine, we began to rate the psychological effects of these drugs on schizophrenic symptoms in some of the later patients in the series. For these purposes we used an interview form of the Modified New Haven Schizophrenia Index (5).

RESULTS

D-amphetamine

D-amphetamine produced an increase in tardive dyskinesia scores in most patients compared to same-day predrug baseline scores, although a few showed only minimal changes (see Fig. 1). Compared to baseline predrug TD scores, 5 to 6 patients showed a clear increase in tardive dyskinesia symptoms after 15–25 mg i.v. d-amphetamine, and one patient, J.G., showed no increase at the standard doses, but a small increase after 40 mg i.v. d-amphetamine.

For a number of patients on the d-amphetamine protocol, we have both an active-drug and placebo-control day (Fig. 2). Change scores for maximum postdrug dyskinesia in the drug versus the placebo days showed that i.v.

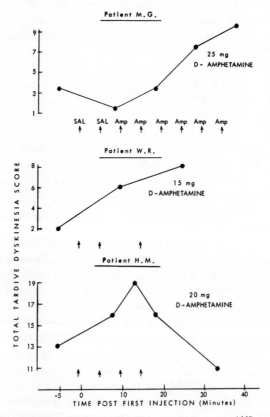

Figure 1.   Effects of d-amphetamine on tardive dyskinesia. Each ↑ or ↑^AMP indicates time of the injection of approximately 5 mg d-amphetamine through the i.v. line, and ↑^SAL indicates the time of saline injection.

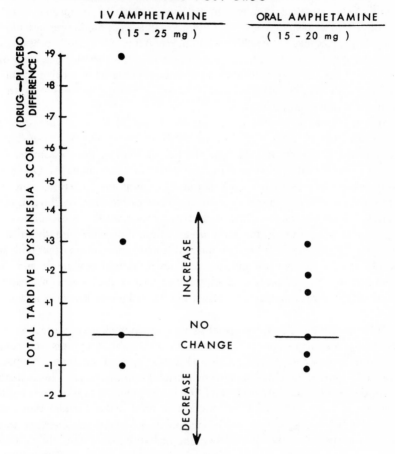

Figure 2.   Effects of i.v. or oral amphetamine, as compared to saline placebo on tardive dyskinesia. Each point represents the maximum postdrug score on the active amphetamine day, minus the maximum postinjection score on the saline placebo day.

amphetamine increased symptoms of tardive dyskinesia substantially in 3 of 5 patients, and no patient showed a substantial decrease in symptoms of tardive dyskinesia on d-amphetamine. Oral amphetamine had a smaller effect on increasing tardive dyskinesia symptoms. The results showing greater effectiveness of i.v. versus oral amphetamine for increasing symptoms for tardive dyskinesia are similar to the results of Davis and Janowsky, who showed significant changes in psychotic symptoms after i.v. amphetamine, but no marked exacerbation of symptoms with single doses of oral amphetamine.

The effects of d-amphetamine on blood pressure were not directly related to its effect on increasing dyskinetic symptoms. Although the patients who showed the smallest increase in tardive dyskinesia symptoms after i.v. d-amphetamine also had only small or no increases in blood pressure after the drug (e.g., patient J.G. had about 10mm Hg increase in systolic pressure after the 40 mg dose, but returned to baseline with a few minutes), several of the other patients who showed more pronounced increases in tardive dyskinesia scores also had relatively small blood pressure increases with i.v. d-amphetamine administration.

It is of interest to note that 2 patients, W.R. and M.B., who were reported to have a history of tardive dyskinesia, showed no or only very questionable subclinical TD symptoms while in the hospital before the i.v. amphetamine test (i.e., total tardive dyskinesia scores of 0–2 on different days). On the basis of the extent of severity of their baseline TD symptoms, questions were raised among the staff about the accuracy of the history of tardive dyskinesia. In both patients, however, an i.v. amphetamine test produced an intensification of the dyskinesia symptoms in the body areas where they were already present at marginal levels, and also brought out additional symptoms in other body areas where there had been no indication of even a mild dyskinetic movement abnormality. The increase in symptoms of tardive dyskinesia in these areas remitted to their low baseline levels within 1½ to 3 hours after drug administration.

In most patients, psychological effects of amphetamine were also noted clinically, and in later patients in the series, psychotic symptoms were rated by brief interview on the Modified New Haven Schizophrenia Index. No patients showed a marked increase in psychosis after d-amphetamine. This is different from the results that Janowsky and Davis (6) reported in more acute schizophrenic patients, where i.v. amphetamine produced a marked transient increase in psychosis; only a few of our patients showed any increase in their psychosis scores on the NHSI. The one or two patients who did show some increase in psychosis scores after oral or i.v. d-amphetamine were the less chronic patients, whereas the psychopathology scores of chronic schizophrenic patients were unaffected by d-amphetamine.

Apomorphine

Contrary to our initial expectations, apomorphine did not increase symptoms of tardive dyskinesia. In some patients, one or more doses of the drug produced a mild to marked decrease in TD scores, while in other patients there was little or no change in dyskinetic symptoms. Figure 3 presents the results of total dyskinesia scores for several patients. Since there was no simple dose-response relationship for the effect of apomorphine on dyskinetic symptoms in the dose range we tested, we computed mean scores on the apomorphine and

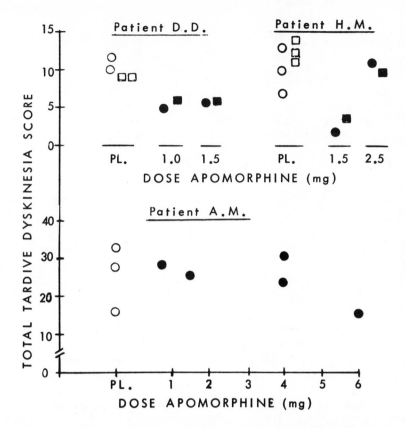

Figure 3.   Effects of several doses of apomorphine (s.c.) or saline placebo (s.c.) on tardive dyskinesia; 3 representative patients. Symbols: ○ □ placebo days, ○ ■ apomorphine days; ○ • observational ratings; □ ■ TV tape ratings.

the placebo days, and took the difference between the drug and placebo means. These drug-placebo-difference scores are presented in Figure 4. At a rating of 20 minutes post apomorphine, 5 patients showed a decrease in tardive dyskinesia scores (mean, 24% decrease), and at the TV tape ratings conducted at 40 minutes, 6 patients showed moderate to marked decrease in dyskinesia scores (mean, 39% decrease). Two patients showed more than a 60% decrease at the 40 minute point. At both points there were 2 or 3 patients who showed essentially no change or a small questionable increase in TD symptoms.

Most patients experienced emetic effects of apomorphine (nausea and/or vomiting) at some drug dose, although the maximum dose that patients tolerated without side effects varied from 1.5 to 6.0 mg. However, there was no consistent relationship between the effects of apomorphine on emesis and movement symptoms.

No patient showed any substantial increase in psychosis on apomorphine,

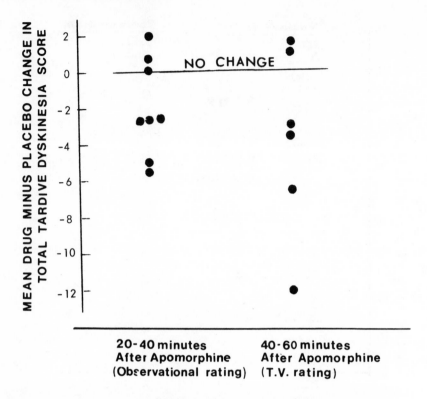

20-40 minutes   40-60 minutes
After Apomorphine   After Apomorphine
(Observational rating) (T.V. rating)

Figure 4.   Effects of apomorphine versus saline placebo on tardive dyskinesia. Each point represents the mean TD symptom score on several apomorphine days, minus the mean score on several saline placebo days.

and several patients showed a decrease in psychotic symptoms. These results were also contrary to what might be predicted on the basis of a dopamine supersensitivity theory of schizophrenia. These apparently ''therapeutic'' effects of apomorphine on psychotic symptoms have been discussed in more detail elsewhere (7, 8).

DISCUSSION

The behavioral effects of i.v. d-amphetamine, which increased symptoms of tardive dyskinesia, are consistent with the data from animal models and with the interpretation that abnormalities in brain catecholamines are involved in the pathophysiology of tardive dyskinesia. Amphetamine acts primarily through its effect on presynaptic neurons, by releasing and blocking reuptake of brain dopamine and norepinephrine rather than by directly stimulating postsynapatic receptors. The effects of i.v. amphetamine on TD that we report compliment the results of some previous studies which show that chronic administration of another indirectly acting dopamine agonist, L-dopa, increased symptoms of tardive dyskinesia, and a drug, reserpine, which depletes presynaptic biogenic amines, also decreased symptoms of tardive dyskinesia (3, 4).

The effects of apomorphine in patients with tardive dyskinesia, on the other hand, did not seem to parallel the behavioral effects that apomorphine has been reported to have in the animal models that have been proposed as possible analogues of this human clinical syndrome. In rats withdrawn from chronic administration of neuroleptics, apomorphine produces greater stereotyped movements than in saline controls; these pharmacological effects have been interpreted as evidence for postsynaptic dopamine receptor supersensitivity. In human patients with tardive dyskinesia, on the other hand, apomorphine tended to reduce dyskinetic movements. The behavioral effects of apomorphine in tardive dyskinesia that we have reported in this paper are similar to the effects of this drug in two other movement disorders, Huntington's chorea (9) and dyskinesia induced by chronic administration of L-dopa in patients with Parkinson's disease (10). Some of the pathophysiology of these other two diseases have also been hypothesized to involve supersensitivity of postsynaptic dopamine receptors. It is also interesting to note that in their monkey model of tardive dyskinesia, Gunne and Barany (11) have also reported that similar doses of apomorphine reduced symptoms of tardive dyskinesia in monkeys who had developed these symptoms after chronic administration of neuroleptic drugs.

The paradoxical behavioral effects of apomorphine in man, which seem to run counter to initial predictions based on the supersensitivity hypothesis, may be due to several factors. The use of apomorphine to test the postsynaptic supersensitivity hypothesis was based on its action as a direct postsynaptic dopamine-receptor stimulator (12, 13). However, recent experimental findings have indicated that apomorphine also has important effects on presynaptic dopamine neurons and receptors, as well as on its previously established postsynaptic receptor action (14, 15). These presynaptic effects of apomorphine result in a decrease in tyrosine hydroxylase activity and dopamine synthesis, with a consequent decrease in functionally available dopamine. At low doses of apomorphine (.03–.10 mg/kg in animal studies), these presynaptic effects are the predominant effects of the drug, whereas at higher doses (e.g., 0.5–2 mg/kg), the direct postsynaptic stimulating effect of the drug may account for most of its behavioral effects within the first hour after drug administration. The doses of apomorphine that we gave to patients (.75–6 mg s.c.), when converted to a mg/kg basis, are about .01 to .14 mg/kg in our subjects; these are more similar to the doses at which the inhibitory effects of apomorphine have been found to predominate in rats and mice (15), and they are lower than most of the doses (.25–2 mg/kg) at which supersensitivity to apomorphine has been shown in animals after termination of chronic neuroleptic administration. The effects of apomorphine which we have shown in patients with tardive dyskinesia, as well as similar effects of apomorphine previously reported in patients with other choreiform movement disorders, might, therefore, be due to the presynaptic inhibitory effect of apomorphine rather than its effect of directly stimulating dopamine receptors. This interpretation of the reasons for apomorphine's effect on reducing TD symptoms *is* consistent with our observation that apomorphine also decreased psychosis scores in a few of these patients. If dopamine overactivity plays a role in the pathogenesis or activation of schizophrenic symptoms, as has been suggested by several investigators (16), then the effect of low doses of apomorphine on decreasing presynaptic dopaminergic activity might therefore lead to a reduction in the patients' psychosis scores. These clinical effects of apomorphine in reducing psychosis have been confirmed in later studies, in which we showed a synergistic effect of apomorphine in chronic schizophrenic patients who were concurrently treated with low or standard doses of neuroleptic medication (7, 8).

Most of our patients experienced emetic effects of apomorphine at some dose, and these emetic effects have been attributed to the postsynaptic action of the drug. It is possible, however, that there may be different dopamine receptors mediating the emetic versus the motor effects of the drug. Recent research in dogs (17), for example, has reported that a higher dose of apomorphine was required to produce stereotyped behavior than emesis in this species.

An unambiguous interpretation of our behavioral results on the effects of apomorphine in patients with tardive dyskinesia in regard to the postsynaptic supersensitivity hypothesis of this disorder is, therefore, more difficult, because of the dose of apomorphine we used and the recent research demonstrating inhibitory effects of this drug on presynaptic dopamine neurons. To more adequately test the postsynaptic supersensitivity hypothesis, we might have to go to much higher doses of apomorphine, similar to those doses at which agonist effects have been seen clinically in patients with Parkinson's disease (18). An alternate strategy would be to use another dopamine agonist drug that had a direct action on stimulating postsynaptic dopamine receptors but did not have much potent presynaptic effect at the usual clinically administered doses. One recent report (19) has indicated that bromocriptine, an ergot drug with some properties of a direct dopamine agonist, did increase symptoms of Huntington's chorea, whereas it had previously been shown that apomorphine decreased these symptoms (9). Very preliminary results of a trial conducted by one of the authors (Tamminga) indicates that bromocriptine may increase symptoms of tardive dyskinesia.

Our positive results with d-amphetamine have implications for theory and clinical testing. Since amphetamine exerts its effects primarily through release and blockade of reuptake of biogenic amines in the presynaptic neuron, our results suggest that more attention should be given to possible defects in the functioning of presynaptic neurons in tardive dyskinesia. The results reported in Chapter 5 demonstrate that chronic administration of neuroleptic drugs in the rat do produce changes in some of the biochemical processes associated more closely with presynaptic neurons. Of greater clinical significance, however, is our finding that amphetamine could elicit recognizable symptoms of tardive dyskinesia in some patients who had very minimal or subclinical signs of the disease. Since the symptoms of tardive dyskinesia vary considerably from day to day, routine clinical evaluations might easily miss the diagnosis in some of the patients. In cases in which there is some reason (clinical history or length of neuroleptic administration) to presume the possibility of tardive dyskinesia, an i.v. amphetamine test might be a useful additional diagnostic method to help uncover early cases of this disorder. For those patients who demonstrate symptoms of tardive dyskinesia during the provocative test, a more careful evaluation can be pursued, and remedial measures such as reduction of neuroleptic drugs, extended drug holidays, or therapeutic trials with drugs that might decrease tardive dyskinesia symptoms could then be instituted to try to prevent progression of the disease.

ACKNOWLEDGMENTS

Supported in part by fellowships from the Foundations Funds for Research in Psychiatry to Dr. Smith (FFRP 74-578) and Dr. Tamminga (FFRP 74-592).

REFERENCES

1. Burt, D.R., Cresse, I., Snyder, S. Dopamine receptor binding predicts clinical and pharmacological potencies of anti-schizophrenic drugs. *Science, 192*:481–483, 1976.
2. Kazamatsuri, H., Chien, C.P., Cole, J.O. Long-term treatment of tardive dyskinesia with haloperidol and tetrabenzaine. *Am. J. Psychiatry, 130*:479–482. 1973.
3. Villineuve, A., Boszarmeyi, Z. Treatment of drug-induced dyskinesias. *Lancet, 1*:353–354, 1970.
4. Gerlach, J., Reisby, N., Randrup, A. Dopaminergic hypersensitivity and cholinergic hypofunction in the pathophysiology of tardive dyskinesia. *Psychopharmacology, 34*:21–35, 1974.
5. Schaffer, M.H., Tamminga, C.A., Davis, J.M. Modified New Haven Schizophrenia Scale. Mimeograph, 1977.
6. Janowsky, D.S., Davis, J.M. Methylphenidate, dextroamphetamine, and levafetamine. *Arch. Gen. Psychiatry, 33*:304–308, 1976.
7. Smith, R.C., Tamminga, C.T., Davis, J.M. Effect of apophorphine on schizophrenic symptoms. *J. Neural Transm., 40*:171–176, 1977.
8. Tamminga, C.T., Shaffer, M.H., Smith, R.C., Davis, J.M. Schizophrenic symptoms improve with apomorphine. *Science, 200*:567–568, 1978.

9.   Tolosa, E.S., Sparber, S.B. Apomorphine in Huntington's chorea: clinical observations and theoretical considerations. *Life Sci., 15*:1371–1380, 1975.

10. Duby, S.E., Cotzias, G.C., Papavasiliov, P.S. Injected apomorphine and orally administered levodopa in parkinsonism. *Arch. Neurol., 27*:474–480, 1972.

11. Gunne, L.M., Barany, S. Haloperidol-induced dyskinesia in monkeys. *Psychopharm., 50*:237–240, 1976.

12. Ernst, A.M. Mode of action of apomorphine and amphetamine in gnawing compulsion in rats. *Psychopharmacologia, 10*:316–323, 1967.

13. Andén, N.E., Rubenson, A., Fuxe, K., Hökfelt, T. Evidence for dopamine receptor stimulation by apomorphine. *J. Pharm., Pharmacol., 14*:627–629, 1968.

14. Walters, J.R., Bunney, B.S., Roth, R.H. Piribedil and apomorphine pre- and post-synaptic effects of dopamine synthesis and neurological activity. In *Advances in Neurology*, vol. 9. Calne, D.B., Chase, T.N., Barbeau, A. (eds.). New York: Raven Press, pp. 273–284, 1975.

15. Carlsson, A. Receptor mediated control of dopamine metabolism. In *Pre- and Post-Synaptic Receptors*. Usdin, E., Bunney, W.E. (eds.). New York: Dekker, pp. 49–65, 1975.

16. Snyder, S.H. Cathecolamines in the brain as mediators of amphetamine psychosis. *Arch. Gen. Psychol., 27*:169–179, 1972.

17. Nymark, M. Apomorphine provoked stereotypy in the dog. *Psychopharmacologia, 26*:361–368, 1972.

18. Cotzios, G.C., Papavasiliov, P.S., Tolosa, E.S., Mendez, S.S., Bell-Midura, M. Treatment of Parkinson's disease with apomorphines. *N. Eng. J. Med., 294*:567–572, 1976.

19. Kartzinel, R., Hunt, R.D., Calne, D.B. Bromocriptine in Huntington's chorea. *Arch. Neurol., 33*:517–518, 1976.

32

A Neuroendocrine Study of Supersensitivity in Tardive Dyskinesia

CAROL A. TAMMINGA
ROBERT C. SMITH
GHANSHYAM PANDEY
JOHN M. DAVIS
and LAWRENCE A. FROHMAN

Recent methodologic advances have allowed an increasingly precise description of the central neurotransmitter control of pituitary hormone secretion. Neuropharmacologic probes have been used by various investigators in an attempt to assess brain activity of specific transmitter systems in humans. These techniques generally involve administration of a drug with a described pharmacologic action to an experimental group, with the subsequent measurement of a target pituitary hormone. The present study explores the use of this technique to obtain biochemical evidence of the purported pathophysiology of tardive dyskinesia.

Tardive dyskinesia, the hyperkinetic movement disorder that develops as a side effect of long-term neuroleptic drug treatment, is thought to result from supersensitive central dopamine (DA) receptors in the corpus striatum. It has been proposed that supersensitivity develops following prolonged "chemical denervation" by DA-receptor antagonists such as those used in the treatment of schizophrenia (1). This hypothesis is supported by the pharmacologic observations that levodopa and amphetamine intensify the involuntary movements of tardive dyskinesia (2,3), and antipsychotic drugs known to block DA receptors diminish dyskinesias (4,5). A long-recognized phenomenon, denervation hypersensitivity was initially used to explain certain pharmacologically mediated responses noted to be enhanced following surgical denervation in the peripheral nervous system (6–8). Sharpless and Halpern subsequently proposed that supersensitivity could account for the increased brain excitability that follows depressant-drug use (9). More recently, Ungerstedt reported that following peripheral apomorphine administration, rats with chemically induced unilateral caudate nucleus lesions showed a unilaterally augmented motor response (circling behavior), and he inferred supersensitivity (10). Subsequent reports by other investigators have provided considerable behavioral and biochemical data supporting the concept that the DA receptors in the brain become hypersensitive following both denervation and chronic neuroleptic treatment (11–15).

The present study has focused on two hormones, growth hormone (GH) and prolactin (Prl), for which clear dopaminergic control is recognized (16,17). Studies in experimental animals and human subjects suggest that prolactin release is controlled primarily by an inhibitory factor, the secretion of which is stimulated by DA-containing neurons in the tuberoinfundibular neuronal tract (18–21). It is not yet clear whether dopaminergic synapses within the hypothalamus contribute to the regulation of prolactin release, or whether DA acts directly on pituitary DA receptors (22,23). Irrespective of the site of DA action, DA antagonists briskly elevate plasma Prl levels, and DA agonists inhibit Prl release. In contrast to the effects on Prl, plasma GH is consistently elevated in response to a variety of drugs that augment DA-mediated nerve transmission (24). Basal GH levels are generally too low for a suppressant effect to be detected. Following administration of pharmacologic agents that alter DA-mediated neural transmission, measurement of these hormones would theoretically be expected to reveal an augmented hormonal response in schizophrenic patients with tardive dyskinesia if indeed increased DA-receptor sensitivity occurred with chronic antipsychotic-drug use and accompanied tardive dyskinesia.

METHODS

The patients used in this study were diagnosed as having chronic schizophrenia (CS), according to the Research Diagnostic Criteria of Spitzer and Endicott (25). The 8 patients with tardive dyskinesia (TD) exhibited persistent, involuntary, and irregular movements of the oral-buccal-lingual region and of the extremities, often including gait. All patients were free from neuroleptic drugs for at least 5 days, and the patients with tardive dyskinesia were drug-free for 1 to 3 months at the time of endocrine testing. Specific characteristics of this population are indicated in the Table 1.

Subjects were studied at 9 A.M. in a fasting state while resting in bed. Baseline blood samples were collected for 1 hour prior to drug administration; 0.75 mg. of apomorphine or 500 mg. levodopa was given after this baseline period. Heparinized blood samples were collected at frequent intervals for 3 hours and kept at 4°C until the plasma was separated and frozen at -20°C.

Table 1
Characteristics of Patients and Controls

Group 1. Chronic schizophrenia with tardive dyskinesia

Patient	Age	Sex	Duration of Neuroleptic Treatment (years)	Major Clinical Symptoms
1	33	F	4	Oral smacking, facial grimaces
2	39	F	12	Oral smacking, jerky extremity movements
3	34	M	15+	Irregular Lip & finger movements
4	63	F	15+	Persistent oral & finger movements
5	25	M	3	Severe facial & extremity movements
6	52	M	10	Heel-walking gait, extremity movements
7	49	F	8	Extremity movements, irregular oral tics
8	59	F	12	Oral tics, fly-catching tongue movements

Group 2. Chronic schizophrenia without tardive dyskinesia

n = 10	(mean ±SD) 26.2	5F 7M	4.7±1.2	Hallucinations, delusions, and/or thought disorders present continually for >1 year

Group 3. Controls

n = 12	25.8 ±2.0	3F 7M		

Prl and GH were measured by a homologous double antibody radioim-munoassay (26), using purified hormone obtained from the Pituitary Hormone Distribution Service of the NIAMDD. Significance of the data was analyzed with the Fisher exact test, which was used to compare the number of abnormal responses in the patient group with those found in the control group (27).

RESULTS

The mean baseline Prl values for the three groups of subjects were similar to those of controls, and all groups were within normal limits for this laboratory. In response to levodopa, Prl levels in all groups were suppressed from the predrug stable baseline, but a consistently blunted Prl response to levodopa was present in both patient groups. All chronic schizophrenic patients had a decreased response compared to that of the control group, which consisted of a diminution greater than 50% in plasma Prl levels during a period of 120 minutes (Fig. 1). These differences between the control group and the TD and CS groups were highly significant (P <.01 and P <.005, respectively).

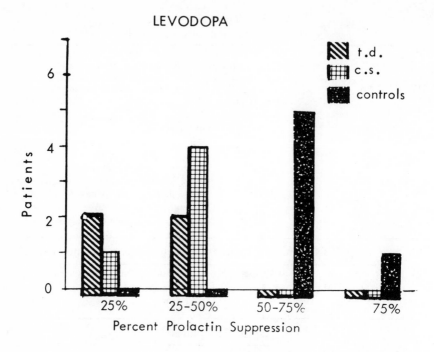

Figure 1.   Percent prolactin suppression from a stable baseline in response to levodopa (500 mg orally). Patient groups have tardive dyskinesia (t.d.), chronic schizophrenia (c.s.) or are normal controls. Peak suppression, which occurs 60–120 minutes following drug administration, is less than 50% in all subjects of both patient populations, greater than 50% in all controls.

After apomorphine administration, serum Prl values were suppressed in all groups. Eight of the 11 CS patients had less than 20% suppression from baseline, whereas the controls all responded to apomorphine with a suppression greater than 20% (Fig. 2). When the total chronic schizophrenic group (TD + CS) was compared to controls, the difference was statistically significant (P<.02).

The baseline values for GH were less than 1 ng/ml in all groups. Plasma GH levels rose in all subjects in response to levodopa (Fig. 3). The peak GH response in the TD and in the CS group was not significantly lower than that in the controls when tested individually (P<.14 and P<.07, respectively). However, within the combined schizophrenia group (TD + CS), 7 of 9 patients had an abnormally low GH response to levodopa, whereas only 2 of 11 normal subjects failed to increase GH levels above 5 ng/ml. The difference between the controls and the combined patient group was statistically significant (P<.02).

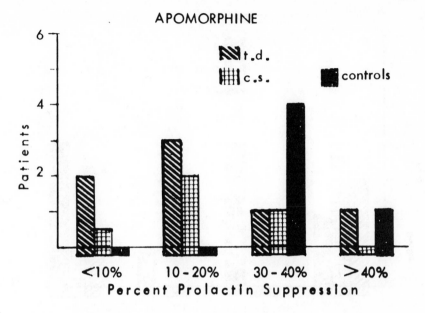

Figure 2.   Percent prolactin suppression from a stable baseline following administration of apomorphine (.75 mg subcutaneously). Patient groups as in Figure 1. Significantly more patients failed to suppress adequately, compared with controls who suppressed 30% or more.

Following apomorphine administration, the mean GH response of the schizophrenic group showed a trend toward hyporesponsiveness (Fig. 4), but the differences did not reach statistical significance.

DISCUSSION

In summary, these studies do not demonstrate an endocrine supersensitivity in patients who have tardive dyskinesia, as would have been predicted by the purported nigrostriatal supersensitivity. On the contrary, a significant hyporesponsivity was found to dopaminergic drugs in all the schizophrenic patients. These results can be explained in several ways. Since DA receptors differ pharmacologically and physiologically between and/or within DA tracts in the brain (28–31), these data can be interpreted to further support the hypothesis that DA receptors in the pituitary have their own distinguishing characteristics. Receptor characteristics may well vary considerably among central DA tracts. Just as psychosis (purportedly DA-mediated) does not intensify with prolonged neuroleptic use, so endocrine parameters affected by DA may not be augmented following long-term DA-receptor blockade. How-

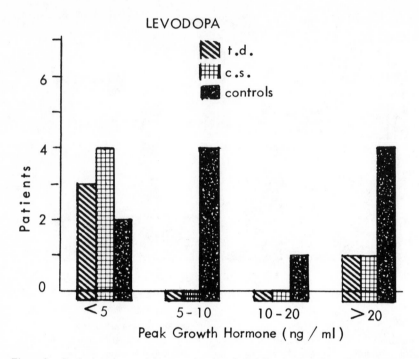

Figure 3.   Peak plasma growth hormone level (ng/ml) following levodopa administration (500 mg orally). Patient groups as in Figure 1. Significantly more patients (t.d. and c.s.) had peak GH levels below 5 ng/ml than did controls.

ever, it cannot be forgotten that some studies have already shown that neuroendocrine hypersensitivity occurs in animals following denervation or blockage of the tuberoinfundibular pituitary system. The dose of apomorphine required to decrease Prl levels in rats chronically treated with haloperidol is lower than that required in saline-treated controls (32), and an increased inhibition of Prl has been observed in response to apomorphine administration 14 days after hypothalamic deafferentation (33). One can argue for the presence of a mechanism other than receptor supersensitivity to account for the symptoms in tardive dyskinesia. Altered responses in the nigrostriatum could, for example, be due to defects in feedback sensitivities and mechanisms rather than alteration in the DA receptor itself.

In addition to the failure to confirm hypersensitivity in patients with TD, a significant hyporesponsiveness of the two pituitary hormones, GH and Prl, was also found in the chronic schizophrenic patient group without TD. This diminished hormonal responsiveness could occur in the tuberoinfundibular neurons secondary to chronic drug administration. However, patients were neuroleptic-free from 5 days to 3 months, and responsivity was not correlated

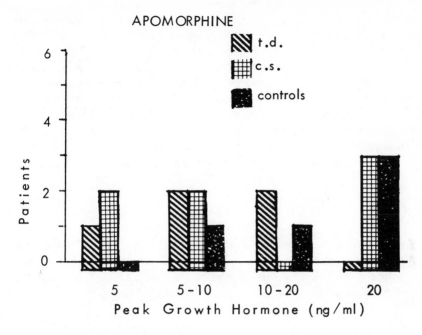

Figure 4.   Peak plasma growth hormone levels (ng/ml) following apomorphine administration (.75 mg subcutaneously). Patient groups as in Figure 1. There was a tendency, although not statistically significant for patients to have lower GH peaks than normal controls.

with duration of drug-free period. Alternatively, the changes observed could indicate a central regulatory abnormality associated with chronic schizophrenia.

An indirect effect of chronic neuroleptics on the endocrine system may result in blunted hormonal responses. It is well documented that Prl levels are elevated in patients receiving neuroleptic medication (34–37). Perhaps a (yet unidentified) compensatory hormone feedback loop may participate in blunting the Prl responses to dopaminergic agonists, due to the constant neuroleptic–induced stimulation of Prl. Alternately, since alterations in the phasic secretion of LH and disruptions in cyclic gonadal steroid secretion occur in certain schizophrenic females chronically treated with neuroleptics, these changes could be responsible for blunting of both the GH and Prl response. Both in laboratory animals and in man, estrogen levels clearly alter baseline secretion of GH and Prl and their response to drugs (38–41). A simultaneous demonstration of decreased estrogen secretion accompanied by blunted GH or Prl responses to drugs in drug-free schizophrenic patients who had been chronically medicated would be required to establish this as an accountable mechanism.

The finding of hormonal hyporesponsiveness to dopaminergic stimulation, whether due to an abnormality intrinsic to chronic schizophrenia or to direct or indirect effects of chronic antipsychotic drugs, thus warrants further study, both of other hormones and of possible alterations in monoamine systems in schizophrenia. The present results do not support the hypothesis of supersensitivity in the tuberoinfundibular neurons following chronic antipsychotic drugs in schizophrenic patients with or without tardive dyskinesia, but do suggest possible pharmacologic differences in central DA receptors. The data do demonstrate a simultaneous hyporesponsiveness of GH and prolactin to dopaminergic stimulation in a chronic schizophrenic population.

ACKNOWLEDGMENTS

This investigation was supported in part by fellowships FFRP 74–592 and FFRP 73–578 from the Foundations Fund for Research in Psychiatry to Drs. Tamminga and Smith, respectively, and by grant AM 18722 from the Public Health Service to Dr. Frohman.

REFERENCES

1. Rubovitz, R., Klawans, H.L. Implications for amphetamine-induced stereotyped behavior as a model for tardive dyskinesia. *Arch. Gen. Psychiatry, 27*:502–507, 1972.
2. Gerlach, J., Reisby, N., Randrup, A. Dopaminergic hypersensitivity and cholinergic hypofunction in the pathophysiology of tardive dyskinesia. *Psychopharmacologia, 24*:21–35, 1974.
3. Smith, R.C., Tamminga, C.A., Haraszti, J., Pandey, G.N., Davis, J.M. Effects of dopamine agonists in tardive dyskinesia. *Am. J. Psychiatry, 134*:763–768, 1977.
4. Klawans, H.L. The pharmacology of tardive dyskinesia. *Am. J. Psychiatry, 130*:82–85, 1973.
5. Kobayaski, R.M. Drug therapy of tardive dyskinesia. *N. Engl. J. Med., 296*:82–85, 1977.
6. Cannon, W.B., Rosenblueth, A. *The Supersensitivity of Denervated Structures: A Law of Denervation*. New York: Macmillan, 1949.
7. Trendelenburg, U. Supersensitivity and subsensitivity to sympathomimetic amines. *Pharmacol. Rev., 15*:225–276, 1963.
8. Fleming, W.W., McPhillips, J.J., Westfall, D.P. Postjunctional supersensitivity of excitable tissues to drugs. *Ergeb. Physiol., 68*:55–119, 1973.
9. Sharpless, S.K., Halpern, L.M. The electrical excitability of chronically isolated cortex studied by means of permanently implanted electrodes. *Electroencephalogr. Clin. Neurophysiol., 14*:244–255, 1962.
10. Ungerstedt, U. Postsynaptic supersensitivity after 6-hydroxydopamine induced degeneration of the nigrostriatal dopamine system. *Acta Physiol. Scand., 367* (suppl):69–93, 1971.
11. Iverson, S.D., Creese, I. Behavioral correlates of dopaminergic supersensitivity. In *Advances in Neurology*, Calne, D.B., Chase, T.N., Barbeau, A. (eds.). New York: Raven Press, pp. 81–92, 1975.
12. Brown, G.M., Garfinkel, P.E., Warsh, J.J. Effect of carbidopa on prolactin, growth hormone and cortisol secretion in man. *J. Clin. Endocrinol. Metab., 43*:236–239, 1976.

13. Smith, R.C., Davis, J.M. Behavioral supersensitivity to apomorphine and amphetamine after chronic high-dose haloperidol treatment. *Psychopharmacol. Comm., 1*:285–288, 1975.

14. Smith, R.C., Varies, J.M. Behavioral evidence for supersensitivity after chronic administration of haloperidol, clozapine, and thioridazine, *Life Sci., 19*:725–732, 1976.

15. Moore, K.E., Thronburg, J.E. Drug-induced dopaminergic supersensitivity. In *Advances in Neurology,* Calne, D.B., Chase, T.N., Barbeau, A. (eds.). New York: Raven Press, pp. 93-104, 1975.

16. Frohman, L.A., Stachura, M.E. Neuropharmacologic control of neuroendocrine function in man. *Metabolism, 24*:211–234, 1975.

17. DeWeid, D., DeJong, W. Drug effects and hypothalamic-anterior pituitary function. *Annu. Rev. Pharmacol. Toxicol., 7*:389–412, 1974.

18. Kleinberg, D.L., Noel, G.L., Frantz, A.G. Chlorpromazine stimulation and L-dopa suppression of plasma prolactin in man. *J. Clin. Endocrinol. Metab. 33*:873–876, 1971.

19 Friesen, H.,Guyda, H., Hwang, P. Functional evaluation of prolactin secretion: A guide to therapy. *J. Clin. Invest., 51*:706–709, 1972.

20. Saito, S., Abe, K., Nagata, N. Effect of L-dopa on anterior pituitary hormone release in man. *Endrocrinol Jpn., 19*: 435–442, 1972.

21. Brown, W.A., Van Woert, M.H., Ambani, L.M. Effect of apomorphine on growth hormone release in humans. *J. Clin. Endocrinol. Metab., 37*:463–465, 1973.

22. MacLeod, R.M. Regulation of prolactin sectetion. In *Frontiers in Neuroendocrinology,* Martini, L., Ganong, W.F. (eds.) New York: Raven Press, pp. 169–194, 1976.

23. Diefenbach, W.P., Carmel, P.W., Frantz, A.G. Suppression of prolactin secretion by L-dopa in the stalk sectioned rhesus monkey. *J. Clin. Endocrinol. Metab., 43*:636–642, 1976.

24. Martin, J.B., Brain regulation of growth hormone secretion. In *Frontiers of Neuroendocrinology,* Martini, L., Ganong, W.F. (eds.). New York: Raven Press, pp. 129–168, 1976.

25. Spitzer, R.K., Endicott, J., Robins, E. Prelininary report of reliability of research diagnostic criteria applied to psychiatric case records. In *Predictability in Psychopharmacology,* Sudilousky, A., Gershon, S., Beer, R., (eds.). Raven Press, pp. 245–258, 1975.

26. Sinha, Y.N., Selby, F.W., Lewis, U.J., Vander Laan, W.P. A homologous radioimmunoassay for human prolactin. *J. Clin. Endocrinol. Metab., 36*:509–512, 1973.

27. Segal, S. *Nonparamaetric Statistics for the Behavioral Sciences.* New York: McGraw-Hill, 1956.

28. Cools, A.R. Two functionally and pharmacologically distinct dopamine receptors in the rat brain. *Adv. Biochem. Psychopharmacol., 16*:215–225, 1977.

29. Kitae, S.T., Sugimoti, M., Kocsis, J.D. Dopamine eliciting excitatory and inhibitory effects on striatal neurons. *Exp. Brain Res., 24*:351–354, 1976.

30. Rick, J., Payne, P., Cannon, J., Frohman, L.A. Evidence for differences in pituitary dopamine (DA) receptors from those in the kidney, based on the prolactin (Prl) suppressive effects of 2-aminotetalin analogs. *Clin. Res., 25*:566A, 1977.

31. Friend, W.C., Brown, G.M., Lee, T. Neuroleptic receptors in pituitary and striatum. Read before the New Research Program of the 130th annual meeting of the American Psychiatric Association, Toronto, May 1977.

32. Lal, H., Brown, W., Drawbaugh, R. Enhanced prolactin inhibition following chronic treatment with haloperidol and morphine. *Life Sci., 20*:101–106, 1977.

33. Cheung, C.Y., Weiner, R.I. Supersensitivity of anterior pituitary dopamine receptors involved in the inhibition of prolactin secretion following destruction of the medical basal hypothalamus. *Endocrinology, 99*:917–941, 1976.

34. Wilson, R.G., Hamilton, J.R., Boyd, W.D., Forrest, A.P.M., Cole, E.N. Boyns, A.R., Griffths, K. The effect of long-term phenothiazine therapy on plasma prolactin. *Br. J. Psychiatry, 127*:71–75, 1975.

35. Kolakowska, T., Wiles, D.H., McNeilly, A.S., Gelder, M.G. Correlation between plasma levels of prolactin and chlorpromazine in psychiatric patients. *Psychol. Med.*, 5:214–216, 1975.
36. Beaumont, P.J.U., Gelder, M.G., Friesen, H.G., Harris, G.W., MacKinnon, P.C.B., Mandelbrote, B.M., Wiles, D.H. The effects of phenothiazines on endocrine function. *Br. J. Psychiatry*, 124:413–419, 1974.
37. Meites, J., Lu, K.H., Wutteke, W., Welsch, C.W., Nagasawan, H., Quadpi, S.K. Recent studies on functions and control of prolactin secretion in rats. *Recent Prog. Horm. Res.*, 28:527–590, 1972.
38. Frantz, A.G., Kleinberg, D.L., Noel, G.L. Studies on prolactin in man. *Recent Prog. Horm. Res.*, 28:527–590, 1972.
39. Carlson, H.E., Jacobs, L.S., Daushday, W.H. Growth hormone, thyrotropin and prolactin responses to thyrotropin-releasing hormone following diethylstilbestrol pretreatment. *J. Clin. Endocrinol. Metab.*, 37:488–491, 1973.
40. Buckman, M.T., Peake, G.T. Estrogen potentiation of phenothiazine-induced prolactin secretion in man. *J. Clin. Endocrinol. Metab.*, 37:977–980, 1973.
41. Wiedemann, E., Schwartz, E., Frantz, A.G. Acute and chronic estrogen effects upon serum somatomedian activity, growth hormone, and prolactin in man. *J. Clin. Endocrinol. Metab.*, 42:942–951, 1976.

33

Pathophysiological Aspects of Reversible and Irreversible Tardive Dyskinesia

J. GERLACH
and A. FAURBYE

Tardive dyskinesia has been the object of clinical as well as pharmacological research at the Sct. Hans Hospital for more than two decades, beginning with a systematic study by Uhrbrand and Faurbye (1) in 1960, and followed up in 1964 by a study of 109 patients with tardive dyskinesia, which attempted to elucidate the predisposing factors and the therapeutic possibilities (tetrabenazine and orphenadrine) (2). In the 1970's, these clinical studies were extended into more comprehensive pharmacological manipulations of tardive dyskinesia by means of various drugs, such as haloperidol, thioridazine, and clozapine (3,4), alphamethyl-p-tyrosine (AMPT) (5,6), baclofen (7), L-dopa (5), biperiden (6), scopolamine and physostigmine (5), and lithium (8). Studies of the relationship between hyperkinesia and hypokinesia were also carried out (9). Concurrently, neuropathological studies were instituted: in 1970 the first systematic examination of the brains of patients with tardive dyskinesia was published by Christensen, Moller, and Faurbye (10). The methodological problems of working with *post-mortem* brains resulted in subsequent efforts concentrating on studies of rat brains after long-term exposure to neuroleptics (see Fog and Pakkenberg elsewhere in this volume [11]). Finally, basic pharmacological, anatomical, and biochemical studies of various forms of dyskinesia in lower animals were carried out over a period of years in the Pharmacological Research Laboratory, Sct. Hans Hospital, by Fog, Munkvad, Randrup, and Scheel-Krüger (for reviews see 12,13,14).

The term *tardive dyskinesia* was introduced by Faurbye and coworkers in 1964 (2) and has gained international acceptance. It seems appropriate in connection with the hyperkinetic movement disturbances arising during or after long-term neuroleptic treatment. It should be noticed, however, that hyperkinetic movements—sometimes quite similar to tardive dyskinesia—may occur at any stage in the neurological treatment, initially in association with acute dystonia (15), subsequently in connection with parkinsonism and akathisia (16), and relatively late in the course of treatment in the form of the proper tardive dyskinesia syndrome. This state of affairs has undoubtedly contributed to the confusion which has been prevailing in the classification of neurological side effects, and which may still be a problem in the daily clinical work and research (17).

In the following, a brief account will be given of some aspects of the dyskinesia research at Sct. Hans Hospital, particularly concerning the possible pathophysiological mechanisms underlying reversible and irreversible tardive dyskinesia. Emphasis will be laid on observations suggesting reduced dopaminergic neurotransmission to be the primary pathogenic factor of tardive dyskinesia, but secondary dopaminergic hyperfunction and/or cholinergic hypofunction, and the possibility of neuronal degeneration as a basis for irreversible tardive dyskinesia, will be mentioned briefly. But first, we will mention the rating scale developed by us for the recording of tardive dyskinesia.

TARDIVE DYSKINESIA RATING SCALE

Originally, a relatively simple scale was used in which the frequency of the oral tardive dyskinetic movements was scored (5). The final form of our rating scale is more detailed (see pp. 267), meeting the problems we have encountered along the road. Among these rating problems the following should be emphasized:

1. An estimate of the intensity of hyperkinesia gives a more valid assessment than a score of the frequency. The latter is a built-in constituent of the individual dyskinesia pattern, and as such is only partly susceptible to pharmacological therapy. To a large extent, the qualitative individuality of the dyskinesia, including the frequency of movement, is preserved.

2. The use of video recordings makes it possible to employ a scale of scores ranging from 0 to 6, and not as previously from 0 to 3.

3. In addition to the hyperkinetic movement element, recording should include a more detailed description of the pattern of oral dyskinesia, including the amplitude and duration of each mouth opening and/or tongue protrusion, together with the signs of parkinsonism, dystonia if present, and the mental state.

4. The hyperkinesias may vary very considerably during the course of an observation period. This variation may be summed up in a global estimate, but

in this way you lose information about details in the picture of dyskinesia. This is also the case if the patient is only recorded in one definite situation, e.g. when he is not being directly observed or when he is making a drawing. The problem can be solved by using two (or more) sets of scores: (1) when the patient is unoccupied and not directly observed, and (2) when the patient is distracted and activated by voluntary hand movements, or otherwise. The two sets of scores may then be put together into a mean.

5. Sedation may result in a nonspecific antihyperkinetic effect. If the sedation is slight, its effect may be eliminated by activating the patient by means of voluntary hand movements. Just in this connection the above two sets of scores have shown their usefulness (see also [18]).

Using the rating scale shown in Figure 1, you may obtain a relatively finely graduated recording of the overall picture in tardive dyskinesia. Still, it must be admitted that the more detailed and sensitive the scale, the greater the demands made on the raters if a high degree of reliability is to be obtained. In this connection we consider research on tardive dyskinesia still to be at a stage where explorative studies of pathogenic mechanisms should be given priority over pragmatic studies concerning more or less subtle differences in the antihyperkinetic effect of the various drugs. The problem is more one of understanding the mechanisms underlying this potentially irreversible neurological complication than of studying quantitative differences between symptomatic, and in the long run, possibly aggravating forms of treatment. So, primarily, the recording of tardive dyskinesia has to be both detailed and valid. This may be the best contribution to our understanding of the pathogenic mechanisms of the syndrome and may prospectively make the dyskinesia rating procedure no longer necessary.

PRIMARY REDUCED DOPAMINERGIC NEUROTRANSMISSION

Reduced dopaminergic neurotransmission seems in some way to be a primary and integrated factor in the pathogenesis of tardive dyskinesia. This assumption is supported by the following observations:

1. Tardive dyskinesia is more liable to develop in patients who have shown parkinsonism initially in the neuroleptic treatment than in patients who have not presented such a reaction (19). Similar observations have been made during long-term treatment of monkeys (20).

2. Associated with anticholinergic treatment, Parkinson symptoms (e.g. tremor of the tongue) may be seen to gradually change into slow, writhing movements (= tardive dyskinesia [21]). Correspondingly, patients with Parkinson's disease under treatment with L-dopa may tend to develop hyperkinesia in those body segments where Parkinson symptoms were most pronounced before the treatment (9). The morbid process in parkinsonism seems

to favor the development and to determine the character of these involuntary movements (22).

3. L-dopa treatment of persons without parkinsonism does not lead to hyperkinesia (23).

4. Antidopaminergic treatment with synthesis inhibitors (6) or receptor blockers (3) usually reduces the involuntary movements in oral tardive dyskinesia, but often elicits prolonged mouth opening. The hyperkinetic movements are reappearing on anticholinergic treatment.

5. At the commencement of neuroleptic treatment, and on intensifying a treatment which is already going, a few patients (16) and monkeys (24) show hyperkinetic movements which in appearance and localization correspond to tardive dyskinesia. This may be related to reduced dopaminergic neurotransmission and increased dopamine turnover induced by the neuroleptic treatment.

6. Preliminary results suggest that tardive dyskinesia may be more pronounced after treatment with haloperidol (a powerful blocker of dopaminergic receptors) than after treatment with thioridazine (a weaker blocker of dopaminergic receptors [3]).

7. Christensen et al. (10), in a nonblind study, found cell degeneration in the substantia nigra in 27 out of 28 brains from patients with tardive dyskinesia, compared to 7 out of 28 brains from control patients matched with regard to age, sex, and diagnosis.

8. Elderly subjects, especially those predisposed to the development of tardive dyskinesia, show reduced activity in the dopaminergic neurons (25). This reduced dopaminergic neurotransmission seems in one way or another to sensitize patients for the development of tardive dyskinesia, and to determine its location. So far, the exact biochemical mechanisms underlying this sensitization are unknown, but increased sensitivity of certain dopaminergic receptors and/or reduced activity in certain cholinergic neurons appear to play a role.

SECONDARY RELATIVE DOPAMINERGIC HYPERACTIVITY—CHOLINERGIC HYPOFUNCTION

There is considerable evidence of a relative dopaminergic hyperactivity being a pathogenetic factor underlying the hyperkinetic movement element in the tardive dyskinesia syndrome (for references, see [26]). For one, it may be pointed out that the hyperkinetic movement element itself becomes manifest or is intensified on withdrawal of long-term neuroleptic treatment (whereby dopaminergic receptors become accessible to the available dopamine) or on intensive L-dopa or amphetamine treatment. Conversely, the hyperkinesias are reduced by dopamine antagonists, without the patient necessarily showing any sign of parkinsonism.

This relative dopaminergic hyperactivity may depend on the following: (1) a shift in the equilibrium between the dopaminergic and the cholinergic transmitter systems (16), (2) a postsynaptic dopaminergic receptor hypersensitivity (26,27), or (3) a displaced balance between the activity in different dopaminergic receptors (28).

There is still uncertainty as to the significance of these factors for the development of tardive dyskinesia. This also holds for the significance of the GABA-ergic transmitter system. A phenomenon which has been particularly discussed is so-called postsynaptic dopaminergic receptor hypersensitivity. The phenomenon is well accounted although not fully clarified in animal experiments, and is presumably implicated in the pathogenesis of *reversible* tardive dyskinesia. In the development of *irreversible* tardive dyskinesia, however, other factors appear to play a part.

REDUCED BIOLOGICAL BUFFER CAPACITY—IRREVERSIBLE TARDIVE DYSKINESIA

While subjects who are mentally and neurologically healthy usually tolerate a pharmacological influence on the dopaminergic, cholinergic, and GABA-ergic systems without any alteration in their mental and neurological state, pronounced changes appear under such treatment in patients with Parkinson's disease and tardive dyskinesia. The further the disease has proceeded, the more intense is the pharmacological response. So it may be said that in the affections of the above-mentioned basal ganglia, the pathological process involves a reduced biological buffer capacity, i.e., the inability, in response to outer stimuli or to disturbances of the inner homeostatic systems, to execute adequate compensatory actions (5).

This reduced buffer capacity presumably constitutes an essential part of the background for irreversible tardive dyskinesias, as these cases display a considerable sensitivity to pharmacological influences. However, the defect behind this reduced buffer capacity is still not known. Neuropathological studies of post-mortem brains from patients with tardive dyskinesia have shown cell degeneration in the basal ganglia, but the results are still not conclusive (29). In itself, however, the irreversibility makes permanent morphological or biochemical changes more likely.

Both age and neuroleptics can cause irreversible oral dyskinesia, but tardive dyskinesia is rarely irreversible before the age of 50 years. It therefore seems reasonable to assume that neuroleptics accentuate those age-dependent cerebral changes which by themselves may lead to hyperkinesia, particularly in the oral region (2,10).

The following factors are to be underlined as possible pathogenic elements in *irreversible* tardive dyskinesia:

1. Initially, the blockade of dopaminergic receptors by neuroleptic drugs leads to an increased synthesis and turnover of dopamine and acetylcholine in

the basal ganglia (30,31). Later, tolerance phenomena develop, associated with a fall in the synthesis and turnover of the two transmitter substances, often to a level below the initial one (32,33,34). This long-term effect may be irreversible and may accentuate that defect which appears with age, particularly in the dopaminergic transmitter system but also in the cholinergic and GABA-ergic transmitter systems (35).

2. Neuronal destruction can be observed as a consequence of precipitation of neuromelanine. This process is related to both age (35) and treatment with certain neuroleptics (e.g., thioridazine [36]). The neuromelanine precipitation is localized, especially to those neurons involved in the monoaminergic neurotransmission, in particular the dopaminergic neurons of the substantia nigra.

3. Neuronal destruction may also be due to localized cerebral hypoxia, which is likewise associated with both age (35) and neuroleptic treatment (2). These hypoxic changes mainly affect the diencephalon and thereby the basal ganglia. Furthermore, Lyon (37) has drawn our attention to the fact that the ventrolateral part of the striatum, which may be associated with the innervation of the oral musculature, has a poorer vascular supply than the rest of the striatum. In consequence, this region in particular may be more sensitive to the sequelae of arteriosclerotic-thrombotic changes. This is in accordance with the finding of a 10% cell loss ($p < 0.01$) in the ventrolateral striatum in rats following long-term (36 weeks) treatment with flupenthixol decanoate 4 mg/kg weekly. (For further discussion, see 11,38.)

A reasonable approach to the elucidation of this problem would consist of, first, the production of irreversible tardive dyskinesia in experimental animals, preferably monkeys (cf. [24]); then, with the aid of autoradiographic technique, localization of those regions which offer the greatest possibility of finding pathological changes, i.e., those elements of the basal ganglia which influence the innervation of the oral musculature; and finally, application of morphological and biochemical methods of investigation to this tissue. This approach would provide a reasonable chance of demonstrating the possible pathophysiological process underlying tardive dyskinesia. A project along these lines has been initiated at Sct. Hans Hospital, Roskilde, in collaboration with Ferrosan, Malmö, Sweden.

SUMMARY

Reversible tardive dyskinesia appears to depend on a primary reduced dopaminergic neurotransmission and a secondary relative dopaminergic hyperactivity, the latter depending on (a) a shift in the equilibrium between the dopaminergic and the cholinergic transmitter systems, (b) a postsynaptic dopaminergic receptor hypersensitivity, and/or (c) displaced balance between the activity in functionally different dopaminergic receptors.

Irreversible tardive dyskinesia, occurring almost exclusively in elderly patients and appearing in continuation of reversible tardive dyskinesia, seems above all to depend on a reduced biological buffer capacity, i.e., the inability, in response to external pharmacological influences and internal disturbances in the homeostatic systems, to provide adequate compensatory action to maintain normal neurological and mental functions. As result of such a reduced buffer capacity, even small shifts in the equilibrium between the activity of various types of neurons and receptors lead to persistent tardive dyskinesia. The defect underlying this reduced buffer capacity may be degenerative changes in dopaminergic, cholinergic, and/or GABA-ergic systems, possibly cell loss related both to age and to neuroleptic treatment.

Please refer to the table in Chapter 24, where all the Tardive Dyskinesia scales are.

REFERENCES

1. Uhrbrand, L., Faurbye, A. Reversible and irreversible dyskinesia after treatment with perphenazine, chlorpromazine, reserpine and electroconvulsive therapy. *Psychopharmacologia* (Berl.), *1*:408–418, 1960.
2. Faurbye, A., Rasch, R.J., Petersen, P.B., Brandborg, G., Pakkenberg, H. Neurological symptoms in pharmacotherapy of psychosis. *Acta Psychiatr. Scand.*, *40*:10–27, 1964.
3. Gerlach, J., Simmelsgaard, H. Tardive dyskinesia during and following treatment with haloperidol, haloperidol + biperiden, thioridazine and clozapine. *Psychopharmacology*. (In press).
4. Gerlach, J., Thorsen, K., Fog, R. Extrapyramidal reactions and amine metabolites in cerebrospinal fluid during haloperidol and clozapine treatment of schizophrenic patients. *Psychopharmacologia* (Berl.), *40*:341–350, 1975.
5. Gerlach, J., Reisby, N., Randrup, A. Dopaminergic hypersensitivity and cholinergic hypofunction in the pathophysiology of tardive dyskinesia. *Psychopharmacologia* (Berl.), *34*:21–35, 1974.
6. Gerlach, J., Thorsen, K. The movement pattern of oral tardive dyskinesia in relation to anticholinergic and antidopaminergic treatment. *Int. Pharmacopsychiatry*, *11*:1–7, 1976.
7. Gerlach, J., Rye, T., Kristjansen, P. Effect of baclofen on tardive dyskinesia. *Psychopharmacology*. (In press), 1978.
8. Gerlach, J., Thorsen, K., Munkvad, I. Effect of lithium on neuroleptic-induced tardive dyskinesia compared with placebo in a double-blind cross-over trial. *Pharmakopsychiatr. Neuropsychopharmakol.*, *8*:51–56, 1975.
9. Gerlach, J. Relationship between tardive dyskinesia, l-dopa-induced hyperkinesia and parkinsonism. *Psychopharmacologia*, *51*:259–263, 1977.
10. Christensen, E., Møller, J.E., Faurbye, A. Neuropathological investigations of 28 brains from patients with dyskinesia. *Acta Psychiatr. Scand.*, *46*:14–23, 1970.
11. Fog. R., Pakkenberg, H. Anatomical and Metabolic Changes After Long and Short-Term Treatment With Perphenazine in Rats. In *Tardive Dyskinesia*, Fann, W.E., Smith, R.C., Davis, J.M., Domino, E.F. (eds). New York: Spectrum Publications, (this vol.).

12. Fog, R. On stereotypy and catalepsy: studies on the effect of amphetamines and neuroleptics in rats. *Acta Neurol. Scand.* (Suppl. [50]), *48*:1–66, 1972 (Thesis).

13. Scheel-Krüger, J., Christensen, A.V., Arnt, J. Muscimol differentially facilitates stereotypy but antagonizes motility induced by dopaminergic drugs: a complex gaba-dopamine interaction. *Life Sci., 22*:75–84, 1978.

14. Randrup, A., Scheel-Krüger, J., Fog, R., Munkvad, I. A short survey of animal psychopharmacology. 1st World congress of ethology applied to zootechniques (in press).

15. Delay, J., Deniker, P. Drug-induced extrapyramidal syndromes. In Diseases of the Basal Ganglia. *Handbook of Clinical Neurology,* Vol. 6, Wenken, P.J., Bruyn, G.W. (eds.). Amsterdam: North Holland Publishing Company, pp. 248–266, 1969.

16. Casey, D.E., Denney, D. Original investigations: pharmacological characterization of tardive dyskinesia. *Psychopharmacologia, 54*:1–8, 1977.

17. Faurbye, A. The structural and biochemical basis of movement disorders in treatment with neuroleptic drugs and in extrapyramidal diseases. *Compr. Psychiatr., 11*:205–225, 1970.

18. Tamminga, C.A., Smith, R.C., Ericksen, S.E., Chang, S., Davis, J.M. Cholinergic influences in tardive dyskinesia. *Am. J. Psychiatry, 134*:769–774, 1977.

19. Crane, G.E. Pseudoparkinsonism and tardive dyskinesia. *Arch. Neurol., 27*:426–430, 1972.

20. Gunne, L-M., Barany, S. Haloperidol-induced tardive dyskinesia in monkeys. *Psychopharmacologia, 34*:21–35, 1974.

21. Crane, G.E. Tardive Dyskinesia: A Review. In *Neuropsychopharmacology.* Boissier, J.R., Hippius, H., Pichot, P. (eds.). New York: Elsevier, pp. 346–354, 1975.

22. Cotzias, G.C. Levodopa in the treatment of parkinsonism. *JAMA, 218*:1903–1908, 1971.

23. Quaade, F., Pakkenberg, H., Juhl, E. Levodopa as a treatment of obesity. *Acta Med. Scand., 195*:129–130, 1974.

24. Gunne, L-M., Bárány, S. A primate model for tardive dyskinesia. In *Tardive Dyskinesia.* Fann, W.E., Smith, R.C., Davis, J.M., Domino, E.F. (eds.). New York: Spectrum Publications (this vol.).

25. Carlsson, A., Winblad, B. Influence of age and time interval between death and autopsy on dopamine and 3-methoxytyramine levels in human basal ganglia. *J. Neural Transm., 38*:271–276, 1976.

26. Tarsy, D., Baldessarini, R.J. The pathophysiologic basis of tardive dyskinesia. *Biol. Psychiatry, 12*:431–450, 1977.

27. Smith, R.C., Davis, J.M. Behavioral evidence for supersensitivity after chronic administration of haloperidol, clozapine, and thioridazine. *Life Sci., 19*:725–732, 1976.

28. Cools, A.R. Two functionally and pharmacologically distinct dopamine receptors in the rat brain. *Biochem. Psychopharmacol., 16*:215–225, 1977.

29. Jellinger, K. Neuropathologic Findings after Neuroleptic Long-Term Therapy. In *Neurotoxicology.* Roizin, L., Shiraki, H. Grcević. (eds.). New York: Raven Press, pp. 25–42, 1977.

30. Bartholini, G., Stadler, H., Gadea-Ciria, M., Lloyd, K.G. The Effect of Antipsychotic Drugs on the Release of Neurotransmitters in Various Brain Areas. In *Antipsychotic Drugs: Pharmacodynamics and Pharmacokinetics.* Sedvall, G., Uvnäs, B., Zotterman, Y. (eds.). Stockholm: Pergamon Press, pp. 105–116, 1974.

31. Sedvall, G., Bjerkenstedt, L., Fyrö, B., Härnryd, C., Wode-Helgodt, B. The Use of Mass Fragmentography to Study Effects of Antipsychotic Drugs on Brain Dopamine Metabolism. In *Antipsychotic Drugs: Pharmacodynamics and Pharmacokinetics.* Sedvall, G., Uvnäs, B., Zotterman, Y. (eds.). Elmswood, N.Y.: Pergamon Press, pp. 331–342, 1974.

32. Scatton, B., Glowinski, J., Julou, L. Neuroleptics: effects on dopamine synthesis in the nigro-neostriatal, meso-limbic and meso-cortical dopaminergic systems. In *Antipsychotic Drugs: Pharmacodynamics and Pharmacokinetics.* Sedvall, G., Uvnäs, B., Zotterman, Y. (eds.). Stockholm: Pergamon Press, pp. 243–255, 1974.

33. Hyttel, J. Changes in dopamine synthesis rate in the supersensitivity phase after treatment with a single dose of neuroleptics. *Psychopharmacologia, 51*:205–207, 1977.

34. Sethy, V.H. Effects of chronic treatment with neuroleptics on striatal acetylcholine concentration. *J. Neurochem., 27*:325–326, 1976.

35. Barbeau, A. Aging and the extrapyramidal system. *J. Amer. Geriatr. Soc., 21*:145–149, 1973.

36. Forrest, F.M. Evolutionary origin of extrapyramidal disorders in drug-treated mental patients, its significance, and the role of neuromelanin. In *Phenothiazines and Structurally Related Drugs*. Forrest, I., Carr, C.J., Usdin, E. (eds.). New York: Raven Press, pp. 255–268, 1974.

37. Lyon, M. Personal communication with reference to *Brain Vascular System*, Kaplan, Ford (eds.). New York: Elsevier, 1966.

38. Nielsen, E.B., Lyon, M. Evidence for cell loss in corpus striatum after long-term treatment with a neuroleptic drug (flupenthixol) in rats. *Psychopharmacology,* (in press).

34

Neuromuscular Pathophysiology in Tardive Dyskinesia

J. W. CRAYTON

The intensity of research interest in tardive dyskinesia (TD) in recent years has highlighted the importance of this side effect of neuroleptic drug treatment and focused attention on the disabling effect of TD on psychotic patients (1). Despite this intensified interest, there is as yet no consensus concerning the basic neuropathological mechanisms involved in this disorder. Research findings to date are difficult to integrate into one simple organizing scheme. Part of the difficulty with determining basic neuropathological mechanisms stems from the inconsistent relationship of tardive dyskinesia to neuroleptic drug treatment. Although the emergence of TD is roughly correlated with length and amount of drug treatment (2), there are significant exceptions to this rule. Some patients develop tardive dyskinesia after only a few weeks or months on drug treatment at relatively low dosages (3). Further complicating hypotheses about tardive dyskinesia is its inconsistent response to treatment. A wide variety of pharmacological agents have been employed in the treatment of TD (4), but none has shown universal efficacy. Agents which reduce the efficacy of dopaminergic transmission, such as haloperidol (5), reserpine (6), and manganese (7), all have been effective in *some* patients with tardive dyskinesia. Similarly, agents which enhance cholinergic activity, such as physostigmine (8), deanol (9), and choline (10), are also effective in some, but not all, patients. The exceptions to these rules—i.e., the numerous patients who fail to respond to dopaminergic-cholinergic balance treatments—suggest that the syndrome of tardive dyskinesia may be associated with a wide variety of basic neurophysiological mechanisms. There is frequent mention in the literature, for example, of the important predisposing effect of various organic brain lesions in TD patients (11–14).

In the studies to be described, we have undertaken an exploration of neurophysiological measures in patients with tardive dyskinesia. The aim of these studies has been to precisely define the disordered neuronal mechanisms in this condition and, perhaps, the subpopulations of patients which would be more or less responsive to one or another treatment modality. Our report describes abnormalities of neuromuscular physiology in this disorder and also emphasizes the neurophysiological heterogeneity of tardive dyskinesia.

SUBJECTS

Patients with TD, all of whom had also been diagnosed as schizophrenic, were studied at one of two locations: the Illinois State Psychiatric Institute, on the research units administered by Dr. John Davis, and the Clinical Investigation Unit at Manteno Mental Health Center. The Unit of MMHC is a research ward established to study problems of the treatment of long-term schizophrenic patients and the assessment and treatment of drug side effects in such patients. Control subjects included chronic schizophrenic patients without tardive dyskinesia at the Illinois State Psychiatric Institute and Manteno Mental Health Center, and normal volunteer controls.

METHODS

Patients were evaluated as to their symptomatology and severity of tardive dyskinesia by the scale developed by Smith and associates (15). According to this scale, patients with "high" scores received a score of 10 or more, "medium" 5–9, and "low" less than 5. Spinal monosynaptic reflex testing was carried out by procedures described in detail in another publication (16). Briefly, the patient reclined in a large easy chair with his leg extended and flexed at an angle of approximately 30 degrees. 1A afferent sensory fibers were stimulated with a bipolar surface electrode placed in the popliteal fossa, and the reflex activity was recorded by surface electrodes placed over the distal tendon and belly of the soleus muscle. Electrode placement was adjusted so that a maximal reflex response could be elicited at the lowest possible stimulus intensity. If no reflex response was elicited, the stimulating and recording electrodes were adjusted to be certain that no reflex response could be elicited from another site. In addition, the search for the H reflex was extended through the entire range of the M, or direct muscle, response, which ordinarily has a higher threshold than the H response and plateaus at a stimulus intensity higher than that necessary to elicit an H reflex. If no discernible H reflex was obtained at the point where the M response plateaued, the patient was considered to have no H response.

The recovery curve of alpha motor-neuron excitability was also determined by methods described previously (16) by giving paired stimuli at interstimulus intervals between 50 msec and 5 sec at a stimulus intensity which gave a near-maximal H response with the smallest possible M response. The muscle potentials were fed into a PDP-8 computer, and five values for each S_1–S_2 delay were averaged. We focused on three principal features of the recovery curve for this study: H_0, defined as the S_1–S_2 delay time at which there was an initial return of excitability of at least 10%; H_x, the maximum H_2–H_1 value between 100 and 300 msec; and H_y, the lowest value for H_2–H_1 in the epoch between 300 and 600 msec delay. In a few subjects, H_x and H_y fell outside of the usual epoch, and in those situations, the maximal or minimal value for H_x and H_y was chosen as the inflexion points on the curve, regardless of where they occurred.

Single fiber electromyography was carried out by methods described by Eckstedt and Stalberg (17). This method permits a measure of the density of muscle fibers belonging to the same motor neuron within the uptake area of the electrode. An increased fiber density (FD) is found in conditions characterized by motor neuron degeneration followed by collateral reinnervation. The measure is a physiological analogue of the terminal innervation ratio determined in structural studies of muscle innervation in muscle biopsy specimens. FD is increased in a variety of peripheral neuropathies and in patients with functional psychosis. Fiber density, defined as the mean number of muscle fibers recorded from a given site in the muscle, was determined for each subject. In addition, in a few subjects the pattern of electromyographic jitter was measured. Jitter was determined by measuring the range of interspike intervals for pairs of muscle fiber responses (fibers innervated by two branches of a motor neuron), and these values for range were converted to mean consecutive differences for pairs of responses by the methods described by Stalberg (18).

RESULTS

Since the absence of an H reflex has been found to be more prevalent in patients with peripheral neuropathies (19), and also in patients with Huntington's chorea (20), we determined the proportion of our subjects with tardive dyskinesia who failed to have an H reflex. In all but one of the 31 subjects, we were able to decide unequivocally whether the subject had a H reflex or not, and all of the subjects were then classified according to whether their tardive dyskinesia scores were high, moderate, or low. One subject had such a small (20–40 uv) and inconstant H reflex that it was difficult to classify it as present or absent; thus this patient was not included in the data analysis. For the 30 subjects in whom the presence or absence of an H reflex could be

unequivocally determined, the absence of H-reflex activity was highly correlated with tardive dyskinesia score (Table 1). Eight of the nine subjects who
lacked an H reflex had high TD scores, while all of the patients with low
tardive dyskinesia scores had H reflexes (2 × 3 Chi-square = 8.0555, p <
0.02). All efforts to elicit an H reflex, whether by facilitation maneuvers, such
as the Jendrassic maneuver, or by electrode movement, failed to elicit an H
reflex. Each of the subjects who failed to show an H reflex was studied on a
second occasion, but on each trial we failed to elicit an H reflex.

H-REFLEX RECOVERY CURVES

Recovery cycles of motor-neuron excitability were studied in 22 patients.
Comparative analysis of Ho, Hx, and Hy between these patients and 19 control
subjects is shown in Table 2, and the value of Hx is displayed in Figure 1.
Examples of H-reflex curves of 4 schizophrenic patients with high tardive
dyskinesia scores are shown in Figure 2. The curves in low TD-score subjects,
all of whom had minimal signs of TD, are similar to those previously recorded
in some chronic schizophrenic patients (16). The values for Hx, the peak of
secondary facilitation, were significantly higher in patients with high TD
scores than in either patients with chronic schizophrenia alone or normals.

Table 1
Presence or Absence of H Reflex in Tardive Dyskinesia

TD Status	H Reflex	
	Absent	Present
Low Scores (7)	0	7
Moderate Scores (8)	1	7
High Scores (15)	8	7

Chi-square = 8.056, p<0.02

Table 2

	Ho (msec)	Hx%	Hy%
Normal Controls (19)	83.2 ± 20.8	86.7 ± 20.7	38.5 ± 20.8
Chronic Schizophrenics (11)	- ± -	55.7 ± 29.3	34.6 ± 32.7
Tardive Dyskinesia (23)	91.8 ± 78.5	86.7 ± 37.3*	27.1 ± 29.8
High	55.3 ± 67.8	109.3 ± 46.8*	18.4 ± 34.2
Moderate	100.8 ± 31.7	80.8 ± 30.0	34.5 ± 19.5
Low	162.5 ± 87.6†	72.3 ± 28.7	35.0 ± 29.2

*p<0.05, compared with chronic schizophrenic (t-test)
†p<0.05, compared with normals (t-test)

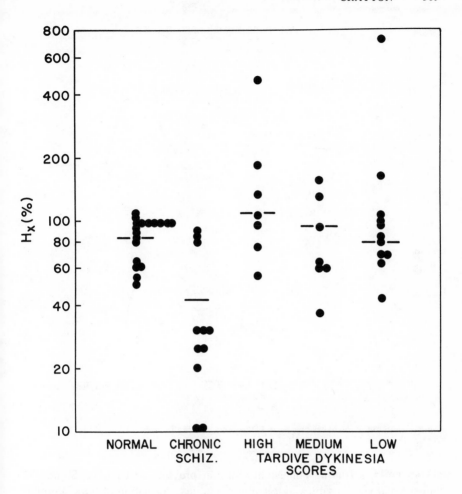

Figure 1.   Scattergram of values for Hx in controls and patients with TD. Horizontal bars indicate group means. The two extreme values of 747 and 488 are excluded from the determination of the means. There is a trend toward an association of higher values for Hx with higher TD scores.

SINGLE FIBER ELECTROMYOGRAPHY

Fiber density, the mean number of muscle potentials belonging to the same motor unit within the uptake area of the electrode, was determined in the extensor digitorum longus muscle in voluntarily activated muscles of 8 TD patients, and the values were compared with schizophrenic (26) and normal (19) subjects (Fig. 3). The TD patients had significantly higher values for FD than either of the other two groups. Schizophrenic subjects had significantly

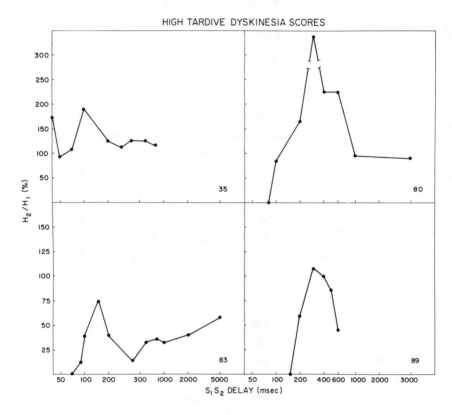

HIGH TARDIVE DYSKINESIA SCORES

Figure 2.   H-reflex recovery curves in TD patients with high scores.

elevated FD, a finding consistent with our previous study (21). Some TD patients had very complex motor-unit potentials, consisting of 5 to 7 components, while normally only 1 or occasionally 2 components are found in the majority of recording sites. An example of a complex motor-unit response from a TD subject is illustrated in Figure 4, where a motor unit response with 6 components is illustrated.

SF EMG jitter is defined as the variability of latency of responses between two components of a motor unit. This jitter is thought to represent uncertainty of neural and neuromuscular transmission in distal nerve twigs and at the neuromuscular junction (18). Higher values for jitter are characteristic of denervation-reinnervation processes. In one TD subject, we found extreme values for jitter. In Figure 5, it can be seen that jitter of the second component is on the order of 1000 microsec., whereas the normal jitter between two components in a healthy motor unit is usually less than 50 microsec. Another extreme example of neurotransmission deficits is illustrated in Figure 6. In the left panel, a large amount of jitter is present between the two components when

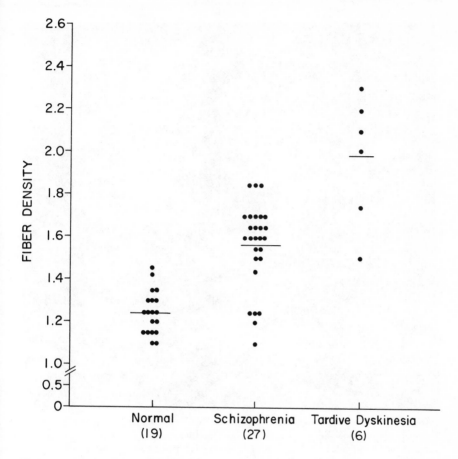

Figure 3.   Distribution of values for fiber density in normal controls, schizophrenic patients and TD subjects. Horizontal bar indicates group means.

the firing rate for the pair is 3/sec. When the firing rate is increased to 10/sec. (right panel), the second component drops out completely. This patient represents an exceptional case, however, with an absent H reflex, increased FD (2.05), and increased jitter. In most cases, TD patients did not differ from non-TD schizophrenics or normals in the frequency or extent of jitter values.

DISCUSSION

Three types of abnormalities have been found in TD subjects: a high incidence of absent H reflexes, increased secondary facilitation in the H-reflex recovery curve, and increased fiber density.

An unexpected finding in this study was the absence of an H reflex in a

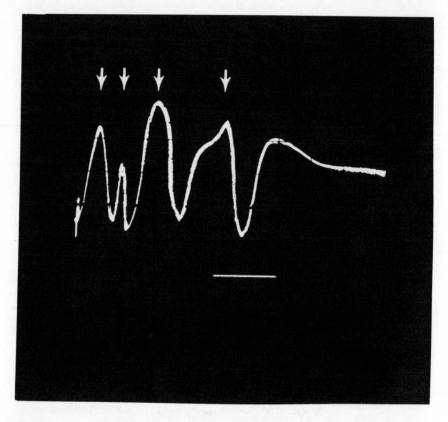

Figure 4. Single-fiber electromyographic recording from a patient with TD, illustrating a complex motor unit potential. The oscilloscope sweep is triggered by the first component. Superimposed sweeps. Normally only one or occasionally two potentials are seen.

significant proportion of the patients with TD. To date, we have studied nearly 100 normal control subjects and approximately 300 schizophrenic patients without TD and have yet to find a subject in whom we could not elicit an H reflex. The absence of an H reflex has been found in other neurologic conditions. Moniga (19) found that a significant percentage of patients with peripheral neuropathies had small or absent H reflexes. Others have found a high incidence of absent H reflexes in patients with Huntington's chorea (20) and suggested that the absence of an H reflex might provide a basis for the early diagnosis of Huntington's chorea. Our findings suggest that the absence of an H reflex is probably more generally related to choreiform movement disorders or to the presence of significant organic pathology.

This conclusion is supported by the SF EMG findings where TD patients were found to have the highest values for fiber density among the three groups

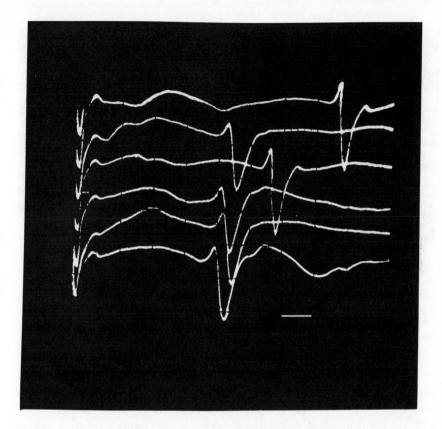

Figure 5.   Increased jitter between two components of a motor-unit potential in a patient with TD. Bar indicates 1 msec. Normally the range of potential variability is 50 microsecs.

studied. Increased fiber density is usually associated with motor-neuron degeneration followed by collateral reinnervation. In one TD subject we found an extraordinarily high value for electromyographic jitter. Increased jitter has been found in degenerative disease of peripheral motor neurons (22). Stalberg's studies of the electrophysiological correlates of neuronal degeneration and reinnervation suggest that an immature collateral sprout formed during the process of reinnervation of denervated muscle will show high values for jitter, while more mature collateral branches will show normal values for jitter. In this way, the process of regeneration can be monitored by repeated measurements of jitter. This same patient had no demonstrable H reflex. It seems possible that when neuronal transmission is compromised to the point where jitter increases to the value seen, then an H reflex may no longer be able to be elicited. Further studies would be required to substantiate this point, however.

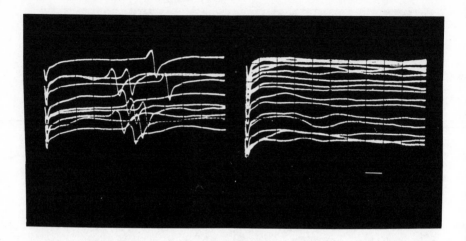

Figure 6.   Tardive dyskinesia subject. Single-fiber electromyographic recordings from a pair of muscle fibers belonging to the same motor unit. In the left panel, the frequency of neuron firing is 3/sec. Variability is increased, compared with normal, but both components of each pair are present. In the right panel, the patient increases neuron firing to 10/sec. The second component fails to follow at this increased rate. This failure to follow indicates unstable transmission in distal motor-nerve twigs.

The correlation between severity of TD and magnitude of Hx, the value for the peak of secondary facilitation in the H-reflex recovery curve, is further evidence for the presence of neurological impairment in TD patients.

There is considerable discussion about the factors influencing the height of this secondary facilitation peak. Gassel has proposed that both intrinsic spinal-cord mechanisms and descending facilitation "long-loop" pathways are involved (23).

Either of these systems could be involved in producing the elevated value for Hx in TD subjects. The role of descending supraspinal facilitation is especially interesting in the light of the proposed alteration in dopaminergic neuronal activity in TD. Evidence from various studies suggests that the value for Hx is at least partially affected by dopaminergic tone. Hx is increased in parkinsonian subjects (24), in whom thalamic surgery (25) or treatment with L-dopa (26) produces a reduction in Hx. Some schizophrenic subjects have significantly low values for Hx, which are increased by dopamine-receptor blockade (16). A simple way of organizing this data is to hypothesize that low dopaminergic activity is associated with increased secondary facilitation, while high dopaminergic activity is associated with decreased secondary facilitation. If this scheme held true for TD, the high values of Hx in TD would reflect lower dopamine activity. Such a conclusion would not be easily reconcilable with "dopamine receptor supersensitivity" models of TD (27), but are consistent with findings of improvement in TD in some subjects with dopaminergic agents such as apomorphine.

Each of the three types of neurophysiological abnormalities described here has been associated with an anatomical lesion in the neuromuscular regulatory system, and it is of interest to explore further the possibility of a structural lesion of the brain in TD. Such a putative lesion could be either preexisting and predisposing or a concomitant of the neuroleptic treatment thought to be causal in TD. An anatomical lesion underlying TD has been suggested previously (17), although neuropathological studies have not yet demonstrated any characteristic pathological lesion. It has been a frequent finding among clinicians that patients who develop tardive dyskinesia have a higher incidence of neurological organic brain syndromes than non-TD controls (3). This may be especially true of those younger patients who, after treatment with neuroleptic medication for relatively short periods of time, develop tardive dyskinesia. Simpson describes a young woman with a previous history of encephalitis who developed persistent and irreversible TD after a brief course of neuroleptic treatment. A growing current in our understanding of the relationship of central to peripheral processes would suggest that one possibility for explaining the peripheral neuropathic findings is that they are secondary to central neuropathology. There is good evidence that cortical lesions can produce neuropathology in the peripheral nervous system (29). The central and peripheral aspects of the neuropathology of TD might also be related as two separate manifestations of a single neuropathic process. The pattern of neuronal degeneration followed by collateral sprouting suggested by the increased fiber density values prompts an exploration of the possible effects of a process of neuronal degeneration and regeneration occurring in the central nervous system. There are several reports now about this sort of ''neuronal plasticity'' in various model systems, and the evidence suggests that the central nervous system as well as the peripheral system is actively involved in neuronal plastic events (30). If there were a lesion in the dopamine system, which could conceivably be produced by prolonged neuroleptic drug treatment, the compensatory process in the nervous system would be an increase in the collateral branching of dopaminergic neurons and an increase in the dopaminergic receptors in the brain. The effect of this process would not necessarily be an increase in receptor supersensitivity in the brain, as proposed by Klawans and others (31), but it would be an increase in dopaminergic tone when the neuroleptic was withdrawn, because of the increase in the number of dopamine receptors, not because of their sensitivity. Supporting evidence for such a hypothesis has been obtained by Snyder et al. (32), who found that the increase in sensitivity to dopamine agonist compounds following prolonged haloperidol treatment was due not to alterations in receptor affinity or sensitivity, but to an increase in the number of dopamine receptors. In fact, the result of such an increased collateral branching of dopamine fibers could be a *reduction* in dopaminergic tone in the nervous system, since the stimulus to feedback excitation to dopaminergic neurons would be reduced. Such a model is consistent with the finding of extremely high excitability values of the H-reflex recovery curve for the H reflex (which in other conditions is associated with reduced dopamine activity), together with evidence for dopamine-receptor "supersensitivity," which may actually represent increased numbers of receptors. Collateral reinnervation would provide a basic mechanism for understanding these apparently discrepant results.

Although other mechanisms may be influential in the production of TD, our data implicates structural alterations in the nervous system as playing a key role. While not answering the question of how the structural alterations are related to TD, the findings tend to reinforce the clinical impression that those with neurological disorders are at high risk in developing TD when given neuroleptics, and they warrant special attention to the emergence of this condition.

REFERENCES

1. Baldessarini, R.J., Tarsy, D. Mechanisms underlying tardive dyskinesia. In *The Basal Ganglia*, Yahr, M.D. (ed.). *Res. Publ. Assoc. Res. Nerv. Ment. Dis.* New York: Raven Press, pp. 433–446, 1976.
2. Ey, H., Faure, H., Rappard, P. Les reactions d'intolerance vis-a-vis de la chlorpromazine. *Encephale, 45*:790–796, 1956.
3. Simpson, G.M., Kline, M.S. Tardive dyskinesia: manifestations, incidence, etiology, and treatment. In *The Basal Ganglia*, Yahr, M.D. (ed.). *Res. Publ. Assoc. Res. Nerv. Ment. Dis.* New York: Raven Press, pp. 427–432, 1976.
4. Tarsy, D., Baldessarini, R.J. The tardive dyskinesia syndrome. In *Clinical Neuropharmacology*, vol. 1. Klawans, H. (ed.). New York: Raven Press, pp. 29–61.
5. Kazamatsuri, H., Chien, C., Cole, J. Treatment of tardive dyskinesia. II. Short-term efficacy of dopamine blocking agents, haloperidol and thiopropazate. *Arch. Gen. Psychiatry, 27*:100–103, 1972.
6. Crane, G.E. Mediocre effects of reserpine on tardive dyskinesia. *N. Engl. J. Med., 288*:104–105, 1973.
7. Kunin, R.A. Manganese and niacin in the treatment of drug-induced dyskinesias. *J. Orthomolecular Psychiatry, 5*:4–27, 1976.
8. Klawans, H.L., Jr., Rubovits, R. Effect of cholinergic and anticholinergic agents on tardive dyskinesia. *J. Neurol. Neurosurg. Psychiatr., 27*:941–947, 1974.
9. Casey, D.E., Denney, D. Deanol in the treatment of tardive dyskinesia. *Am. J. Psychiatry, 132*:864–867, 1975.
10. Davis, K.L., Berger, P.A., Hollister, L.E. Choline for tardive dyskinesia. *N. Engl. J. Med., 293*:152, 1975.
11. Poursines, Y., Alliez, J., Toga, M. Syndrome parkinsonien consecutif a la prise prolongee de chlorpromazine avec ictus morte intercurrent. *Rev. Neurol., 100*:745–751, 1959.
12. Forrest, F.W., Forrest, I.S., Roizin, L. Clinical biochemical and postmortem studies on a patient treated with chlorpromazine. *Agressologie, 4*:259–265, 1963.
13. Hunter, R., Blackwood, W., Smith, M.C., Cumings, J.N. Cases of persistent dyskinesia following phenothiazine medication. *J. Neurol. Sci., 7*:763–773, 1968.

14. Christensen, E., Moller, J.E., Faurbye, A. Neuropathological investigations of 28 brains from patients with dyskinesia. *Acta Psychiatr. Scand.*, *46*:14–23, 1970.
15. Smith, R.C. This volume.
16. Crayton, J.W., Meltzer, H.Y., Goode, D.J. Motoneuron excitability in psychiatric patients. *Biol. Psychiatry*, *12*:545–561, 1977.
17. Ekstedt, J., Stålberg, E. Single fibre electromyography for the study of the microphysiology of the human muscle. In *New Developments in Electromyography and Clinical Neurophysiology*, vol. 1, Desmedt, J.E. (ed.). Basel: Karger, pp. 84–112, 1973.
18. Stålberg, E., Ekstedt, J., Broman, A. The electromyographic jitter in normal human muscles. *Electroencephalogr. Clin. Neurophysiol.*, *31*:429–438, 1971.
19. Moniga, S.K. Significance of certain evoked responses in cases of neurogenic disorders. *Electromyography*, *12*:191–211, 1972.
20. Johnson, E.W., *et al.* Huntington disease: early identification by H-reflex testing. *Arch. Phys. Med. Rehabil.*, *58*:162–166, 1977.
21. Crayton, J.W., Stålberg, E., Hilton-Brown, P. The motor unit in psychotic patients; a single fiber electromyographic study. *J. Neurol. Neurosurg. Psychiatry*, 1977.
22. Stålberg, E., Schwartz, M.S., Trontelj, J.V. Single fiber electromyography in various processes affecting the anterior horn cell. *J. Neurol. Sci.*, *24*:403–415, 1975.
23. Gassel, M. A critical review of evidence concerning long loop reflexes excited by muscle afferents in man. *J. Neurol. Neurosurg. Psychiatry*, *33*:358, 1970.
24. Takamori, M. H-reflex study in upper motoneurone diseases. *Neurology*, *17*:32–40, 1967.
25. Laitinen, L.V., Ohno, Y. Effects of thalamic stimulation and thalamotomy on the H-reflex. *Electroencephalogr. Clin. Neurophysiol.*, *28*:586–591, 1970.
26. McLeod, J.G., Walsh, J.C. H-reflex studies in patients with parkinson's disease. *J. Neurol. Neurosurg. Psychiatry*, *35*:77, 1972.
27. Implications of amphetamine-induced stereotyped behavior as a model for tardive dyskinesias. *Arch. Gen. Psychiatry*, *27*:502–507, 1972.
28. Smith, R.C., Tamminga, C.A., Haraszti, J., Pandy, G.N., Davis, J.M. Effects of dopamine agonists in tardive dyskinesia. *Am. J. Psychiatry*, *134*:763–768, 1977.
29. Raisman, G. Neuronal plasticity in the septal nuclei of the adult rat. *Brain Res.*, *14*:25–48, 1969.
30. Guth, L. Axonal regeneration and functional plasticity in the central nervous system. *Exp. Neurol.*, *45*:606–654, 1974.
31. Klawans, H.C. The pharmacology of tardive dyskinesia. *Am. J. Psychiatry*, *130*:82–86, 1973.
32. Snyder, S.H. This volume.

35

Status of Deanol as a Cholinergic Precursor—Experimental Evidence and Clinical Uses in Tardive Dyskinesia

EDWARD F. DOMINO
and BEVERLY KOVACIC

EXPERIMENTAL EVIDENCE

DuVigneaud *et al.* (1) found that dimethylaminoethanol (deanol) could substitute for choline in preventing fatty livers in rats. They also showed that deuterated deanol was converted in vivo to deuterated choline. They suggested that deanol was a precursor for choline in rat tissue. Their specific evidence was for rat liver. Pfeiffer (2) postulated that free choline had difficulty penetrating the blood-brain barrier because it was a quaternary nitrogen analogue with a positive charge. He suggested that deanol could readily penetrate the blood-brain barrier because it was a tertiary nitrogen derivative and in the brain it could be methylated to choline. In this way it should enhance brain acetylcholine levels. Pfeiffer, Jenney, Gallagher *et al.* (3) showed that deanol in large doses had stimulant properties consistent with a role as a precursor of brain acetylcholine. These findings were further elaborated in comparison with choline (4). Pfeiffer and his associates initiated a controversy which is still unresolved. It is hoped that this review will provide a perspective. One of us (Domino) was trained in pharmacology in Pfeiffer's department at the University of Illinois at the time deanol was still a postulated potential drug. It excited a number of people formerly with that department to do research on deanol. Deanol has always been controversial both clinically and experimentally.

Pepeu, Freedman, and Giarman (5) provided the first negative experimental study. They were unable to show a clear-cut increase in rat brain acetylcholine following deanol. Unfortunately, a small series of only seven animals was studied, and a slight but not statistically significant increase in brain acetylcholine was seen after deanol. The rats were killed by guillotine, a procedure now known to result in relatively low brain acetylcholine. Those who believed deanol was an acetylcholine precursor could still disagree with Pepeu *et al.* that no change in brain acetylcholine was found. Years later Pedata, Wieraszko, and Pepeu (6) extended their studies to include the effects of choline, phosphorylcholine as well as deanol, on rat brain acetylcholine, using focused microwave irradiation sacrifice. This method is now widely accepted as the best for measuring brain acetylcholine. Acetylcholine was measured by the frog rectus abdominis assay. Equimolar doses of all three potential precursors given i.p. had no effect on rat brain acetylcholine. When given intraventricularly, both choline and phosphorylcholine antagonized hemicholinium-induced depletion of brain acetylcholine; deanol was without any effect. Very large doses of phosphorylcholine given i.p. partially antagonized hemicholinium-induced depletion of striatal acetylcholine. Because parenteral phosphorylcholine was more effective in this respect than parenteral choline or deanol, it was postulated that phosphorylcholine penetrated into the brain better or that it provided phosphate for ATP, necessary to synthesize acetylcholine (7).

Details of how the brain receives its source of choline for the synthesis of acetylcholine are still far from clear. Measurements of free choline in recent years, particularly using special quick-freezing or microwave irradiation to the head, indicate very low levels, on the order of 8.4 nmol/g (8). Mann (9) and Mann and Bennett (10) showed, using rats, that ^{3}H-choline given i.p. is rapidly incorporated into the liver and appears in the plasma as a labeled lipid or lipoprotein complex. Free plasma choline does not seem to readily penetrate the brain; rather, it appears as though the labeled lipid choline entered the brain. ^{3}H-choline-labeled lecithin injected i.v. did not enter the brain, but like free ^{3}H-choline, entered the liver. Plasma containing labeled lipid was isolated after i.p. ^{3}H-choline, in which the free choline was removed on a cation-exchange column. When this plasma lipid, which had no free choline, was given i.v., it was rapidly incorporated into the brain, and after a short time appeared as free choline in the plasma. If a quick-freezing cold extraction process was used to prevent post-mortem release of free choline, most of the isotope in the brain was in the form of phospholipid (80%), with the rest as free choline and as acetylcholine. When no attempt was made to control post-mortem release of free choline, more than 50% of the total isotope in the brain was as free choline, suggesting that phospholipid breakdown is the source of the post-mortem increase in brain choline. Dahlberg and Schuberth (11) showed that aminoethanol, methylaminoethanol, and serine, but not proline (as a control), given i.p. to rabbits increased plasma choline within ½ to 1 hr postinjection for about 4 hr. Neither aminoproponal nor proline increased plasma choline. Deanol, given orally to rabbits and humans, had a similar action. They suggested that nitrogen base exchange occurred in which the choline moiety of phospholipids in the liver and other organs was displaced by these endogenous nitrogen compounds. The effect of serine was of special interest because it can participate in base exchange in the brain.

There is some evidence in vitro that choline uptake by nervous tissue involves two kinetically different components referred to as the high- and low-affinity uptake systems. Cornford et al. (12) were unable to demonstrate a high-affinity uptake system for choline across the blood-brain barrier of the rat. Instead, they found that brain choline uptake is via a single carrier-mediated process coupled with diffusion at high concentrations, a conclusion compatible with Diamond (13), Sparf (14), Freeman et al. (15), Freeman and Jenden (16), and Schuberth et al. (17), but not Dross and Kewitz (18) or Kewitz et al. (19,20). Cornford et al. found that hemicholinium-3, deanol, tetramethylammonium, tetraethylammonium, 2-hydroxyethyltriethylammonium, carnitine, normal rat serum, and to a lesser extent, lithium and spermidine all inhibited choline uptake across the rat blood-brain barrier. Deanol had 5 to 10 times greater affinity for choline transport into the brain than choline itself. Hence, if deanol is methylated in the brain, it should be an excellent source of choline. On the other hand, if deanol is not methylated in the brain it would actually inhibit the active transport of free choline into the brain. Whether it would inhibit the transport of the choline containing the lipid or lipoprotein complex described by Mann is unknown. Yamamura and Snyder (21,22) have emphasized that what they call the high-affinity uptake of choline is easily saturated and therefore is an obvious obstacle to increasing brain acetylcholine.

Although twenty-five years ago we did not know about an active transport system for choline through the blood-brain barrier, Pfeiffer's idea of trying to get a precursor of acetylcholine which penetrated easily the blood-brain barrier is still very seductive and as yet elusive. A number of investigators have shown that the stepwise methylation of ethanolamine, which results in the synthesis of choline in the liver, does not occur in the brain (23,24,25,26). If the brain cannot methylate deanol, then its administration to enhance brain acetylcholine will be counterproductive, for the transport of choline will be reduced. It appears that free choline, possibly phosphorylcholine, serine, the plasma lipid of Mann, and lysophosphatidylcholine (27) are the most suitable precursors of brain acetylcholine. But what about deanol? Is or is not deanol a precursor of brain acetylcholine? Danysz et al. (28) found that chronic administration of deanol in daily doses of 175 and 350 mg/kg i.p. markedly elevated brain acetylcholine in mice in 8 to 14 days. Strangely, by 23 days of treatment brain acetylcholine levels returned to control levels, which were very low. These investigators used decapitation for killing the animals and the frog rectus bioassay for measuring acetylcholine. Goldberg and Silbergeld (29) and Goldberg (30) found that both lead-treated and control mice showed 60% elevated acetylcholine levels following deanol administration. Brain acetylcholine was measured using the choline kinase assay. Haubrich et al. (31) also reported that both deanol and choline elevated rat brain acetylcholine. The animals were killed by focused microwave irradiation to the head. Both choline and acetylcholine were isolated by high voltage paper electrophoresis and measured by the choline kinase assay. These investigators specifically pointed out that although deanol is a substrate for choline kinase, it did not interfere with their assay. Both i.p. choline and deanol as well as its acetamidobenzoate salt (Deaner) were highly effective in elevating striatal acetylcholine.

In sharp contrast to the Goldberg and Haubrich studies are those of Zahniser, Shih, Kopp, and Hanin (32), Zahniser, Chou, and Hanin (33), and Zahniser et al. (34). In mice, deanol rapidly elevated plasma and red-cell choline. However, the increases in blood choline after deanol did not increase total brain choline or acetylcholine. In a subsequent study these investigators showed that only after a massive dose of deanol were striatal acetylcholine levels elevated. No other brain areas showed any change. Zahniser et al. (34) also studied the effects on newborn rat pups of mothers fed a choline-deficient diet, a choline-deficient diet supplemented with N-methylaminoethanol and deanol, and a choline-supplemented diet. The diets were given from 15 days before to 15 days after delivery. All pups of mothers fed the N-methyl-aminoethanol and most of the pups whose mothers were fed the deanol diet died even though brain choline and acetylcholine were elevated compared to those on a choline-deficient diet. There was a shift of brain phospholipids in the animals on a N-methylaminoethanol and deanol diet with phosphatidylcholine deficient, and phosphatidyl N-methylaminoethanol and phosphatidyl N-dimethylaminoethanol elevated. Surprisingly, pups whose mothers were given a choline-supplemented diet showed no elevation in brain choline or acetylcholine. The latter findings are surprising because of the evidence that choline administration elevates brain acetylcholine. Nagler et al. (35) and Cohen and Wurtman (36,37) have emphasized that rat brain choline and acetylcholine levels are influenced by the amount of choline in their diet. In addition, dietary lecithin elevates serum-free choline (38).

Hanin et al. (39) demonstrated that 1 gm of deanol p-acetamidobenzoate (deaner) given to 1 normal subject orally dramatically elevated both plasma and red-cell choline and acetylcholine. Within 1 hr a 1200% elevation in plasma choline was observed, which decreased over the next 23 hrs. Even 24 hrs later a 50% elevation in plasma choline was seen. In this subject, the predeanol plasma choline level was 10 nmol/ml. It rose to 119.6 nmol/ml 1 hr after deanol, and was 15.2 nmol/ml 24 hrs later. These startling findings must be elaborated and confirmed, for they indicate a remarkable ability of deanol to elevate blood choline and acetylcholine in man. Ceder and Schuberth (40) have described a new GCMF assay for deanol. Especially important would be to measure deanol, choline, and acetylcholine levels simultaneously in man in both plasma and red cells, and in addition, in brains of animals. The striatum would especially be important and would probably be the most likely area to show changes. In addition, turnover studies are essential.

CLINICAL USE OF DEANOL IN TARDIVE DYSKINESIA

The rationale behind the use of deanol for the treatment of tardive dyskinesia is based on the assumption that normal movement requires a balance between acetylcholinergic and dopaminergic activity of the striatum. Prolonged use of neuroleptics disrupts this balance by producing long-term blockade of post-synaptic striatal dopamine receptors, causing them to become supersensitive to dopamine. This results in a functional excess of dopamine activity and a relative deficit of acetylcholine activity of the striatum. Deanol may restore the balance by being converted first to choline, then to acetylcholine, elevating striatal levels and activity of acetylcholine and counterbalancing dopamine-receptor supersensitivity.

Deanol was first used for the treatment of tardive dyskinesia in 1974. Initial reports (41,42) were highly encouraging, and since then at least 161 patients have been evaluated in 28 studies. Results are summarized in Table 1. Patient characteristics are listed in Table 2. (The first 16 references listed in the tables have recently been reviewed in detail by Casey [57].) Of the 161 patients in Table 1, 59 improved (37%), 1 worsened (0.006%), and 101 (63%) showed only a mild response or no change. If the results of blind, placebo-controlled studies are considered separately, the success rate drops to 16% improved (16 of 101 patients).

In the crossover study of Simpson et al. (63, improvement occurred in all patients during the first treatment phase, regardless of which drug (placebo or deanol) the patients received. The authors concluded that deanol may have contributed to the decline, but other explanations had to be considered, such as the fact that symptoms of tardive dyskinesia fluctuated in severity during the day as well as over time, generally. This was especially apparent in patients who had received neuroleptics immediately prior to the study. There was an upsurge in their symptoms when they came off the neuroleptics, and their decline was somewhat more dramatic than that seen in patients who had been off medication for longer periods.

From the paper of Stafford and Fann (65), only 9 of the 29 patients discussed in that paper are listed under that reference in Table 1; 10 of the patients were the subjects of another publication (46), and it is not clear if the remaining 10 patients are the same as those of Reference 58.

Table 1
Deanol for Tardive Dyskinesia

Ref.ª	First Author—Year	Pts.ᵇ	Designᶜ	Mg/Day, Duration	Results	Comment
41	Miller—1974	2	Open	600, 1 week	Improved	Improved in first week
42	Casey—1974	1	Open	1600, 8 weeks	Improved	Improved in first week
43	Escobar—1975	2	Open	1200, 2 weeks	No change	
44	Crane—1975	11	Open	1200–1600, 18 days	No change	
45	Curran—1975	1	Open	500, 8 weeks	Improved	Improved in first week
46	Fann—1975	10	Open	500, 5 days	Improved	Improved in first week
47	DeSilva—1975	4	Open	800–1000, 2 weeks	Improved	Improved in first week
48	Laterre—1975	1	Open	225–900, 14 weeks	Improved, worsened	Improved with low dose; worsened with high dose
49	Davis—1975	4	Open	1600–2000, 3–8 weeks	No change	Eventually responded to choline
50	Widroe—1976	2	Open	200–300, 3–8 weeks	1 improved 1 no change	Many drugs changed at the same time
51	Nesse—1976	1	Open	1500, 19 days	No change	Peripheral cholinergic side effects
52	Cole—1976	12	DB, PC	1500, 5 weeks	No change	No significant change in global rating of dyskinesias
53	Kumar—1976	1	Open	1200, 12 weeks	Improved	Dyskinesia did not return
54	Bockenheimer—1976	11	DB, PC	1500, 5 weeks	7 improved 4 unchanged	Orofacial dyskinesia improved; limb dyskinesia unchanged
55	Tamminga—1976	6	DB, PC	1500, 3 weeks	No change	Insignificant variable effect of slight improvement to slight worsening
56	Casey—1977	6	SB, PC	800–2000, 4 weeks	3 improved 2 unchanged 1 worsened	Response correlated with physostigmine response
57	Casey—1977	1		6000	No change	Peripheral cholinergic side effects
58	Fann—1976	10	SB	Up to 1800, 3 mos.	Improved	Subjects on no neuroleptics almost completely relieved

Ref.[a]		Pts.[b]		Dose	Results	
59	Mehta—1976	1	Open	600, 3 mos.	No change	Marked sialism, bronchospasm, rigidity
			Open	800, 5 mos.	No change	
60	Ray—1977	1	Open	600	great imp.[d]	Concomitant with lithium, which in toxic doses appeared to worsen TD
61	Crews—1977	1	Open	300	Improved	
62	Tarsy—1977	1	Open		No change	Discontinued due to increased obsessive symptoms
		1	Open	3000	Improved	
63	Simpson—1977	10	DB, PC, CO	200–1000, 5 weeks then 1200, 3 weeks	Mild imp.	Improvement *may* have been due to deanol; not dramatic; placebo improved
64	Tarsy—1977	4	DB, PC, CO	1000, 4 weeks; 2000, 4 weeks	2 Improved / 2 No change	No significant effects; placebo improvement
65	Stafford—1977	1	PC	1000, 11 days	1 No change / 1 Moderate imp.	Dropped out due to psychotic break
		9		1200, 2 weeks	4 Slight imp. / 4 No change	
66	Jus—1978	29	DB, PC, CO	500–1000, 8 weeks	2 Total imp. / 1 Marked imp. / 23 No change	No significant effect. Imp. stable with deanol, unstable with placebo
					2 Dropouts	Due to excitement, overactivity
					1 Dropout	Due to increased delusions and hallucinations
67	Pickar—1978	1	Open		No imp.	
68	Penovich—1978	14	DB, PC, CO	2000, 4 weeks	3 Mild imp.	Three patients with both subjective (mild) and objective (32–44%) imp.; significant imp. over baseline, but not over placebo scores

[a]Ref. = Reference number
[b]Pts. = Number of patients
[c]Abbreviations: CO = Crossover; DB = Double blind; PC = Placebo-controlled; SB = Single blind
[d]imp. = Improvement

Table 2
Characteristics of Patients Listed in Table 1

Ref.	First Author—Year	Pts.	Sex, Age	Type TD*	Duration TD
41	Miller—1974	1	M 66	BLM, LE	3 months
		1	F 57	BLM	8 months
42	Casey—1974	1	M 59	BLM, UE, LE, T	4 months
43	Escobar—1975	1	M 68	BLM, UE, LE, T	1 month
		1	F 55	BLM	12 months
44	Crane—1975	11	M,F 58†	BLM, UE, LE, T	
45	Curran—1975	1	M 42	BLM, T	120 months
46	Fann—1975	10		BLM, UE, LE	
47	DeSilva—1975	1	F 46	BLM	Years
		1	F 62	BLM	Years
		1	M 21	T	Years
		1	F 74	BLM, LE, UE, T	Years
48	Laterre—1975	1			
49	Davis—1975	1	M 39	BLM	
		3			
50	Widroe—1975	1	F 68	BLM	3 months
		1	F 43	BLM	1 month
51	Nesse—1976	1	F 37	BLM	48 months
52	Cole—1976	12	F	BLM, UE, LE, T	
53	Kumar—1976	1	F 17	BLM, UE, LE, T	
54	Bockenheimer—1976	11	F 55†	BLM, LE, UE	Years
55	Tamminga—1977	6	M,F 56†	BLM, T, UE, LE	
56	Casey—1977	6		BLM, T, LE, UE	Years
57	Casey—1977	1	M		
58	Fann—1976	10			
59	Mehta—1976	1	M 89	BLM, UE	Years
		1	F 80	BLM	Years
60	Ray—1977	1	F 77	BLM, LE	
61	Crews—1977	1	F 46	BLM, T, UE	
62	Tarsy—1977	1	M 25	BLM, E, T, UE	Years
		1	M 28	T, E, UE, LE, To	Years
63	Simpson—1977	10	M,F 59†	All pts.: To, UE Most: BLM, LE	
64	Tarsy—1977	4	M	All 5 pts.: M, F	
		1	M	variable T, UE, LE	
65	Stafford—1977	9			
66	Jus-1978	29	M,F 51†	15 pts.: BL 14 pts.: BLM	18 pts. years 11 pts. unknow
67	Pickar—1978	1	F 23	All body parts	
68	Penovich—1978	14	M,F 56†		6 pts. years 5 pts. < 1 yea 3 pts. unknow

*Type of tardive dyskinesia: BL = bucco-lingual; BLM = bucco-linguo-masticatory; UE = upper extremity; LE = lower extremity; T= trunk; To = tongue; M = mouth; F = face
†Average age

Jus *et al.* (66) report that although statistical analysis did not reveal any significant changes in their population as a whole, 3 of their 29 patients experienced considerable relief from their symptoms of tardive dyskinesia during treatment with deanol. Improvement was of a stable character and lasted throughout the administration of the drug. Positive results obtained with placebo were transient and unstable and frequently disappeared when patients were still on placebo.

The factors of age, sex, dose of deanol, and duration of treatment do not seem to correlate with a positive deanol response. Casey (57) tabulated data suggesting that average months of tardive dyskinesia symptoms seen inversely correlated with a deanol effect. The number of patients, however, was too small to draw a conclusion. Unfortunately, additional data from recent studies is not presented in a way that lends itself to addressing this question. Perhaps if in future studies such parameters for individual patients were presented in tabulated form rather than as averages or ranges for patient populations, data could be accumulated which would assist in the identification of potential deanol respondents.

Doses of deanol usually employed range from 200 to 2000 mg/day. Tarsy *et al.* (62) report the use of 3000 mg/day in a single patient, and Penovich *et al.* (68) mention, but do not elaborate on, successful use of 3000 mg/day. The highest dose that has been reported (57) is 6000 mg/day in a patient whose symptoms of tardive dyskinesia remained unaffected although he developed excessive peripheral cholinergic symptoms.

Onset of beneficial effects has been reported to occur within the first week of treatment (41,42,45,46,47,56). Many authors report sustained benefit after discontinuation of deanol (41,53,54,56,64,66,69,70). Further investigations are needed to ascertain if this is a genuine long-term effect of deanol or if it can be accounted for by such factors as spontaneous fluctuation of symptom severity. A possible long-term effect of deanol argues against pooling placebo data collected in periods preceding and following a period of deanol treatment (as in the study of Penovich *et al.* [68]). Topographic differences in response to deanol have been noted, with oro-facial dyskinesia being preferentially improved (54,56,63).

Side effects of deanol seen in patients treated for tardive dyskinesia include increase in mental symptoms (4 patients [62,66]); mild insomnia, irritability, and mood changes (4 patients [56]); severe peripheral cholinergic effects (3 patients [51,57,59]); occipital headache (1 patient [69]); and severe increase in systolic blood pressure (3 patients [46]). Fann *et al.* (46) recommend that daily blood-pressure determinations be made on patients being evaluated on deanol. The side effect of excessive cholinergic activity provides indirect evidence that deanol is acting as a precursor of acetylcholine.

An increase in symptoms of parkinsonism in patients on deanol has been observed (44,46,50). This is compatible with the hypothesis that etiologically, parkinsonism represents an opposite state from tardive dyskinesia. Parkinsonism is believed to be due to a deficit of striatal dopaminergic activity and an excess of acetylcholinergic activity. A shift from tardive dyskinesia to parkinsonism in deanol-treated patients may be the clinical manifestation of "overshooting the mark" in an attempt to restore neurotransmitter balance by increasing acetylcholine activity.

Although blind, placebo-controlled studies indicate that the success rate of deanol as a treatment for tardive dyskinesia is not large, it appears that a small percentage of patients benefit greatly from the drug. Perhaps these patients represent a subgroup with an underlying pathophysiology different from that of most tardive dyskinesia patients. Another possibility is that deanol respondents absorb, distribute, and metabolize the drug differently from nonrespondents. Pharmacokinetic studies of deanol in the two types of patients would be worthwhile. Deanol did not elevate plasma choline levels in 9 tardive dyskinesia patients: 1 patient improved moderately, 4 improved slightly, and 4 showed no change in symptom severity (65). Aside from this, little else has been done in the area of biochemical studies of deanol-treated tardive dyskinesia patients.

Currently, *challenge* drugs are being assessed for their ability to delineate subgroups of tardive dyskinesia patients and to predict outcome of therapy with deanol or choline. A challenge drug is one which would be expected to temporarily enhance or reduce dopamine-acetylcholine imbalance and thus temporarily enhance or reduce tardive dyskinesia movements. Casey and Denney (56) recently evaluated 6 patients with single challenge doses of a dopamine agonist (levodopa) and antagonist (droperidal), as well as with an acetylcholine agonist (physostigmine) and antagonist (benztropine). A blind trial with placebo and deanol followed. The pattern of response to the challenge drugs suggested a division of the patients into two groups. Three patients (Group I) who improved with a dopamine antagonist or an acetylcholine agonist also improved while taking deanol. The other 3 patients (Group 2) were made worse with a dopamine antagonist or acetylcholine agonist, and became worse or showed no change while taking deanol. The results of Group I are clearly consistent with models of dopamine excess and acetylcholine deficit. Results of Group 2, however, do not fit the model, and for these patients another explanation of underlying neuropathology must be sought. It would be interesting to examine the effects of amphetamine and apomorphine (both dopamine agonists) in the two groups of patients, since it has been reported (72) that consistent with the dopaminergic theory, amphetamine increased dyskinetic movements in most tardive dyskinesia patients, but that apomorphine, contrary to the dopamine theory, reduced them substantially in some patients. The ability of apomorphine to block presynaptic dopamine receptors (thus inhibiting dopamine release) may account for its observed effect, but it is also possible that different subgroups of tardive dyskinesia patients were being dealt with. The study of Casey and Denney (56) supports

Table 3
Challenge Drugs and Deanol

Ref.[a]	First Author—Year	Challenge Drug	Dose; Route	Pts.[b]	Challenge Response	Deanol Response	
49	Davis—1974	Physostigmine	3 mg; i.v.	1	Good imp.[c]	No change	Unresponsive to Valium; imp. on choline
55	Tamminga—1977	Physostigmine	Up to 2 mg; i.v.	2 1 1	Good imp. Mild imp. Moderate imp.	No change No change No change	Unresponsive to choline imp. on choline
56	Casey—1977	Physostigmine Benztropine Levodopa Droperidol	1.0 mg; i.v. 2.0 mg; i.v. 500 mg; p.o. 2.5 mg; i.v.	6	See text See text See text See text	See text	6 patients in study
62	Tarsy—1977	Physostigmine Benztropine Diphenhydramine	i.v. i.v. i.v.	1	No change No change No change	No change No change No change	Case report; imp. on Haloperidol
64	Tarsy—1977	Benztropine Physostigmine	i.v. i.v.	5	No change; minor variable change	2 imp. 3 no change	5 patients in study
71	Carroll—1977	Physostigmine Amphetamine Placebo Apomorphine	1 mg; i.v. 10 mg; p.o. 2–6 mg; s.c.	1	Worse Worse No change Marked imp.	No change	Case study; same patient as in reference 51. 14 other drugs tried; only apomorphine and Haloperidol helped

[a]Reference
[b]Number of Patients
[c]Improvement

the notion that there may be subtypes of tardive dyskinesia patients. The response to physostigmine correlated with the response to deanol. Tamminga *et al.* (55), however, found no correlation or present evidence that positive responses to physostigmine may be due to the drug's sedative properties. Other studies in which challenge drugs were given before a trial of deanol therapy are presented in Table 3. More controlled studies in this area are needed before any conclusions can be drawn regarding the ability of a challenge drug to predict response to deanol. Deanol is not the answer to the need for a drug to treat tardive dyskinesia; however, in the absence of any satisfactory treatment, a trial of deanol seems warranted.

REFERENCES

1. DuVigneaud, V., Chandler, J.P. Simmonds, S. *et al.* The role of dimethyl- and monomethylaminoethanol in transmethylation reactions *in vivo. J. Biol. Chem., 164*:603–613, 1946.
2. Pfeiffer, C.C. Parasympathetic neurohumors; possible precursors and effect on behavior. *Int. Rev. Neurobiol., 1*:195–244, 1959.
3. Pfeiffer, C.C., Jenney, E.H., Gallagher, W. *et al.* Stimulant effect of 2-dimethylaminoethanol—a possible precursor of brain acetylcholine. *Science, 126*:610–611, 1957.
4. Pfeiffer, C.C., Broth, D.P., Bain, J.A. Choline versus dimethylaminoethanol (deanol) as possible precursors of cerebral acetylcholine. In *Biological Psychiatry*, Wortis, J. (ed.). New York: Grune and Stratton, pp. 259–272, 1959.
5. Pepeu, G., Freedman, D.X., Giarman, N.J. Biochemical and pharmacological studies of dimethylaminoethanol (deanol). *J. Pharmacol. Exp. Ther., 129*:291-295, 1960.
6. Pedata, F., Wieraszko, A., Pepeu, G. Effect of choline, phosphorylcholine and dimethylaminoethanol on brain acetylcholine level in the rat. *Pharmacol. Res. Commun., 9*:755–761, 1977.
7. Berry, J.F., Stotz, E. Role of phosphorylcholine in acetylcholine synthesis. *J. Biol. Chem., 218*:871–874, 1956.
8. Eade, I.V., Hebb, C.O., Mann, S.P. Free choline levels in the rat brain. *J. Neurochem., 20*:1499–1502, 1973.
9. Mann, S.P. The supply of choline from the circulating plasma to the brain. In *Synapses*, Cotrell, G.A., Usherwood, P.N.R. (eds.). New York: Academic Press, pp. 361–362, 1977.
10. Mann, S.P., Bennett, R.C. The fate of choline in the circulating plasma of the rat. In preparation, 1978.
11. Dahlberg, L., Schuberth, J. Regulation of plasma choline by base exchange. *J. Neurochem., 29*:933–934, 1977.
12. Cornford, E.M., Braun, L.D., Oldendord, W.H. Carrier mediated blood-brain transport of choline and certain choline analogues. *J. Neurochem., 20*:299–308, 1978.
13. Diamond, I. Choline metabolism in brain. The role of choline transport and the effects of phenobarbital. *Arch. Neurol., 24*:333–339, 1971.
14. Sparf, B. On the turnover of acetylcholine in the brain. *Acta Physiol. Scand. Suppl., 397*:1–47, 1973.
15. Freeman, J.J., Choi, R.L., Jenden, D.J. Kinetics of plasma choline in relation to turnover of brain choline and formation of acetylcholine. *J. Neurochem., 24*:735–741, 1975.

16. Freeman, J.J., Jenden, D.J. The source of choline for acetylcholine synthesis in brain. *Life Sci.*, *19*:949–962, 1976.

17. Schuberth, J., Sundwall, A., Sorbo, B., Lindell, J.O. Uptake of choline by mouse brain slices. *J. Neurochem.*, *13*:347–352, 1966.

18. Dross, K., Kewitz, H. Concentration and origin of choline in the rat brain. *Naunyn Schmiedebergs. Arch. Pharmacol.*, *274*:91–106, 1972.

19. Kewitz, H., Dross, K., Pleul, O. Choline and its metabolic successors in brain. In *Central Nervous System—Studies on Metabolic Regulation and Function*, Genazzani, E., Kerken, H. (eds). New York: Springer, pp. 21–32, 1973.

20. Kewitz, H., Pleul, O., Dross, K. *et al.* The supply of choline in rat brain. In *Cholinergic Mechanisms*, Waser, P.G. (ed.). New York: Raven Press, pp. 131–135, 1975.

21. Yamamura, H.I., Snyder, S.H. Choline: high-affinity uptake by rat brain synaptosomes. *Science*, *178*:626–628, 1972.

22. Yamamura, H.I., Snyder, S.H. High affinity transport of choline into synaptosomes of rat brain. *J. Neurochem.*, *21*:1355–1374, 1973.

23. Marshall, E.F., Chojnacki, T., Ansell, G.B. The methylation of [^{32}P] phosphatidyl-monomethylaminoethanol by S-adenosyl-L-[Me-^{14}C] methionine in liver preparations. *Biochem. J.*, *95*:30–31P, 1965.

24. Bjornstadt, P., Bremer, J. *In vivo* studies on pathways for the biosynthesis of lecithin in the rat. *J. Lipid Res.*, *7*:38–45, 1966.

25. Ansell, G.B., Spanner, S. The metabolism of labelled ethanolamine in the brain of the rat *in vitro. J. Neurochem.*, *14*:873–885, 1967.

26. Ansell, G.B., Spanner, S. The metabolism of [Me-^{14}C] choline in the brain of the rat *in vivo. Biochem. J.*, *110*:201–206, 1968.

27. Illingworth, D.R., Portman, O.W. The uptake and metabolism of plasma lysophos-phatidylcholine *in vivo* by the brain of the squirrel monkey. *Biochem. J.*, *130*:557–567, 1972.

28. Danysz, A., Kocmierska-Grodzka, D., Kostro, B. Pharmacological properties of 2-dimethylaminoethanol (bimanol-DMAE). *Diss. Pharm. Pharmacol.*, *19*:469–477, 1967.

29. Goldberg, A.M., Silbergeld, E.K. Neurochemical aspects of lead-induced hyperactivity. *American Society of Neurochemists 5th Annual Meeting Abstracts*, p. 185, 1974.

30. Goldberg, A.M. Is deanol a precursor of acetylcholine? *Dis. Nerv. Syst.*, *38*:16–20, 1977.

31. Haubrich, D.R., Wang, P.F.L., Clody, D.E., *et al.* Increase in rat brain acetylcholine induced by choline or deanol. *Life Sci.*, *17*:975–980, 1975.

32. Zahniser, N.R., Shih, T.M., Kopp, U., Hanin, I. Extent of 2-dimethylaminoethanol (deanol) biotransformation to choline (Ch) and acetylcholine (ACh) in blood and brain: a gas chromatograph/mass spectrometric (GC/MS) analysis. *Society for Neuroscience Abstracts*, 1977.

33. Zahniser, N.R., Chou, D., Hanin, I. Is 2-dimethylaminoethanol (deanol) indeed a precursor of brain acetylcholine? A gas chromatographic evaluation. *J. Pharm. Exp. Ther.*, *200*:545–559, 1977.

34. Zahniser, N.R., Katyal, S.L., Shih, T.M., *et al.* Effects of N-methylaminoethanol and N,N-dimethylaminoethanol in the diet of pregnant rats on neonatal rat brain cholinergic and phospholipid profile. *J. Neurochem.* (Submitted for publication, 1978.)

35. Nagler, A.L., Dettbarn, W.D., Seifter, E., *et al.* Tissue levels of acetylcholine and cholinesterase in weaning rats subjected to acute choline deficiency. *J. Nutrition*, *94*:13–19, 1968.

36. Cohen, E.L., Wurtman, R.J. Brain acetylcholine: increase after systemic choline administration. *Life Sci.*, *16*:1095–1102, 1975.

37. Cohen, E.L., Wurtman, R.J. Brain acetylcholine: control by dietary choline. *Science*, *191*:561–562, 1976.

38. Wurtman, R.J., Hirsch, M.J., Growden, J.H. Lecithin consumption raises serum-free choline levels. *Lancet*, :68–69, 1977.

39. Hanin, I., Kopp, U., Zahniser, N.R., *et al*. Acetylcholine and choline in human plasma and red blood cells: a gas chromatograph mass spectrometric evaluation. In *Cholinergic Mechanisms and Psychopharmacology*, Jenden, D.L. (ed.). New York: Plenum Press, pp. 181–195, 1978.

40. Ceder, G., Schuberth, J. 2-dimethylaminoethanol (deaner) in body fluids. *J. Pharm. Pharmacol.*, *29*:373–374, 1977.

41. Miller, E. Deanol: a solution for tardive dyskinesia? *N. Engl. J. Med.*, *291*:796–797, 1974.

42. Casey, D.E., Denney, D. Dimethylaminoethanol in tardive dyskinesia. *N. Engl. J. Med.*, *291*:797, 1974.

43. Escobar, J.I., Kemp, K.F. Dimethylaminoethanol for tardive dyskinesia. *N. Engl. J. Med.*, *292*:317–318, 1975.

44. Crane, G.E. Deanol for tardive dyskinesia. *N. Engl. J. Med.*, *292*:926, 1975.

45. Curran, D.J., Nagaswami, S., Mohan, K.J. Treatment of phenothiazine-induced bulbar persistent dyskinesia with deanol acetamidobenzoate. *Dis. Nerv. Syst.*, *36*:71–73, 1975.

46. Fann, W.E., Sullivan, J.L., Miller, R.D., *et al*. Deanol in tardive dyskinesia: a preliminary report. *Psychopharmacologia*, *42*:135–137, 1975.

47. DeSilva, L., Huang, C.Y. Deanol in tardive dyskinesia. *Br. Med. J.*, *3*:466, 1975.

48. Laterre, E.C., Fortemps, E. Deanol in spontaneous and induced dyskinesias. *Lancet*, *1*:1301, 1975.

49. Davis, K.L., Berger, P.A., Hollister, L.E. Choline for tardive dyskinesia. *N. Engl. J. Med.*, *293*:152, 1975.

50. Widroe, H.J., Hiesler, S. Treatment of tardive dyskinesia. *Dis. Nerv. Syst.*, *37*:162–164, 1976.

51. Nesse, R., Carroll, B.J. Cholinergic side effects associated with deanol. *Lancet*, *2*:50–51, 1976.

52. Cole, J.O., Gardos, G., Granacher, R. Drug evaluations in tardive dyskinesia: papaverine and deanol. Presented at the 129th annual meeting of the American Psychiatric Association, Miami Beach, Florida, May 1976.

53. Kumar, B.B. Treatment of tardive dyskinesia with deanol. *Am. J. Psychiatry*, *133*:978, 1976.

54. Bockenheimer, S., Lucius, G. Zur therapie mit dimethylaminoethanol (deanol) bei neuroleptikainduzierten extrapyramidalen hyperkinesen. *Arch. Psychiatry Nervenk.*, *222*:69–75, 1976.

55. Tamminga, C.A., Smith, R.C., Ericksen, S.E., *et al*. Cholinergic influences in tardive dyskinesia. *Am. J. Psychiatry*, *134*:769–774, 1977.

56. Casey, D.E., Denney, D. Pharmacological characterization of tardive dyskinesia. *Psychopharmacology*, *57*:1–8, 1977.

57. Casey, D.E. Deanol in the management of involuntary movement disorders: a review. *Dis. Nerv. Syst.*, *38*:7–15, 1977.

58. Fann, W.E., Stafford, J.R., Thornby, J.I., *et al*. Chronic deanol administration in tardive dyskinesia. *Clin. Pharmacol. Ther.*, *18*:106, 1976.

59. Mehta, D., Mehta, S., Mathew, P. Failure of deanol in treating tardive dyskinesia. *Am. J. Psychiatry*, *133*:1467, 1976.

60. Ray, I. Tardive dyskinesia treated with deanol acetamidobenzoate. *Can. Med. Assoc. J.*, *117*:129, 1977.

61. Crews, E.L., Carpenter, A.E. Lithium-induced aggravation of tardive dyskinesia. *Am. J. Psychiatry*, *134*:933, 1977.

62. Tarsy, D., Granacher, R., Bralower, M. Tardive dyskinesia in young adults. *Am. J. Psychiatry*, *134*:1032–1034, 1977.

63. Simpson, G.M., Voitashevsky, A., Young, M.A., *et al*. Deanol in the treatment of tardive dyskinesia. *Psychopharmacology*, *52*:257–261, 1977.

64. Tarsy, D., Bralower, M. Deanol acetamidobenzoate treatment in choreiform movement disorders. *Arch. Neurol.*, *34*:756–758, 1977.

65. Stafford, J.R., Fann, W.E. Deanol acetamidobenzoate (deaner) in tardive dyskinesia. *Dis. Nerv. Syst., 38*:3–6, 1977.
66. Jus, A., Villeneuve, A., Gautier, J., *et al.* Deanol, lithium and placebo in the treatment of tardive dyskinesia. *Neuropsychobiology, 4*:140–149, 1978.
67. Pickar, D., Davies, R.K. Tardive dyskinesia in younger patients. *Am. J. Psychiatry, 135*:385–386, 1978.
68. Penovich, P., Morgan, J.P., Kerzner, B., *et al.* Double-blind evaluation of deanol in tardive dyskinesia. *JAMA, 239*:1997–1998, 1978.
69. Casey, D.E. Deanol for tardive dyskinesia (concluded). *N. Engl. J. Med., 293*:359, 1975.
70. Davis, K.L., Berger, P.A., Hollister, L.E. Deanol in tardive dyskinesia. *Am. J. Psychiatry, 134*:807, 1977.
71. Carroll, B.J., Curtis, G.C., Kokmen, E. Paradoxical response to dopamine agonists in tardive dyskinesia. *Am. J. Psychiatry, 134*:785–789, 1977.
72. Smith, R.C., Tamminga, C.A., Haraszti, J., *et al.* Effects of dopamine agonists in tardive dyskinesia. *Am. J. Psychiatry, 134*:763–768, 1977.

36

Cholinergic Aspects of Tardive Dyskinesia: Human and Animal Studies

KENNETH L. DAVIS
LEO E. HOLLISTER
ADELA L. VENTO
and PHILIP A. BERGER

Administration of the acetylcholinesterase inhibitor physostigmine to some patients with tardive dyskinesia has been shown to significantly diminish the frequency of their abnormal movements (1–5). These results indicate that drugs which increase central cholinergic activity might be useful in the treatment of tardive dyskinesia. Exploitation of this strategy was restricted by the absence of a long-acting oral cholinomimetic. However, recent reports suggest that large doses of the acetylcholine precursors choline and dimethylaminoethanol (DMAE) can increase brain acetylcholine content, and perhaps cholinergic activity (6–9). Thus, precursor loading with choline or DMAE might increase central cholinergic activity in a manner analogous to the way large doses of levodopa increase central dopaminergic activity. Hence it was proposed that these precursors be given to patients with the diagnosis of tardive dyskinesia (10). Initial reports indicated that choline chloride significantly reduced the frequency of abnormal bucco-lingual-masticatory movements in patients with tardive dyskinesia (4,11). Subsequent studies have confirmed the efficacy of choline chloride in patients with this diagnosis (12–13). This chapter will review our studies with choline chloride and offer additional human and animal data.

METHODS

Human Studies

Subjects. Eight male patients between age 35 and 65 and with a diagnosis of tardive dyskinesia gave their informed consent to participate in this study. Seven had an abnormal involuntary movement of 3 to 24 months duration, and 7 patients had not received any neuroleptic medication for the same length of time. One patient had been symptomatic- and neuroleptic-free for only 2 weeks. One patient was on a low dose of haloperidol that had been constant for 3 months.

Drug Administration

Physostigmine. Five patients received 3.0–4.0 mg of physostigmine by gradual intravenous infusion. Twenty to 30 minutes prior to this procedure, all patients were premedicated with 0.5 to 1.0 mg of methscopolamine given subcutaneously. Patients knew that physostigmine might affect their movements, but they were told that either a worsening or improvement was possible.

Dimethylaminoethanol (DMAE). Four patients received DMAE in a dose of 1600 to 2000 mg per day for 21 to 56 days. At the end of this period patients were given a placebo for 14 to 21 days. Patients did not know if they were receiving placebo or DMAE.

Choline Chloride. Five patients received choline chloride. Following a baseline period of 2 to 4 weeks, patients were started on a dose of 4g of choline chloride per day. This was gradually increased to a maximum dose of 20g per day, which was maintained for 3 to 8 weeks. A 4-week placebo period followed. Whenever possible, patients received a second trial of choline chloride lasting 4 weeks following the placebo period. Patients were given 20g of choline chloride per day during this second trial.

Clinical Evaluation

Videotape recordings were made prior to, throughout, and after the physostigmine infusion. During choline chloride, DMAE and placebo-administration patients were videotaped 3–5 times per week. Whenever possible, taping sessions were conducted at the same time each day. Tapes were evaluated by an independent rater blind to the study design, who counted the number of movements throughout each session. Movement frequencies were recorded per 45-second epoch. The Mann-Whitney test for nonparametric data was used for the statistical analysis.

Animal Studies

Sprague-Dawley rats were exposed to haloperidol for 28 consecutive days. Animals received 0.5 mg/kg of haloperidol by subcutaneous injection. Haloperidol was discontinued on day 29. On days 36–39, animals were challenged with 0.125 mg/kg to 1.0 mg/kg of apomorphine given subcutaneously. In addition to apomorphine and haloperidol, these animals were given either 375 mg of choline chloride or water by gavage according to varying schedules. Table 1 outlines the procedures used in these animal studies. There were 10 to 20 rats in each group.

Severity of apomorphine-induced stereotypy was rated by a modification of the scale proposed by Costall and Naylor (14). Two raters, who were blind to the drug condition, evaluated the severity of stereotypy. Interrater reliability exceeded r = .9. The procedures involved in each of these studies are presented in greater detail elsewhere (4,15,16).

RESULTS

Human Studies

Physostigmine. All 5 patients who received physostigmine had a significantly lower frequency of involuntary movements for a 30-minute period 15 to 90 minutes after receiving physostigmine than they had during the baseline, predrug period and the period from 2½ to 24 hours after the physostigmine infusion. These results are summarized in Figure 1.

Dimethylaminoethanol. Three of the 4 patients who received DMAE had no improvement in the frequency of their abnormal movements from the predrug to the DMAE period. One patient had a total disappearance of all abnormal movements. However, his movements did not reappear on placebo, and this

Table 1
Procedures of Haloperidol—Choline Experiment

Group	Days 1–28	Days 29–35	Days 36–39
1	haloperidol	drug free	apomorphine and choline chloride
2	haloperidol	drug free	apomorphine and water
3	haloperidol	choline chloride	apomorphine and choline chloride
4	haloperidol	water	apomorphine and water
5	haloperidol and choline chloride	choline chloride	apomorphine and choline chloride

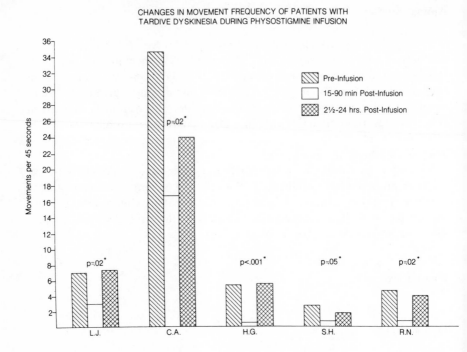

Figure 1.

patient had dyskinetic movements for only 2 weeks prior to the trial of DMAE.

Choline Chloride. All 5 patients who received choline chloride had a significantly lower frequency of abnormal movements while receiving 16g to 20g of choline chloride than during the preceding baseline period. Two of these patients had an exacerbation in the frequency of their involuntary movements when placebo was substituted for choline chloride. However, the remaining 3 patients had essentially no change in the frequency of their oral-facial movements when placebo was substituted for choline chloride. These data are summarized in Figure 2.

Animal Studies

Rats in Groups 1 and 2 tested the acute effects of choline chloride on the animal model of tardive dyskinesia. The animals who received choline chloride by gavage 20 minutes prior to the apomorphine challenge did not significantly differ from animals who received water by gavage 20 minutes before the apomorphine challenge. However, administration of choline chloride on days 28 through 39 (or 1 through 39, as occurred in Groups 3 and 5 respectively), significantly decreased the severity of apomorphine-induced

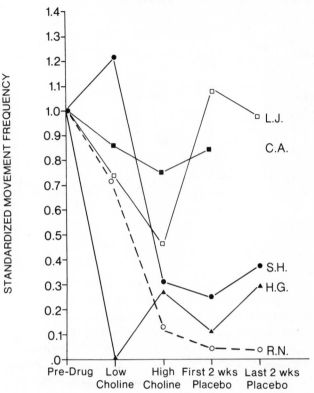

CHANGES IN MOVEMENT FREQUENCIES DURING CHOLINE
CHLORIDE AND PLACEBO TREATMENT

Figure 2.

stereotypy. Thus, Group 3 had significantly less severe stereotypy than Group 4, the water control group, and an analysis of variance indicates a significant effect of the duration of choline chloride administration on the severity of stereotypy in rats. These results are described in Figure 3.

DISCUSSION

In this study, physostigmine significantly suppressed the abnormal involuntary movements of patients with tardive dyskinesia. These results are consistent with other reports of the effect of increasing central cholinergic activity in patients with tardive dyskinesia, and suggest the value of developing a long-acting oral cholinomimetic for the treatment of this condition.

In an attempt to increase brain acetylcholine activity more chronically, all

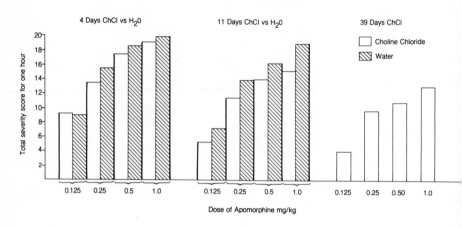

Figure 3.

patients who received physostigmine participated in a therapeutic trial of choline chloride. Every patient who was significantly improved by choline chloride had previously improved during the physostigmine infusion. Thus, there was a perfect correlation between the response to choline chloride and the response to physostigmine. These results suggest that choline chloride, like physostigime, increases central cholinergic activity, and that this cholinergic activity decreases the frequency of involuntary oral-facial movements in patients with tardive dyskinesia. However, this conclusion may be premature.

Three of the 5 patients who responded to choline chloride with a significantly lower movement frequency during choline chloride treatment than the preceding baseline period did not get worse when placed on placebo. It is possible that these 3 patients may have had a slowly remitting tardive dyskinesia that gradually improved after the discontinuation of neuroleptic medications. However, this is unlikely since these patients had a stable oral-facial dyskinesia for 3 to 6 months before beginning choline chloride treatment.

Choline chloride was also tested in an animal model that had been suggested to reflect human tardive dyskinesia (17). The results of the studies are consistent with experiments of the efficacy of choline chloride in the treatment of tardive dyskinesia. However, both human and animal studies suggest that choline chloride does not eliminate all the symptoms of tardive dyskinesia. Rather, it produces a statistically significant reduction in abnormal movement frequency, but patients retain a clinically noticeable dyskinesia. The mechanism of action of both choline chloride and physostigmine on tardive dyskinesia remains speculative. A relationship between increased cholinergic activity and dopaminergic transmission in the substantia nigra and corpus striatum mediated by a GABA-ergic neuron has been proposed (18). This proposed relationship is illustrated in Figure 4. According to this model, increased cholinergic activity would result in decreased dopaminergic transmission. This hypothesis should be further investigated because it raises the possibility that chronic treatment with a cholinomimetic could ultimately produce a hypersensitive dopaminergic receptor. This action on the dopamine receptor would be a consequence of the prolonged diminution in dopaminergic activity secondary to increased cholinergic activity.

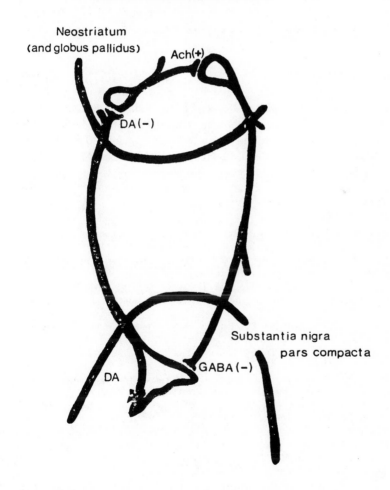

Figure 4.

There was no evidence from this study that DMAE was an effective treatment for patients with tardive dyskinesia. However, the dose of DMAE used in this investigation was considerably below the dose of choline chloride that reduced the movements of patients with tardive dyskinesia. Since DMAE must be converted to choline in the liver before it can increase brain levels of choline or phosphatidylcholine, it would seem that much larger doses of DMAE would be required to elevate brain acetylcholine levels (19).

These early human and animal studies with choline chloride and DMAE have pointed out some of the potential advantages and limitations of a precursor loading strategy which attempts to increase brain acetylcholine to treat patients with tardive dyskinesia. Further studies with these drugs, and other potential cholinomimetic agents such as lecithin and oxotremorine, will determine the extent that pharmacological manipulation of the cholinergic nervous system can be utilized in the treatment of tardive dyskinesia.

ACKNOWLEDGMENTS

We appreciate the support of the staff of the Stanford Psychiatric Clinical Research Center. This research was supported by the Medical Research Service of the Veterans Administration, NIMH Specialized Research Center Grant MH 30854 and U.S. Public Health Service Grant MH 03030.

REFERENCES

1. Klawans, H.L., Rubovits, R. Effect of cholinergic and anticholinergic agents on tardive dyskinesia. *J. Neurol. Neurosurg. Psychiatry, 37*:941–947, 1974.
2. Fann, W.E., Lake, C.R., Gerber, C.J., Cholinergic suppression of tardive dyskinesia. *Psychopharmacologia, 37*:101–107, 1974.
3. Gerlach, J., Reisby, N., Randrup, A. Dopaminergic hypersensitivity and cholinergic hypofunction in the pathophysiology of tardive dyskinesia. *Psychopharmacologia, 34*:21–35, 1974.
4. Davis, K.L., Hollister, L.E., Barchas, J.D., Choline in tardive dyskinesia and Huntington's disease. *Life Sci., 19*:1507–1516, 1976.
5. Casey, D.E., Denny, D. Dimethylaminoethanol in tardive dyskinesia. *N. Engl. J. Med., 291*:797, 1974.
6. Haubrich, D.R., Wang, P.F.L., Clody, D.E., Increase in rat brain acetylcholine induced by choline or deanol. *Life Sci., 17*:975–980, 1975.
7. Cohen, E.L. Wurtman, R.J. Brain acetylcholine: Increase after systemic choline administration. *Life Sci., 16*:1095–1102, 1975.
8. Cohen, E.L. Wurtman, R.J. Brain acetylcholine control by dietary choline. *Science, 191*:561–562, 1976.
9. Ulus, I.H., Wurtman, R.J. Choline administration: Activation of tyrosine hydroxylase in dopaminergic neurons of rat brain. *Science, 194*:1060, 1976.
10. Davis, K.L., Berger, P.A., Hollister, L.E. Tardive dyskinesia and depressive illness. *Psychopharmacol. Commun., 2*:125–131 1976.

11. Davis, K.L., Berger, P.A., Hollister, L.E. Choline for tardive dyskinesia (a letter). *N. Engl. J. Med., 293*:152, 1975.
12. Tamminga, C.A., Smith, R.C., Ericksen, S.E. Cholinergic influences in tardive dyskinesia. *Am. J. .Psychiatry, 134*:769–774, 1977.
13. Growdon, J.H., Hirsch, M.J., Wurtman, R.J. Oral choline administration to patients with tardive dyskinesia. *N. Engl. J. Med., 297*:524–527, 1977.
14. Costall, B., Naylor, R.J. The role of telencephalic dopaminergic systems in the mediation of apomorphine stereotyped behavior. *Eur. J. Pharmacol., 24*:8–24, 1973.
15. Davis, K.L., Berger, P.A., Hollister, L.E. Deanol for tardive dyskinesia. *Am. J. Psychiatry, 134*(7):807, 1977.
16. Davis, K.L., Hollister, L.E., Vento, A.L. Choline chloride in methylphenidate- and apomorphine-induced stereotypy. *Life Sci.,* (In press).
17. Tarsy, D., Baldessarini, R.J. Pharmacologically induced behavioral supersensitivity to apomorphine. *Nature, 245*:262–263, 1973.
18. Groves, P.M., Wilson, C.J., Young, S.J. Self inhibition by dopaminergic neurons: an alternative to the "normal feed-back loop" hypothesis for the mode of action of certain psychotropic drugs. *Science, 190*:522–529, 1975.
19. Bjornstad, P., Bremer, J. In vivo studies on pathways for the biosynthesis of lecithin in the rat. *J. Lipid Res., 7*:38–45, 1966.

37

Effects of Choline-Containing Compounds on Tardive Dyskinesia and Other Movement Disorders

JOHN H. GROWDON
and RICHARD J. WURTMAN

In 1975, Cohen and Wurtman showed that acetylcholine synthesis could be influenced by the levels of its precursor choline in the diet and in the blood stream (1). This chapter will review the evidence that (1) the amount of choline that is available to the brain determines the amount of acetylcholine that is synthesized and released, and that (2) oral choline can be usefully administered to humans with tardive dyskinesia and other diseases in which physicians may wish to enhance cholinergic tone.

NUTRITIONAL AND PRECURSOR CONTROL OF BRAIN ACETYLCHOLINE SYNTHESIS

When rats receive choline chloride by injection (30–120 mg/kg, i.p. [1]) by stomach tube (2), or via the diet (3), choline and acetylcholine levels in the brain and in peripheral, cholinergically innervated organs increase rapidly. These increases are noted in the hippocampus, an area rich in cholinergic nerve terminals, as well as in all other brain regions examined (4). The consumption of a single meal containing lecithin, the natural source of choline in the diet, also causes major increases in acetylcholine levels within the brain and in such peripheral, cholinergically innervated structures as the adrenal medulla (Hirsch and Wurtman, unpublished observations). That choline-induced increases in neuronal acetylcholine levels are associated with enhanced release of the transmitter was first suggested by the finding that choline administration rapidly activates the enzyme tyrosine hydroxylase in the rat caudate nucleus

(5), and that this effect can be blocked if animals are treated with atropine. (The tyrosine hydroxylase is present in different cells—the terminals of nigro-neostriatal neurons—from those that synthesize acetylcholine from choline; hence the change in its activity must reflect a transsynaptic effect, mediated by acetylcholine.) Additional evidence in support of this relationship has been obtained from experiments on the adrenal medulla. This tissue seems ideally suited for such studies inasmuch as it contains only two types of cells, i.e., epinephrine-synthesizing chromaffin cells and the terminals of cholinergic neurons that reach the adrenal via the splanchnic nerve. First, we showed that the administration of a large dose of choline by stomach tube caused, after 24 or 48 hours, an induction of tyrosine hydroxylase (6). (This was similar to the increase previously observed among animals given reserpine [7,8] and other treatments that enhance acetylcholine release by accelerating the flow of impulses along the splanchnic nerve [8].) Next, we demonstrated that this induction did not occur when rats were pretreated with cyclohexamide, an inhibitor of protein synthesis, or among animals whose adrenals had previously been denervated (6) and thus lacked the enzyme, choline acetyltransferase, needed to convert choline to acetylcholine. If animals received any of a number of treatments that are known to increase the rate at which the splanchnic nerve fires (e.g., reserpine, phenoxybenzamine, intraperitoneal 6-hydroxydopamine, insulin, exposure to the cold), the resulting increases in adrenal tyrosine hydroxylase activity were found to be markedly potentiated by the coadministration of choline (9). This affirmed that choline acts primarily not by changing the firing rate of cholinergic neurons, but by increasing the amounts of neurotransmitter released per nerve impulse (9). Choline administration also markedly increases the secretion of epinephrine from the intact adrenal medulla, but not from the denervated organ (10).

The most pronounced behavioral effect of choline demonstrated thus far in experimental animals involves its ability to suppress the analgesia induced by morphine. If rats placed on a hot plate are given morphine, the number of seconds that pass until they flinch or jump is increased; if they also receive choline, there is a dose-related suppression of morphine's analgesic activity (11). This shows both that choline administration—acting via acetylcholine release—modifies behavior, and that cholinergic neurons are involved in mechanisms of pain sensitivity.

Clinical Effects of Administering Choline or Lecithin

Choline administration by injection (1), stomach tube (2), or dietary supplementation (3) increased serum choline, brain choline, and brain acetylcholine levels in the rat; lecithin consumption also increased brain acetylcholine content. The likelihood that a similar sequence occurs in humans prompted speculation that choline could be used to treat patients with brain diseases, such as Huntington's disease (HD) and tardive dyskinesia (TD), that may be associated with deficient cholinergic tone (12,13). We have given choline to 10 patients with HD (14) and 20 patients with TD (15); also choline chloride and lecithin to 16 normal subjects (16,17). This experience indicates that both choline chloride and lecithin are safe for human consumption; both are well tolerated and significantly increase the amount of free choline in the blood that is delivered to the brain for acetylcholine synthesis.

Ten normal subjects fasted for 12 hours and then consumed a single meal containing 2.3g choline base or an equivalent amount of lecithin. Blood samples were obtained prior to the meal and 30 minutes, 1, 4, 8, and 12 hours later. Choline chloride increased serum choline levels from a mean of 11.7 to 21.3 nmols/ml (p < .01) within 30 minutes; levels approached control values within 4 hours. Lecithin was even more effective: serum levels rose by 265% (p < .001) and stayed elevated for 12 hours. In separate experiments, 6 normal subjects ate 3 daily meals (2500 Kcal/day) for 2 days, that contained *no* choline, and 1 week later a similar isocaloric diet that contained 100g of lecithin/day. Blood samples were obtained every 4 hours on the second day of each test diet. We found that the consumption of the high choline diet significantly elevated serum choline levels throughout the day (i.e., for as long as the food was probably being absorbed). In contrast, serum choline remained at basal levels on days during which the low choline diet was consumed. We concluded that the amount of choline in each day's diet normally exerts a major influence on serum choline levels, and that lecithin is more potent in raising these levels than choline chloride alone. The data also provided a scientific basis for giving choline (and lecithin) to patients with brain diseases that may be associated with deficient cholinergic tone.

Huntington's disease is a chronic progressive neurologic disorder characterized by an autosomal dominant pattern of inheritance, plus personality changes, mental deterioration, slurred speech, involuntary muscular contractions (chorea), and unsteady gait. Acetylcholine synthesis may be impaired in this condition, inasmuch as the activity of choline acetyltransferase, the enzyme that catalyzes the conversion of choline to acetylcholine, is reduced in brains of patients who die with HD (18,19,20). Pharmacologic testing is also consistent with inadequate acetylcholine release in this disease: anticholinergic drugs exacerbate the chorea, whereas cholinergic agonists, such as physostigmine, suppress it (21). Ten patients with HD took choline chloride 150–200 mg/kg/day according to a single-drug, open label protocol. Choline ingestion significantly increased choline levels in serum (from 13.6 to 25.8 nmols/ml; p < .001) and in cerebrospinal fluid (from 1.8 to 3.7 nmols/ml; p < .01) (22). Each patient was examined daily for clinical improvement and for signs of cholinergic toxicity. Speed improved in 1 patient, and balance and gait improved in 5 during choline ingestion. These benefits were, however, transient, and did not persist beyond 1 month despite continued choline administration (14). Very high doses of choline (greater than 300 mg/kg/day) commonly produced lacrimation, anorexia, vomiting, and diarrhea, but no changes in pupil size or heart rate; routine hematologic, hepatic, and renal blood tests remained unchanged as well. These symptoms subsided as the choline dose was decreased; however, each patient developed a fishy body odor that did not disappear until the choline was discontinued.

Tardive dyskinesia is a choreic movement disorder characterized by involuntary twitches in the tongue, lips, jaw, and extremities (23). It is believed to occur in susceptible individuals who have taken neuroleptic drugs (e.g., the antipsychotic drugs, such as Thorazine and Haldol [24]). Pharmacologic testing indicates that the pathophysiology of this disease involves an imbalance in the postulated reciprocal relationship between dopaminergic and cholinergic neurons in the basal ganglia. Thus, drugs that either block dopaminergic neurotransmission or enhance cholinergic transmission tend to suppress TD (25). Choline chloride or placebo was given to 20 patients with severe permanent TD, according to a double-blind crossover protocol (15). During the period that choline was ingested, serum choline levels increased in every patient (from a mean of 12.4 to 33.5 nmols/ml; $p < .001$ and choreic movements decreased in 9 of 20 patients. (Four of these 9 patients improved during choline ingestion even though they continued their usual neuroleptic dose. Moreover, in none of the 20 patients continuing to receive a neuroleptic during choline administration was the therapeutic action of the neuroleptic suppressed.) In contrast, no change in the number of movements was observed during the period of placebo ingestion.

These results indicate that (1) choline ingestion increases the availability of choline for acetylcholine synthesis and release in humans as well as in rats, and (2) choline administration can thus be used to enhance cholinergic tone in a disease—tardive dyskinesia—in which such tone is deficient. These data constitute the first rigorously controlled study to show that a naturally occurring dietary nutrient (choline) can be used to treat a nonnutritional brain disease (TD). Lecithin—or even foods with a high lecithin content—may provide even more effective therapy than choline itself; studies to test this hypothesis are currently in progress. Choline precursor therapy may now be attempted in any disease in which the physician wishes to increase cholinergic tone.

ACKNOWLEDGMENTS

These studies were supported in part by grants from ADAMHA (MH–28783), the National Aeronautics and Space Administration (NGR–22–009–627), and the John A. Hartford Foundation.

REFERENCES

1. Cohen, E.L., Wurtman, R.J. Brain acetylcholine: increase after systemic choline administration. *Life Sci., 16*:1095–1102, 1975.
2. Hirsch, M.J., Ulus, I., Wurtman, R.J. Elevation of brain and adrenal acetylcholine levels and of adrenal tyrosine hydroxylase activity following administration of choline *via* stomach tube. *Neurosci. Abs. II* (2):765, 1976.
3. Cohen, E., Wurtman, R.J. Brain acetylcholine synthesis: control by dietary choline. *Science, 191*:561–562, 1976.
4. Hirsch, M.J., Growdon, J.H., Wirtman, R.J. Increase in hippocampal acetylcholine following choline administration. *Brain Res., 332*:383–385, 1977.
5. Ulus, I., Wurtman, R.J. Choline administration: activation of tyrosine hydroxylase in dopaminergic neurons of rat brain. *Science, 194*:1060–1061, 1976.
6. Ulus, I., Hirsch, M., Wurtman, R.J. Trans-synaptic induction of adrenomedullary tyrosine hydroxylase activity by choline: evidence that choline administration increases cholinergic transmission. *Proc. Natl. Acad. Sci. USA, 74*:798–800, 1977.
7. Ulus, I.H., Scally, M.C., Wurtman, R.J. Choline potentiates the trans-synaptic induction of adrenal tyrosine hydroxylase by reserpine, probably by enhancing the release of acetylcholine. *Life Sci., 21*:145–148, 1977.
8. Thoenen, H. Trans-synaptic enzyme induction. *Life Sci., 14*:223–235, 1974.
9. Ulus, I.H., Scally, M.C., Wurtman, R.J. Potentiation by choline of the induction of adrenal tyrosine hydroxylase by phenoxybenzamine, 6-hydroxydopamine, insulin, or exposure to cold. *J. Pharmacol. Exp. Ther.,* (In press).
10. Scally, M.C., Ulus, I.H., Wurtman, R.J. (Submitted for publication.)
11. Botticelli, L.J., Lytle, L.D., Wurtman, R.J. Choline-induced attenuation of morphine analgesis in the rat. *Communications in Psychopharmacology* (In press).
12. Davis, K.L., Hollister, L.E., Berger, P.A., Cholinergic imbalance hypothesis of psychoses and movement disorders: strategies for evaluation. *Psychopharmacol. Commun., 1*:533–543, 1975.
13. Growdon, J.H., Cohen, E.L., Wurtman, R.J. Treatment of brain diseases with dietary precursors of neurotransmitters. *Ann. Intern. Med., 88*:337–339, 1977.
14. Growdon, J.H., Cohen, E.L., Wurtman, R.J. Huntington's disease: clinical and chemical effects of choline administration. *Ann. Neurol., 1*:418–422, 1977.
15. Growdon, J.H., Hirsch, M.J., Wurtman, R.J., Weiner, W. Oral choline administration to patients with tardive dyskinesia. *N. Engl. J. Med., 297*:524–527, 1977.
16. Wurtman, R.J., Hirsch, M.J., Growdon, J.H. Lecithin consumption raises serum free choline levels. *Lancet, 2*:68–69, 1977.
17. Hirsch, M.J., Growdon, J.H., Wurtman, R.J. (Submitted for publication).
18. McGeer, P.L., McGeer, E.G., Fibiger, H.C. Choline acetylase and glutamic acid decarboxylase in Huntington's chorea. *Neurology* (Minneap.), *23*:912–917, 1973.
19. Bird, E.D., Iversen, L.L. Huntington's chorea: post-mortem measurement of glutamic acid decarboxylase, choline acetyltransferase, and dopamine in basal ganglia. *Brain, 97*:457-472, 1974.
20. Stahl, W.L., Swanson, P.D. Biochemical abnormalities in Huntington's chorea brains. *Neurology* (Minneap.), *24*:813–819, 1974.
21. Klawans, H.L., Rubovits, R. Central cholinergic-anticholinergic antagonism in Huntington's chorea. *Neurology* (Minneap.), *22*:107–112, 1972.
22. Growdon, J.H., Cohen, E.L., Wurtman, R.J. Effects of oral choline administration on serum and CSF choline levels in patients with Huntington's disease. *J. Neurochem., 28*:229–231, 1977.

23. Crane, G.E. Tardive dyskinesia in patients treated with major neuroleptics: a review of the literature. *Am. J. Psychiatry, 124* (8) Suppl. :4–54, 1968.
24. Food and Drug Administration Task Force, American College of Neuropsychopharmacology. Neurological syndromes associated with antipsychotic drug use: a special report. *Arch. Gen. Psychiatry, 28*:463–467, 1973.
25. Kobayashi, R.M. Drug therapy of tardive dyskinesia. *N. Engl. J. Med. 296*:257–260, 1977.

38

The Effects of Cholinergic Drugs on the Involuntary Movements of Tardive Dyskinesia

CAROL A. TAMMINGA
ROBERT C. SMITH
and JOHN M. DAVIS

Extensive clinical evidence would suggest that neural systems containing dopamine (DA) and choline have opposing behavioral effects on involuntary movements (1). While the hypokinetic movement disorder of parkinsonism is alleviated by DA agonists and cholinergic antagonists (2,3), the hyperkinetic movement disorders such as Huntington's chorea and tardive dyskinesia are generally alleviated by DA-diminishing drugs and may be intensified by cholinergic antagonists. Studies in experimental animals substantiate these clinical observations by providing evidence for a mutual antagonism between cholinergic and dopaminergic neurons within the basal ganglia (4–6). Thus, since tardive dyskinesia has been hypothesized to be a dopamine-supersensitive disease (7), pharmacologic manipulation of cholinergic neural pathways may prove therapeutic in patients with tardive dyskinesia.

Several studies provide information about the influence of augmenting or diminishing cholinergic transmission on tardive dyskinesia symptoms. A number of investigators have reported that physostigmine diminishes the involuntary movements of tardive dyskinesia (8,9,10). Two anticholinergic drugs, biperiden and scopolamine, have been found to exacerbate the dyskinetic movements (8–10). Oral choline, believed to augment central cholinergic transmission, has been shown to diminish the oral-facial dyskinesia (11–13), as well as to cause depressive mood changes (22). Deanol, a purported (although controversial) acetylcholine precursor, has been used in the treatment of tardive dyskinesia. Many uncontrolled studies and single case reports detail therapeutic trials of deanol (14–19), some reporting a positive therapeutic effect. At the time we began our studies, there were no double-blind, placebo-controlled studies published that validated the clinical impression that deanol helps tardive dyskinesia.

This paper contains data from double-blind, placebo-controlled trials of three cholinomimetic agents. Physostigmine was used in an acute single-dose trial to assess tardive dyskinesia movement response to a cholinergic agent. The acute effect of an i.v. dose of physostigmine may indicate the potential efficacy of the treatment of tardive dyskinesia symptoms with chronic cholinergic agents. Chronic deanol was evaluated because of the reports of its efficacy and of its purported cholinergic actions. And because of the body of evidence from animal studies that oral choline does indeed increase brain acetylcholine (21–23), we carried out an open therapeutic trial of oral choline.

SUBJECTS AND METHODS

Twelve patients with tardive dyskinesia were included in the present study. The majority came from long-term mental-health facilities; two were referred from the community. Specific characteristics of the population are summarized in Table 1.

Patients were withdrawn from all neuroleptic medication at least 2 weeks prior to testing. Each gave voluntary consent to the procedures. Since a

Table 1

Characteristics of the 12 Tardive Dyskinesia (TD) Patients Studied

Patient	Sex	Age	Psychiatric Diagnosis	Years on Neuroleptic Drugs	Area of Primary Symptom Manifestation
1	Female	68	Chronic schizophrenia	15+	Mouth, tongue, eyes
2	Female	63	Chronic schizophrenia	15+	Hands
3	Female	57	Chronic schizophrenia	15+	Mouth, tongue, waist
4	Female	33	Schizophrenia; mental retardation	4	Face
5	Female	49	Chronic schizophrenia	8	Mouth
6	Female	59	Chronic schizophrenia	15+	Mouth, tongue, face
7	Female	59	Chronic schizo-affective schizophrenia	12	Mouth
8	Female	72	Chronic schizophrenia	15+	Face
9	Female	73	Chronic schizophrenia	15+	Mouth, tongue, face
10	Male	52	Chronic schizophrenia	10	Hands, feet
11	Male	34	Chronic schizophrenia	15	Hands
12	Male	25	Schizo-affective schizophrenia	3	Face

number of different drug trials, both acute and chronic, were included in this study, the sequence of tests was arranged so that there was a 5–7 day drug-free period following any chronic dose medication, and a 2–3 day period following any single-dose drug trial.

Involuntary movements were rated on a scale developed by the Smith Tardive Dyskinesia Scale (see pp. 247–254). During the initial evaluation period, the ratings were performed daily, and videotaping was done twice a week. Videotaping continued to be done during acute and chronic drug trials at critical times, and they were rated in series at a later time.

Physostigmine was administered i.v., 60 minutes after 1 cc of methscopolamine, a peripheral cholinergic blocker. A dose of 0.5 ml i.v. bolus was administered every 5 minutes through a forearm vein; the active drug was preceded by a variable number of sterile saline injections. Up to 2.0 mg physostigmine over 20 minutes was given. Drug injections were stopped when patient discomfort became apparent, as evaluated by the nonblind observer. Using the same clinical method, i.v. Neostigmine and i.v. Brevital were both given as active control drugs, one for peripheral cholinergic action and the other for sedation, respectively.

Deanol was evaluated in a chronic schedule with double-blind, placebo-controlled design in doses beginning at 500 mg a day and increasing to 1250 mg a day over a 3-week period. Daily (morning and afternoon) ratings were done, and twice-weekly videotaped interviews were carried out.

Choline was used in a preliminary nonplacebo trial on a limited number of patients. The drug was given orally in doses beginning at 3g a day, increasing to 18g over a 3-week period. Ratings were done daily, and videotaping done twice weekly. Blood samples were collected for choline levels and prolactin values prior to each dose increase.

RESULTS

Physostigmine

As shown in Figure 1, each patient had a decrease in dyskinetic movements within 10 to 20 minutes following active drug administration, which ranged from 20% to 80% suppression from predrug levels. Neostigmine, a drug which has only peripheral acetylcholinesterase activity, had no effect on the movements. Brevital, a short-acting barbituate, was administered as an active control for the physostigmine-induced sedation. Movements decreased substantially with this drug. However, clinical observations suggested that activating the patients following brevital administration reversed the drug-induced movement diminution; patient activation following physostigmine had less of an effect on the physostigmine-induced decrease in dyskinetic

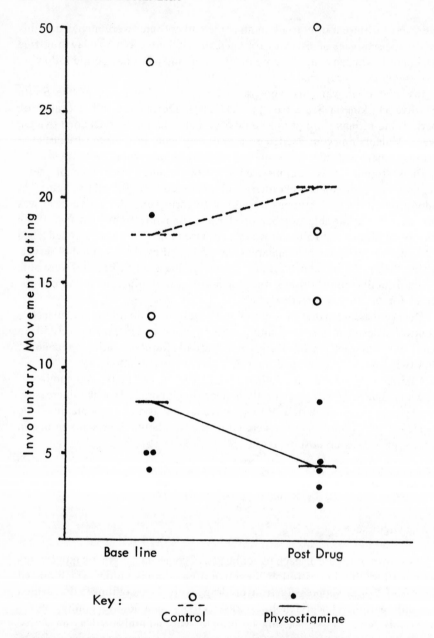

Figure 1.   Change in involuntary movement scores following physostigmine (solid line) and neostigmine (dotted line) administration. Tardive dyskinesia movements were blindly rated pre- and postintravenous physostigmine administration (n = 5). A mean decrease in choreiform movements of greater than 35% occurred. Neostigmine, administered as a peripherally active cholinergic control, was followed by no diminution, rather a small stimulation in the involuntary movements (n = 3).

movements. These observations suggest that sedation controls are important in evaluating physostigmine's effect, but that physostigmine may also decrease dyskinetic movements by other pharmacologic mechanism in addition to any sedating effect.

Deanol

The results fail to show that deanol improved tardive dyskinesia movements to any substantial degree in the 6 patients who received it. Figure 2 illustrates the mean score ($\pm$ SEM) of the average weekly ratings of the tardive dyskinesia patients during the placebo period and the 900 mg and 1250 mg daily dose period. While deanol produced a variable reduction in dyskinesia symptoms in some patients, exacerbation occurred in others. The symptom reduction that did occur in some patients did not persist with continued treatment and did not appear to be dose related. When we looked at primary symptoms alone (bucco-linguo-masticatory), we also found no overall beneficial effect of deanol. Our conclusion is that the effect of deanol on reducing the symptoms of tardive dyskinesia is not great in the doses used in this study.

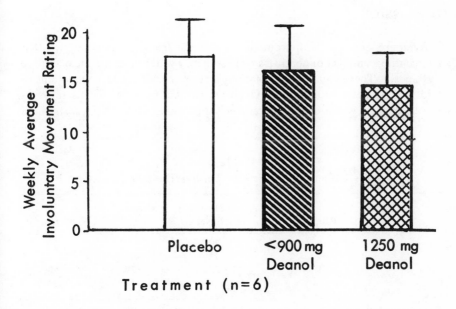

Figure 2.   Mean involuntary movement scores following deanol administration compared with placebo. No significant diminution in involuntary movements occurred in the 6 patients tested when given either a 900 mg or a 1250 mg daily dose for at least a week.

Choline

In a preliminary nonblind trial of oral choline in 4 patients with moderate to severe tardive dyskinesia symptoms, the data indicate some therapeutic effect. Two of the 4 patients showed a trend toward improvement at doses higher than 6g a day (Table 2). Unfortunately, the drug had to be stopped in 2 other patients prior to an adequate dose, due to the onset of depressive symptomatology. In neither of these patients was any substantial improvement noted. Patient B.R. was agitated by the depression, and this could have exacerbated his tardive dyskinesia movements. We have previously suggested (24) that drugs which increase central acetylcholine may cause depression. That this depression was a side effect of oral choline treatment is supported by the observations that the depression remitted with drug withdrawal, and that atropine reduced the depressive symptoms while the patient was on choline. Depression could have been a predicted side effect of cholinomimetic treatment drug, based on the cholinergic-adrenergic balance theory of depression (25). This mood change with choline also tends to confirm the central site of action of choline in humans. Our preliminary findings of therapeutic benefit with choline in tardive dyskinesia supports data found in other controlled series of patients (12,13).

DISCUSSION

Evidence emerges both from this work and from previous studies that augmenting central cholinergic transmission may well be therapeutic in tardive dyskinesia. These data indicate that physostigmine does reduce symptoms of tardive dyskinesia in an action which we suspect goes beyond its sedating effect, because some of the movement-suppressant effect of physostigmine

Table 2
Effects of Choline on Tardive Dyskinesia

| Patient | Choline Daily Dose (gms) | | |
	< 6 gm.	6–12g	12–18g
1	+40% *	–	–
2	+ 12%	+ 40%	–
3	– 25%	– 37%	– 55%
4	+ 7%	– 11%	– 42%

Each % represents percent increase (+) or decrease (–) in TD symptoms (compared to predrug or placebo baseline) with indicated dosage of choline.
*Medication discontinued at this dose because of depression

persists with arousal, whereas this does not occur with the active control, Brevital. The preliminary positive findings with choline tend to further support the position that cholinergic agents are therapeutically effective in TD. These preliminary observations, although insufficient by themselves, are consistent with those reported in the larger controlled studies. Our clinical observation of the severe depression in 2 patients warrants continued careful observation.

The results of deanol administration failed to confirm previous nonblind trials of the drug, which had suggested a treatment effect of deanol in tardive dyskinesia. Certain methodologic artifacts which invariably introduce limitations into the interpretation of results from uncontrolled trials of treatment regimens in tardive dyskinesia may have manifested themselves in the preliminary studies. Placebo effect, spontaneous remissions, activity state, and environmental changes can all alter the expression of dyskinetic movements. In addition, deanol's use as a pharmacologic probe is complicated by the fact that its action as an acetylcholine precursor remains controversial (20). While the results with deanol administration are largely negative, they may not be strong evidence against a cholinergic influence in tardive dyskinesia, because deanol may not be a pure or potent acetylcholine agonist. In summary, while deanol may be effective in treating isolated patients, our results do not confirm its general efficacy in tardive dyskinesia.

Normal regulation of extrapyramidal function depends upon a sensitive balance among the various striatal neurotransmitters, DA and acetylcholine being the two studied in this paper. The results presented here strengthen the previously postulated role of cholinergic transmission in diminishing the choreiform movements of tardive dyskinesia. Cholinomimetic agents may well become of therapeutic use when safe and practical, centrally active cholinergic drugs become available.

ACKNOWLEDGMENTS

1. Barbeau, A., Chase, T.N., Paulson, G.W. Biochemistry of Huntington's chorea. In *Advances in Neurology*, vol. 1., Barbeau, A., Chase, T.N., Paulson, G.W. (eds.). New York: Raven Press, pp. 473–516, 1973.
2. Bernheimer, H., Birkmayer, W., Hornykiewica, Q., Jellinger, K., Seitelberger, E. Brain dopamine and the syndromes of Parkinson and Huntington. *J. Neurol. Sci., 20*:415–455, 1973.
3. Van Woert, M.H., Ambani, L., Bowers, M.B. Levodopa and cholinergic hypersensitivity in Parkinson's disease. *Neurology*, May Suppl., pp. 86–93, 1972.
4. Javoy, E., Agid, Y., Bouvet, D., Glowinski, J. Changes in neostriatal DA metabolism after carbachol or atropine microinjections into the substantia nigra. *Brain Res., 68*:253–260, 1974.
5. Anden, N.E., Bedard, P. Influences of cholinergic mechanisms on the function and turnover of brain dopamine. *J. Pharm. Pharmacol., 23*:460–462, 1971.

6. Nose, T., Takemoto, H. Effect of oxotremorine on homovanillic acid concentration in the striatum of the rat. *Eur. J. Pharmacol., 25*:51–55, 1974.
7. Rubovits, R., Klawan, H.L. Implications of amphetamine-induced stereotyped behavior as a model for tardive dyskinesia. *Arch. Gen. Psychiatry, 27*:502–507, 1972.
8. Gerlach, J., Reisby, N., Randrup, A. Dopaminergic hypersensitivity and cholinergic hypofunction in the pathophysiology of tardive dyskinesia. *Psychopharmacologia, 34*:21–25, 1974.
9. Fann, W.E., Lake, C.R., Gerber, C.J., McKenzie, G.M. Cholinergic suppression of tardive dyskinesia. *Psychopharmacologia, 37*:101–107, 1974.
10. Klawans, H.L., Rubovits, R. Effect of cholinergic and anticholinergic agents on tardive dyskinesia. *J. Neurol. Neurol. Neurosurg. Psychiatry, 27*:941–947, 1974.
11. Davis, K.L., Berger, P.A., Hollister, L.E. Choline for tardive dyskinesia (letter to ed.) *En. Engl. J. Med., 293*:152, 1975.
12. Davis, K.L. Choline chloride in the treatment of Huntington's disease and tardive dyskinesia: a preliminary report. *Psychopharmacol. Bull. 13 (3)*:37–38, 1977.
13. Growdon, J.H., Hirsch, M.J., Wurtman, R.J., Wiener, W. Oral choline administration to patient with tardive dyskinesia. *N. Engl. J. Med., 297*:524–527, 1977.
14. Crane, G.E. Deanol for tardive dyskinesia (ltr to ed.), *N. Engl. J. Med., 292*:292–296, 1975.
15. Curran, D.J., Nagaswami, S., Mohan, K.J. Treatment of phenothiazine induced bulbar persistent dyskinesia with deanol acetamidobenzate. *Dis. Nerv. Syst., 36*:71–73, 1975.
16. DeSilva, L., Huang, C.Y. Deanol in tardive dyskinesia. *Br. Med. J., 3*:466, 1975.
17. Escobar, J.I., Kemp, K.E. Dimethylaminoethanol for tardive dyskinesia (letter to ed.), *N. Engl. J. Med., 292*:317–318, 1975.
18. Fann, W.E., Sullivan, J.L., Miller, R.D., McKenzie, G.M. Deanol in tardive dyskinesia: a preliminary report. *Psychopharmacologia, 42*:135–137, 1975.
19. Laterre, E.C., Fortemps, E. Deanol in spontaneous and induced dyskinesias (letter to ed.), *Lancet, 1*:1301, 1975.
20. Pepu, G., Freedman, D.X., Giarman, W.J. Biochemical and pharmacologic studies of dimethylaminoethanol (deanol). *J. Pharmacol. Exp. Ther., 129*:291–295, 1960.
21. Cohen, E., Wurtman, R. Brain acetylcholine: increase after systemic choline administration. *Life Sci., 16*:1095–1102, 1975.
22. Aquilonius, S.M., Eckernas, S.A. Cortical and striatal *in vivo* uptake and metabolism of plasma choline in the rat: effects of haloperidol and apomorphine. *Acta. Pharmacol. Toxicol. (Kbh), 39*:129–140, 1976.
23. Aquiloniua, S.M., Erikernas, S.A. Plasma concentrations of free choline in patients with Huntington's chorea on high doses of choline chloride. *N. Engl. J. Med., 173*:1105–1105, 1975.
24. Tamminga, C., Smith, R.C., Chang, S., Haraszti, J.S., Davis, J.M. Depression associated with oral choline (letter to ed). *Lancet, 2*:905, 1976.
25. Davis, J.M., Janowsky, D. Cholinergic and adrenergic balance in mania and schizophrenia. In *Neurotransmitter Balances Regulating Behavior*, Domino, E.E., Davis, J.M. (eds.). Ann Arbor: Edward Brothers, p. 135, 1976.

39

Drug Trials in Persistent Dyskinesia

JONATHAN O. COLE
GEORGE GARDOS
DANIEL TARSY
ROBERT P. GRANACHER
CELIA SNIFFIN
BESSEL VANDERKOLK
and ISABELLE TRENHOLM

Over the past 6 years, a series of drug studies in persistent dyskinesia has been carried out by our group at a variety of sites. The work was originally done at Boston State Hospital, but has extended itself into McLean Hospital, the Boston Veterans Administration Hospital, and for a period, a Kentucky state hospital.

Our work began with studies of deanol and papaverine, and has progressed into pilot work with clozapine, cyproheptadine, clonazepam, and dopamine agonists (Sinemet and apomorphine). For all our studies, we have used the Simpson Dyskinesia Rating Scale (DRS) in one of its evolving versions (1) and NIMH-PRB Abnormal Involuntary Movement Scale (AIMS) (2). The DRS is a 33-item scale, which covers a variety of discrete movements (e.g., lipsmacking, bon-bon sign, axial hyperkinesia, foot stamping), each rated on scales of 0 to 4 or higher, depending on the version employed. Data from the DRS is usually analyzed using total scores for various body areas. The AIMS requires more global judgments of the severity of abnormal movements in 7 body areas: face, mouth, jaw, tongue, upper and lower extremities, trunk, and neck), as well as an overall global rating of severity.

PAPAVERINE

Stimulated by a report by Duvoisin (3) that papaverine interfered with the effects of L-dopa in Parkinson's disease and was a dopamine-blocking drug (4), we administered papaverine for 3 weeks in doses of 300 to 600 mg daily to 3 patients rated by both a blind and a nonblind rater. All 3 patients showed some decrease in their dyskinesia, and one also showed some improvement in ward behavior (5). We proceeded to a study of 9 inpatients, using two blind raters who rated all patients over a 3-month period during which patients received papaverine (Pavabid Plateau Caps), 300 mgs b.i.d. for 3 weeks (in 6 new patients) or 6 weeks (in the 3 patients involved in the earlier study). The raters did not know when any given patient was actually receiving papaverine. Overall, a 21.3% decrease in dyskinesia scores on the DRS was observed, but only 2 patients showed enough change to be judged clinically "improved" by the raters. Scores for oral-facial dyskinesia showed significant improvement on both the AIMS and the DRS, while lower extremity movements, specifically toe movements and stamping, showed an unexpected worsening. No side effects were observed. The patients involved in this study had a mean age of 55 and a mean duration of hospitalization of 29 years. During the study, 6 patients were on moderate doses of antipsychotic drugs, while 3 patients received no antipsychotics (6).

A third papaverine study was carried out with a blind crossover design (7). All patients received, randomly, either papaverine for 6 weeks followed by no medication for 6 weeks, or no medication for 6 weeks followed by papaverine for 6 weeks. Papaverine in a slow-release capsule form was used. Patients received 150 mg b.i.d. for the first week, then 300 mg b.i.d. for the next 5 weeks. Regular medication, usually an antipsychotic drug, was held constant for the 12-week study. Patients were rated every 2 weeks by trained raters blind to medication, using the DRS and the AIMS.

At Boston State Hospital, 22 patients completed the study. They were generally older than the 9 patients in the prior study and had relatively severe dyskinesia (DRS total scores averaged 41.2). The 20 Eastern Kentucky State Hospital patients were somewhat younger and had mild dyskinesia (DRS total scores averaged 14.0). For this reason, data from the two studies were analyzed separately. Using analysis of covariance, neither sample showed clear sequence effects, but patients tended to improve more on papaverine when it was given in the first 6 weeks. Neither total scores nor area scores on either the AIMS or the DRS showed much in the way of significant drug effects. In the Boston and Kentucky samples, neck and trunk scores on the DRS showed significantly more improvement on drug, while the AIMS item "neck, shoulders, and hips" showed a trend in this direction. When the data from the first 6 weeks of the study were analyzed as a simple random assignment clinical trial, the Boston papaverine patients showed significantly more improvement than the no-drug group on the AIMS, with a trend ($p < .07$) on the DRS. The Kentucky group did not show this effect.

Four Boston patients had quantitative EEG recordings made, both on and off drug. They showed a significant increase in percent time alpha (8–13 Hz), and a significant decrease in percent time beta 1 (14–26 Hz). Four patients in the Boston sample showed parkinsonian side effects, as did 2 in the Kentucky sample (tremor in 4 patients and rigidity in 3).

Based on the above studies, it appears that papaverine has a modest effect on dyskinetic movements at 600 mgs per day, and shows enough parkinsonism to strengthen the idea that the drug is a dopamine blocker in man. The antidyskinetic effects shown could be helpful in occasional patients.

DEANOL

Ten Boston patients and 6 Kentucky patients completed a double-blind, placebo-controlled 10-week crossover study of deanol in doses up to 1500 mgs a day. The changes in both Simpson and AIMS were trivial in extent—only 3 patients showed any clear improvement on deanol greater than that occurring on placebo. The effects were not statistically significant. No significant changes in psychopathology, as rated on the Brief Psychiatric Rating Scale, were noted in patients completing the study. One McLean patient was dropped from the study because of worsening psychiatric status, and one patient was hospitalized medically for water intoxication; he had had a similar bout of water intoxication 3 years before the study was initiated.

This study conforms to the general conclusions reached by Casey in his recent review (8).

CYPROHEPTADINE

This antihistaminelike drug with reputed effects as an appetite stimulant had been reported by Goldman (9) to markedly reduce dyskinesia in 3 outpatients. On this basis, we assessed the drug in 5 underweight chronic patients with tardive dyskinesia at Boston State Hospital. These patients received 6 weeks of cyproheptadine treatment (4 mgs b.i.d.), with twice-weekly dyskinesia ratings for 14 weeks (4 weeks before and 4 weeks after the 6-week drug trial [10]). We failed to confirm Goldman's positive 3-patient study. Only 2 of our patients showed any improvement, and 1 of these continued to improve at the same rate after cyproheptadine therapy was stopped. The rabbit syndrome present in one of the patients, however, responded dramatically to cyproheptadine, suggesting an anticholinergic antiparkinson drug effect.

CLONAZEPAM

This benzodiazepine is currently marketed for use in epilepsy. It has been reported to favorably affect acute dyskinesias due to phenothiazines (11). A study of the drug in tardive dyskinesia (12) involving 18 patients yielded improvement in 11. However, the dose was rapidly raised to 4 mgs daily, and side effects of ataxia and confusion were observed in some quite elderly patients involved in the study. We have completed a small pilot open study of clonazepam in patients with tardive dyskinesia, beginning with 0.5 mg t.i.d. and increasing the dose by 1.5 mg a week. On this regimen, 6 patients have tolerated the drug well and have shown moderate decreases in dyskinesia scores. One patient who had been previously given clorazepate for his dyskinesia without response showed a remarkable amelioration of his movements on clonazepam.

Although these early results need to be followed up with a double-blind study (which we are now developing), the results are compatible with preliminary reports of decreased dyskinesia after treatment with diazepam (13,14) and clorazepate (15). In the case of these drugs, the problem of disentangling nonspecific sedative or antianxiety effects from a more specific inhibitory effect on dyskinesia possibly mediated through the activation of brain synapses involving GABA is particularly important (16).

CLOZAPINE

Clozapine is an unusual antipsychotic drug. Although chemically similar to loxapine (both being dibenzodiazepines), loxapine has typical neurological side effects, while clozapine does not. Clozapine does not produce catalepsy in animals, and it only weakly antagonizes stereotyped behavior produced by amphetamine or apomorphine, tests on which all other antipsychotics have clear and potent effects (16). It has been studied relatively extensively in Europe and is on the market in many countries. It appears to be an effective antipsychotic free of neurological side effects (18,19).

Work with this drug was initiated at McLean Hospital two years ago on a few pilot patients, and was continued as part of a Sandoz-sponsored study at both McLean and Boston State hospitals from the summer of 1976 until Sandoz, alarmed by reports of agranulocytosis, temporarily suspended the study in May 1977. Subsequently, several new patients had been studied at McLean Hospital in the last few months until Sandoz again required us to halt the admission of new patients to the study in February 1978 because of additional reports of agranulocytosis.

Twenty-seven patients with tardive dyskinesia have now been treated with clozapine. In general, the drug has had a mild to moderate effect in reducing dyskinesia and has had a more positive effect on psychiatric symptomatology (see Table 1). No patient had an exacerbation of his dyskinesia. The best effects on dyskinesia occurred in the 12 patients who remained on the drug for more than 3 months. Of these, 2 showed a complete remission, 1 a marked improvement, and the remainder clear but lesser degrees of improvement, while 1 patient showed no change. Eight patients were taken off the drug when Sandoz discontinued their study of clozapine in May of 1977, and 2 other patients were lost to the study by transfer to a distant hospital and by elopement. Overall results might have been better if these patients had continued on the drug.

Only 3 patients worsened on the drug psychiatrically. One of these appeared to have developed a toxic confusional state; she was confused and disorganized, but cleared very rapidly when the drug was stopped. Six other patients were taken off the drug because of treatment emergent symptoms. One had 2 grand mal seizures; 1 developed a leukopenia of 3,000, possibly due to a viral upper respiratory infection; 2 developed an unusual hypertension with elevated diastolic, but not systolic, pressure; 1 developed leukocytosis; 1 developed persistent asymptomatic tachycardia of 140 beats per minute. Five patients, on the other hand, showed no side effects at all.

The range of side effects shown by the patients is presented in Table 2. As can be seen, no extrapyramidal side effects of the sort seen with conventional neuroleptics occurred. Two patients briefly showed a peculiar slurred speech with difficulty in moving their tongues and jaws. These body parts felt stiff and clumsy, and the patients also felt weak. These symptoms came on abruptly when the dose was raised and remitted rapidly when the dose was slightly lowered. Two other patients noted a restless feeling in their legs just before going to sleep at night for a few nights, but showed no other signs of akathisia.

Table 1

Effects of Clozapine

Improvement in Psychiatric Status (Global Ratings)

Improvement

Change in Dyskinesia		Worse	Unchanged	Minimal	Mild	Moderate	Marked	TOTAL
	Worse							0
	Unchanged	2	2	1			1	6
	Minimal	1	2	1	5	1	2	12
Improvement	Mild				2	2	1	5
	Moderate					2		2
	Marked						2	2
Total		3	4	2	7	5	6	27

Table 2
Side Effects of Clozapine

	# Pts.		# Pts.
Hypersalivation	9	Protuberant abdomen	2
Tachycardia	6	Convulsion	1
Drowsiness	5	Leucopenia	1
Hypotension (postural)	5	Leucocytosis	1
Hypertension	4	Toxic confusion	1
Constipation	3	Blurred vision	1
Slurred speech	2	Nausea & vomiting	1
Dizziness	2	Minor EKG changes	1
Weakness	2	Weight gain	1

Two patients showed a curious protuberance of the abdomen not due to pregnancy or to discernible organic causes. More common troublesome side effects included hypersalivation, leading to wet pillows at night, drowsiness, tachycardia, and postural hypotension.

Eleven patients clearly were more improved psychiatrically on clozapine than they had been on any of several prior antipsychotics. In general, the 8 more chronic patients treated at Boston State Hospital did somewhat less well than the 19 patients at McLean. All the McLean patients but 3 had dyskinesia, probably of less than 6 months' duration, though 10 had been chronically or recurrently psychotic for more than 2 years.

It should also be noted that we raised the dose of clozapine gradually, looking primarily for improvement in psychiatric status rather than attempting to suppress dyskinesia. Most patients mainly received 100–300 mgs a day, though 6 were stabilized in doses over 500 mgs a day. Shopsin et al. (20), who report more favorable effects on dyskinesia, went rapidly to quite high dosages, looking specifically for suppression of dyskinesia.

Our current evaluation of clozapine is that it is a valuable and unique drug, an effective antipsychotic agent essentially free of neurological side effects. It is certainly possessed of other undesirable side effects, however, over and above its risk of agranulocytosis. In dyskinetic patients who required maintenance antipsychotic drug therapy, and who tolerate it well and can have their blood counts regularly monitored, it has a real and valuable place. Clozapine shows every evidence of being the chloramphenicol of psychopharmacology; it has clear risks and real benefits.

DOPAMINE AGONISTS

Recently there has been interest in the possibility that DA agonists may exert "paradoxical" effects, whereby behavioral and motor syndromes, including tardive dyskinesia, normally produced or exacerbated by such agents may actually be suppressed when the drugs are administered in low doses. Although virtually all of the experimental evidence has been accumulated in animal studies, there are indications that similar phenomena may occur in human clinical conditions as well (21).

Since most of the beneficial effects of DA agonists in choreiform syndromes have been described with apomorphine (22–25), it is possible that this drug possesses special and unique properties as a mixed agonist-antagonist at postsynaptic receptors which are not shared by other DA agonists. Although there is no clear evidence for a biphasic effect, one trial of bromocryptine in Huntington's disease at low and high doses produced an increase in chorea at high doses, but no discernible effect at low doses (26), while a second study in Huntington's disease, restricted to low-dose bromocryptine, found improvement (27). Trials of L-dopa in tardive dyskinesia have produced only worsening, but these studies were apparently carried out with high-dose treatment only (28,29). To date, no study has been reported in man in which a biphasic effect on motor behavior has been produced like that observed in animal models of hyperkinetic behavior.

On the basis of the above, we have recently administered Sinemet (a preparation including both L-dopa and carbidopa, a peripheral decarboxylase inhibitor) in separate dosages containing 50, 100, or 250 mgs of L-dopa. These doses are roughly equivalent to 200, 400, and 1,000 mgs of L-dopa given alone. The combination drug was chosen to avoid peripheral side effects. To date, 9 patients have received these doses with the drug administrations separated from each other by at least 2 days. Before and after drug administration, dyskinetic movements were rated at half-hourly intervals using the AIMS and the DRS.

Two patients showed no change in their dyskinesia at any dose, while 4 patients showed a decrease in dyskinesia at one or both of the lower dosages, and 5 patients showed increases in dyskinesia at the 250 mg dose. One additional patient with dyskinesia of very recent onset (about 8 weeks) showed an increase in dyskinesia on the 50 mg dose and was not exposed to higher dosages. All patients had been off antipsychotic medication for at least 2 weeks when the study was initiated. Two of the patients who showed improvement on the lower Sinemet doses were placed on this dose t.i.d. for 1 week. In both patients, the beneficial effect of Sinemet had disappeared by the end of the week. Seven patients also received apomorphine, 1–1.5 mg s.c. One patient showed a marked increase and another patient showed a decrease in dyskinesia; the others showed no apparent changes. Three of the patients also received fusaric acid, a dopamine-beta-hydroxylase inhibitor, 2 hours prior to receiving Sinemet. These combined fusaric-acid–Sinemet administrations followed sessions when that dose of Sinemet was given alone.* Fusaric acid abolished the decrease in score by the lower doses of Sinemet. One patient developed syncope after receiving fusaric acid and the 100 mg Sinemet dose. This pilot study supports the general proposition that low doses of a dopamine agonist can ameliorate dyskinesia, while higher dosages aggravate it. It also suggests that this effect of the low-dose dopamine agonist used in this study is not useful as a longer term therapy.

SUMMARY

We have now looked at a variety of drugs in the treatment of tardive dyskinesia. Of these, cyproheptadine seems of little value, even in uncontrolled study. Controlled studies of deanol and papaverine suggest that papaverine is a bit more effective, probably because of its mild dopamine-blocking activity. Clonazepam had some apparent efficacy in a small open trial. Clozapine appears to be an active antipsychotic drug without neurological side effects. At moderate dosages, its effect on tardive dyskinesia is modest at best, but it may facilitate the gradual fading of dyskinesias. We have reasonable evidence that in single dose trials, low doses of L-dopa reduce dyskinesia in some patients, while higher doses aggravate it in the same patients.

REFERENCES

1. Simpson, G.M., Zoubok, B., Lee, H.J. An early clinical toxicity trial of EX 11-582A in chronic schizophrenia. *Curr. Ther. Res., 19*:87–93, 1976.
2. Abnormal Involuntary Movement Scale. HEW, Alcohol Drug Abuse and Mental Health Administration, Washington, D.C., 1974.
3. Duvoisin, R.C. Antagonism of levodopa by papaverine. *JAMA, 231*:845, 1975.
4. Gonzalez-Vegas, J.A. Antagonism of dopamine-mediated inhibition in the nigrostriatal pathway: a mode of action of some catatonia-inducing drugs. *Brain Res., 80*:219, 1974.
5. Gardos, G., Cole, J.O. Papaverine for tardive dyskinesia? *N. Engl. J. Med. 292*:1355, 1975.
6. Gardos, G., Cole, J.O., Sniffin, C. An evaluation of papaverine in tardive dyskinesia. *J. Clin. Pharmacol., 16*:304–310, 1976.
7. Gardos, G., Granacher, R.P., Cole, J.O., Sniffin, C. The effects of papaverine in tardive dyskinesia. (In preparation.)
8. Casey, D.E. Deanol in the management of involuntary movement disorders: a review. *Dis. Nerv. Syst., 38*:12 (Sect. 2) 7–15, 1977.
9. Goldman, D. Treatment of phenothiazine-induced dyskinesia. *Psychopharmacology, 47*:271–272, 1976.

---

*The fusaric acid portion of the study was conducted with the collaboration of Ernest Hartmann, M.D., Sleep and Dream Laboratory, Boston State Hospital.

COLE, GARDOS, TARSY, GRANACHER, SNIFFIN, KOLK AND TRENHOLM   427

10. Gardos, G., Cole, J.O. Pilot study of cyproheptadine (Periactin) in tardive dyskinesia. *Psychopharmacol. Bull.* (In press).
11. O'Flanagan, P.M. Clonazepam in the treatment of drug-induced dyskinesia. *Br. Med. J.*, *1*:269–270, 1975.
12. Sedman, G. Clonazepam in the treatment of tardive oral dyskinesia. *Br. Med. J.*, *2*:583, 1976.
13. Singh, M.M. Diazepam in the treatment of tardive dyskinesia. *Int. Pharmacopsychiatry*, *11*:232–234, 1976.
14. Jus, K., Jus, A., Gautier, J. Studies on the action of certain pharmacological agents on tardive dyskinesia and on the rabbit syndrome. *Int. J. Clin. Pharmacol. Biopharm.*, *9*:138–145, 1974.
15. Itil, T.M., Unverdi, C., Mehta, D. Clorazepate dipotassium in tardive dyskinesia. *Am. J. Psychiatry*, *131*:1291, 1974.
16. Costa, E., Guidotti, A., Mao, C.C. Evidence for involvement of GABA in the action of benzodiazepines: studies on rat cerebellum. *Adv. Biochem. Psychopharmacol.*, *14*:113–130, 1975.
17. Stille, G., Lauener, H., Eichenberger, E. The pharmacology of 8-chloro-11-(4'-methyl)-piperazino-5-dibenzo (b,e) (1,4) diazepin (clozapine), *Il Farmaco*, 26:603–625, 1971.
18. Simpson, G., Varga, E. Clozapine—a new antipsychotic agent. *Curr. Ther. Res.*, *16*:679–686, 1974.
19. Matz, E., Rick, W., Oh, D., Thompson, H., Gershon, S. Clozapine—a potential antipsychotic agent without extrapyramidal manifestations. *Curr. Ther. Res.*, *16*:687–695, 1974.
20. Shopsin, B., Klein, H., Aaronson, M., Gershon, S., Collora, M. A controlled double-blind comparison between clozapine, chlorpromazine and placebo in acute newly hospitalized schizophrenic patients. (In press.)
21. Carlsson, A. Monoaminergic mechanisms in basal ganglia disease. In *The Basal Ganglia*, M. Yahr (ed.). New York: Raven Press, pp. 181–189, 1976.
22. Düby, S.E., Cotzias, G.C., Papavasiliou, P.S. Injected apomorphine and orally administered levodopa in parkinsonism. *Arch. Neurol.*, *24*:474–480, 1972.
23. Tolosa, E.S., Sparber, S.B. Apomorphine in Huntington's chorea: clinical observations and theoretical considerations. *Life Sci.*, *15*:1371–1380, 1974.
24. Smith, R.C., Tamminga, C., Haraszti, J. Effects of dopamine agonists in tardive dyskinesia. *Am. J. Psychiatry*, *134*:763–768, 1977.
25. Carroll, B.J., Curtis, G.C., Kokmen, E. Paradoxical response to dopamine agonists in tardive dyskinesia. *Am. J. Psychiatry*, *134*:785–789, 1977.
26. Karzinel, R., Hunt, R.D., Calne, D.B. Bromocriptine in Huntington's chorea. *Arch. Neurol.*, *33*:517–518, 1976.
27. Frattola, L., Albizzati, M.G., Sparso, P.F., Trabucci, M. Treatment of Huntington's chorea with bromocryptine. *Acta Neurol. Scand.*, *56*:37–45, 1977.
28. Chase, T.N. Drug-induced extrapyramidal disorders. *Res. Publ. Assoc. Nerv. Ment. Dis.*, *50*:448–471, 1972.
29. Gerlach, J., Reisby, N., Randrup, A. Dopaminergic hypersensitivity and cholinergic hypofunction in the pathophysiology of tardive dyskinesia. *Psychopharmacologia*, *34*:21–35, 1974.

Tardive Dyskinesia: Controlled Studies of Several Therapeutic Agents

TARDIVE DYSKINESIA: THEORETICAL BASIS FOR THERAPEUTIC APPROACH

HISTORICAL BACKGROUND

There was a relatively early recognition and documentation of transient and reversible drug-induced extrapyramidal side effects such as parkinsonism, dystonia, and akathesia, soon after the introduction of phenothiazines in the early 1950's. However, tardive dyskinesia received attention much later in the literature and clinical studies. Sigwald and associates' reports of "Les Accidents Neurologiques des medications neuroleptiques" in 1959 (1) and "Accidents Neurologiques Provoqués par les Drogues Neuroleptiques" in 1960 (2) have often been considered to be the first literature regarding the description of tardive dyskinesia. However, Schönecker (3) described a bucco-lingual syndrome attributed to the use of phenothiazines in 1957, approximately two years before Sigwald's report. Other pioneers in the early sixties who reported on tardive dyskinesia include Faurbye and associates of Denmark (4,5), Degkwitz of Germany (6,7), and Hunter of England (8,9). In the United States, Crane (10,11,12) was one of the early investigators calling attention to this matter in the late sixties. Intriguingly enough, Kline from the United States also published "On the Rarity of 'Irreversible' Oral Dyskinesia Following Phenothiazines" in 1968. He reviewed the world literature on the occurrence of oral dyskinesia persisting for one month or longer after withdrawal of phenothiazines and found that 60 of the 83 reported cases had evidence of prior brain damage. "Since there are less than two dozen reported cases in non-brain damaged patients among 100 million estimated users (of neuroleptic drugs)," he concluded that the syndrome is interesting, but not of great clinical significance (13).

Interest and Importance as Reflected by the Increased Literature

In a review of world literature on tardive dyskinesia published between 1959 and 1968, Crane (12) and Kline (13) cited a total of 26 and 19 studies respectively, roughly two papers per year. However, more than 90% of the cases of dyskinesia were reported after 1964 (12). The search of the literature in relation to tardive dyskinesia in the cumulative Index Medicus and computerized title search in the library (MEDline) revealed a rather striking increase in the number of reports in the last twelve years (see Fig. 1). With some prorated figures in 1976 and 1977, there are a total of 350 articles since 1969 as compared to less than 26 existing prior to 1968. Obviously, with a higher prevalence this drug-induced neurological syndrome has been widely recognized and has not only aroused interest in clinical and research fields, but has also become a social and legal concern.

Various Nomenclature

Despite describing almost identical symptomatologies, the terminology used to describe tardive dyskinesia varies in the literature, depending on the time and mode of onset, duration of medication, course, and outcome. These descriptions include terminal extrapyramidal hyperkinesia (7), irreversible dyskinesia (5), irreversible syndrome of abnormal movements (9), and persistent dyskinesia (14). The most popular term, *tardive dyskinesia*, was first used by Crane (11,15), because of the late occurrence of such a neurological syndrome after long-term neuroleptic treatment. However, with the recent reports that many patients can manifest such a syndrome after only a few months on drug treatment, the term *tardive* may not be relevant. Furthermore, some patients manifest dyskinetic symptoms only at the time when the drug is discontinued; thus a new term *withdrawal dyskinesia* (16) was added to the already complicated terminologies. With close clinical follow-up, some persistent dyskinetic symptoms, once considered to be irreversible, eventually disappear in the course of months or years. Therefore, "irreversible dyskinesia" may inadvertently include some short-lived syndromes. Whether the syndromes described by these different terminologies all share the same pathoetiology or not remains to be seen. The term *persistent dyskinesia* seems

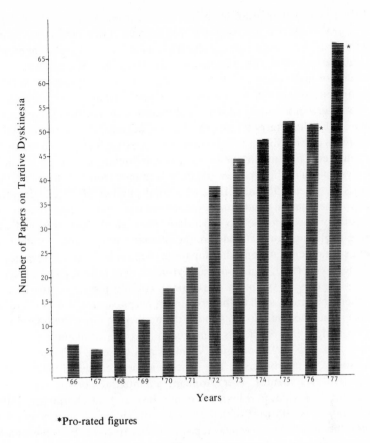

Years

*Pro-rated figures

Figure 1

to be the most adequate terminology since (1) it allows reversible or irreversible outcome, (2) it gives the connotation of a relatively long-term syndrome, and (3) it is not bound by the time of onset as are *withdrawal* and *tardive*. However, for the subtype analysis of the syndrome, some descriptive terms such as *tardive, withdrawal,* or *reversible* may be useful for subclassification and research purposes.

THEORETICAL BASIS FOR THERAPEUTIC APPROACH

Although the number of reports in the literature regarding persistent dyskinesia has increased dramatically as shown in Figure 1, most of the literature in the early era was mainly focused on case reports, descriptions of symptomatology, and demography of the patients. Prevalence studies and postulation on the possible pathoetiology began to appear more frequently in the late 1960's. The therapeutic approach to this syndrome at that period was more or less empirical and anecdotal and hardly based on systematic neuropharmacological concepts at the synapse site. In 1972, Drs. Kazamatsuri, Cole, and this author made an intensive review of therapeutic approaches to tardive dyskinesia, citing more than a hundred references from the previous decade (17). We reviewed a variety of drug and treatment modalities reported to be effective in the short-term treatment of this syndrome. No definite effective treatment was clearly shown to alleviate or reduce dyskinetic symptomatology over a long-term period. In our review, it was found that the prevalence of tardive dyskinesia in the inpatient population ranged from 0.5%, according to 25 reports between 1964 and 1971 of a total number of 27,823 inpatients surveyed. Therapeutic modalities, in our review, were divided into three major categories in order to postulate pharmacological rationale: (1) dopamine-depleting drugs, (2) dopamine-blocking drugs, and (3) other miscellaneous treatment. Among the dopamine-depleting drugs, reserpine, tetrabenazine, oxypertine, and alpha-methyl-dopa were reported to be effective to various degrees in symptom alleviation. Among the dopamine-blocking drugs, phenothiazines, such as thiopropazate, perphenazine, thioproperazine, and chlorpromazine, were used. Among the butyrophenones, haloperidol was the major representative of this family and was tried not only for tardive dyskinesia but also for Huntington's chorea and Gille de la Tourette's syndrome, mostly by neurologists. The miscellaneous treatments include MAO inhibitor (isocarboxazide), L-tryptophan, amantadine, barbiturates, diazepam, chlordiazepoxide, pyridoxine (vitamin B6), and anticholinergic antiparkinson drugs. It is noteworthy that even stereotaxic neurosurgery and dental prosthetic therapy were sometimes reported to be effective. However, most of the studies in the above three major categories were based on a relatively small number of cases, sometimes one or two, and were rarely controlled studies. We concluded that as long as psychiatrists must administer neuroleptic drugs to psychotic patients for many years, this syndrome would pose a continuing problem. It was then clear that further search for the pathoetiology of the syndrome and the corresponding rational treatment were vitally necessary, as was investigation of ways of preventing this distressing iatrogenic complication. The need for standardized diagnostic criteria as well as objective evaluation methods was also evident.

In the early 1970s, we decided to carry out a series of systematic controlled studies based on the hypothesis that tardive dyskinesia was related to hypersensitivity or overactivity of dopamine receptor sites, and therefore could manipulate its symptoms with various chemical agents which would effect activities of neurotransmitters in relation to the dopaminergic receptor activities. The idea was most stimulating to us, because around that time idiopathic Parkinson syndrome began to be treated with L-dopa, a precursor of dopamine, as a result of new knowledge of synaptology and neuropharmacology, which clearly illustrated the relationship between involuntary movement and catecholamine. Our hypothesis was derived from the following observation then available to us: (a) Pathologically, morphological changes in substantia nigra in combination with the midbrain and brain stem were noticed in the majority of the brains of patients who had persistent oral dyskinesia at the time of death (18). These areas have a high concentration of catecholamines, particularly dopamine. (b) Biochemically, excessive administration of L-dopa in the treatment of parkinsonian patients could result in the production of involuntary movements similar to tardive dyskinesia (19,20,21). Since L-dopa is a precursor of dopamine, one can reasonably speculate about the relationship between dyskinesia and the increased activity of catecholamines. (c) Clinically, haloperidol, a strong catecholamine-receptor blocker, was reported to be effective in controlling the involuntary movements manifested in Huntington's chorea (22) and Gilles de la Tourette's syndrome (23). The similarity between the involuntary movements of these syndromes and tardive dyskinesia, and the clinical efficacy of haloperidol, presumably through dopamine-receptor blocking action, further suggested that hyperactivity or hypersensitivity of the dopamine receptor could play an important role in the pathophysiology of tardive dyskinesia.

Our hypothesis was further supported by the reports of Klawans et al. (24,25) and Carlsson (26). They postulated that prolonged blocking of the dopaminergic receptors in the course of antipsychotic therapy might finally produce "chemical denervation" of the dopaminergic receptors. It would be conceivable that after such prolonged denervation, these receptors might develop hypersensitivity to local dopamine with the consequent appearance of dyskinetic movements. Prange et al. (27) also developed the hypothesis that an amine imbalance in the basal ganglia might be present in extrapyramidal motor disorders. He proposed that a preponderance of indolamines (i.e., serotonin and related compounds) in the basal ganglia caused hypertonicity and hypokinesia, while preponderance of catecholamines (i.e., dopamine and related compounds) caused dyskinesia and hypotonicity. He hypothesized that in tardive dyskinesia excessive synthesis of catecholamines overrides the phenothiazine blockade of the receptors on which they act. Prange's hypothesis was similar to ours in terms of hyperactivity of catecholamine, yet he introduced another important concept of balance theory between neurotransmitters.

CLINICAL EFFICACY OF A DOPAMINE-DEPLETING AGENT, TETRABENAZINE (28)

Tetrabenazine was selected as the first drug to study in the treatment of this condition for several reasons. Since tardive dyskinesia appears to be caused by phenothiazines and butyrophenones, drugs with a blocking action on dopaminergic synapses, leading to the hypersensitivity of dopamine receptors, a dopamine-depleting agent, such as tetrabenazine (Nitoman [Great Britain]) (29,30) might well be a more suitable treatment because it would decrease the amount of dopamine activity at the already hypersensitized dopamine-receptor sites. In selecting a dopamine-depleting agent for study, tetrabenazine was preferred to reserpine because of its shorter duration of action and its relative lack of hypotensive effects.

Subjects and Method

Subjects. All patients on the chronic wards of Boston State Hospital were screened for manifestations of clear oral dyskinesia. Thirty patients identified in this preliminary survey were then evaluated in detail by a neurologist to eliminate borderline cases not showing clear oral dyskinesia. All 24 patients identified in this manner were included in the study. There were 13 men and 11 women, ranging in age from 30 to 81 years, with an average age of 55. Their length of psychiatric hospitalization ranged from 10 to 52 years, with an average of 28.8 years. All patients were found to have received various neuroleptic medications for more than 10 years, although 10 were no longer on such medications at the beginning of this study. Their psychiatric diagnoses were as follows: chronic schizophrenia, 17; chronic brain syndrome, 4; mental deficiency, three. Seven of them had been exposed to extensive electroconvulsive therapy in the past, and two had been lobotomized. Eight of the 24 patients manifested the bucco-masticatory type of dyskinesia (one of them also showed choreiform movements of the limbs), and the other 16 showed the bucco-linguo-masticatory type (6 also showed chorea of the limbs).

Treatment Design. *Baseline Period.* All the patients remained for 4 weeks on the same treatment program that they had been on prior to selection for the study. During this period of time, 14 patients were receiving various neuroleptic drugs, while 10 were receiving no neuroleptic medication.

First Placebo Period. At 4 weeks, all patients were placed on placebo, and all the neuroleptic drugs were completely withdrawn for 4 weeks. Drugs other than the neuroleptics, such as anticonvulsant or antidiabetic agents, were continued as before.

Tetrabenazine Period. After the placebo period, the patients were placed on tetrabenazine for 6 weeks. For the first 2 weeks, 50 mg/day of tetrabenazine were given, then 100 mg/day for the next 2 weeks, and 100 or 150 mg/day, for the last 2 weeks. Only those patients whose oral dyskinesia did not respond to 100 mg/day of tetrabenazine received the dosage of 150 mg/day.

Second Placebo Period. The tetrabenazine period was followed by a final 2 weeks of placebo administration.

Medication was adjusted by a psychiatrist who was not involved in the rating of dyskinesia. When a patient required complete discontinuation of tetrabenazine because of side effects, or reinstitution of other antipsychotic medication because of exacerbation of psychotic symptoms, the patient was dropped from the study.

Evaluation. Clinical symptoms of oral dyskinesia were evaluated every week by a psychiatrist who was not involved in the treatment design. Every movement in the oral region, such as chewing, licking, puffing, pursing of the lips, and rolling or protrusion of tongue, was counted for 3 separate 1-minute periods. The mean frequency of dyskinetic movements per minute was calculated at every evaluation. The quantitative observations were carried out at the same time on the same weekday on the patient's ward. The patients were not aware of being watched. This method of measurement was used because it had been observed that the involuntary movements were easily influenced by various situational factors, including direct obvious scrutiny. Reversible extrapyramidal symptoms were also evaluated every 2 weeks using a modified "bilan extrapyramidal" (31). The Nurses' Observation Scale for Inpatient Evaluation, or the NOSIE-30 (32), was recorded biweekly by the ward nurses who were blind to the study design, to see if either placebo or tetrabenazine led to changes in ward behavior.

Results

Fourteen of the 24 patients were receiving phenothiazines or butyrophenones during the baseline period. Antiparkinson drugs (benztropine mesylate or trihexyphenidyl hydrochloride) had also been prescribed for 5 patients. Little change occurred in either oral movements or reversible extrapyramidal symptoms during the 4-week baseline period during which medication was not altered. During the initial 4-week placebo period, the frequency or oral movements did not change significantly, while the reversible extrapyramidal symptoms scores dropped from an average of 4.37 to 3.55 (p<.01, see Table 1).

At the end of the second week on tetrabenazine (50 mg/day), almost complete disappearance of dyskinesia was observed in 3 patients, and a marked reduction of oral dyskinetic movements to less than half of the baseline level was observed in 6 patients. At the end of the fourth week (100 mg/day), complete disappearance of oral dyskinesia was observed in 4 patients, and a marked reduction in 9 patients. The other 11 patients showed only slight decrease in dyskinesia or showed no changes. At the end of the sixth week of

Table 1

Comparison of Different Treatment Conditions on Oral Dyskinesia
and Reversible Extrapyramidal Symptoms (EPS) by Paired t-Test

Comparison	No. of Patients	Oral Dyskinesia Mean Frequency/Minute	t	Reversible EPS Mean Score*	t
Baseline period *vs.* 1st placebo period					
All patients	24	29.6 vs 30.0	0.2011	4.37 vs 3.55	2.8373†
Medicated patients	14	27.4 vs 27.3	0.0244	4.43 vs 3.64	2.7540†
Nonmedicated patients	10	32.9 vs 34.0	0.3663	3.80 vs 3.70	1.000
1st placebo period vs. tetrabenazine 2 weeks	24	30.0 vs 23.2	2.8702‡	3.55 vs 3.55	0.000
1st placebo period vs. tetrabenazine 4 weeks	23	30.0 vs 15.6	4.8019**	3.55 vs 3.43	0.000
1st placebo period vs. tetrabenazine 6 weeks	20	30.0 vs 10.8	6.4986**	3.55 vs 3.60	1.0451

*The score ranges from 1 (no symptoms) to 18 (most intensive symptomatology).

†p<.01   ‡p<.005   **p<.0005

the tetrabenazine period at the dosage of 100 to 150 mg/day, dyskinesia had disappeared in 8 patients (33.3%), was markedly reduced in 6 patients (25.0%), and slightly decreased or remained unchanged in 6 patients. (Nine patients received 150 mg/day because of unsatisfactory response to 100 mg/day.)

There was no sex difference in the response to tetrabenazine. Nine of 13 men, as well as 6 of the 11 women, showed a reduction in abnormal movements. Four patients were dropped from the study during the last 2 weeks of drug administration. Two were dropped because of severe malaise, probably attributable to the high dosage of tetrabenazine, and one was dropped because of a psychotic exacerbation. The other patient left the ward and was not available for evaluation. No patients showed a marked worsening of dyskinesia (Table 2). No other significant side effects attributable to tetrabenazine were observed during the study period.

Two weeks after discontinuance of tetrabenazine, oral dyskinetic movements had almost returned to the frequency observed prior to the institution of tetrabenazine. Comparison of each treatment period by paired t-test revealed that tetrabenazine administration was associated with a marked reduction in the frequency of oral dyskinetic movements. On the other hand, the level of reversible extrapyramidal symptoms did not show any significant change when

Table 2
Efficacy of Tetrabenazine on Tardive Dyskinesia
as Compared to Placebo*

Reduction Rate of Dyskinesia	Tetrabenazine		
	2 wk (50 mg/day)	4 wk (100 mg/day)	6 wk (100–150 mg/day)
100% disappearance	**3** (12.5%)	**4** (16.7%)	**8** (33.3%)
75%–99% reduction	**2** (8.3%)	**8** (33.3%)	**5** (20.8%)
50%–74% reduction	**4** (16.7%)	**1** (4.2%)	**1** (4.2%)
25%–49% reduction	**1** (4.2%)	**4** (16.7%)	**1** (4.2%)
0%–24% reduction or worsening	**14** (58.3%)	**7** (29.2%)	**5** (20.8%)
Dropout	**0** (0.0%)	**0** (0.0%)	**4** (16.7%)
Total	**24**	**24**	**24**

*Figures in bold indicate the number of patients.

tetrabenazine periods were compared with the earlier placebo period (Fig.2). In addition to the improvement in the frequency of oral dyskinesia, changes in intensity of the movements were observed in the majority of the patients. As the frequency of dyskinesia was decreased, it was often noted that facial grimacing became milder, the amplitude of chewing movements was much reduced, protrusion of tongue disappeared, and associated choreic movements of limbs became less prominent.

NOSIE scores did not show any significant changes during the study period. The total patient assets score averaged 55.0 in the first placebo period and 54.8 at the end of the fourth week on tetrabenazine. Although some slight changes in the patients' behavior occurred in the course of the study, no clear deterioration occurred during the placebo period, and no clear improvement occurred during tetrabenazine administration.

Comment

Tardive dyskinesia is a complicated syndrome, which consists of a variety of involuntary movements involving many areas of the body. In order to assess quantitatively changes in involuntary movements, rating scales for dyskinesia have been proposed (33,34). However, they seem unsatisfactory for the purpose of objective quantification, since the rating depends largely on the subjective impression of the examiner. In addition, the quantitative evaluation

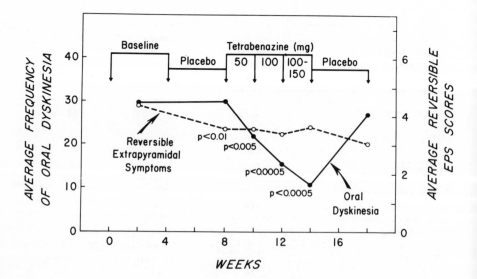

Figure 2. Changes of Oral Dyskinesia and Reversible Extrapyramidal Symptoms (EPS)

of dyskinesia is made difficult by the fact that involuntary movements are markedly affected by many factors (e.g., conversation, stress, drowsiness). For these reasons, only the frequency of oral dyskinetic movements was measured in the present study. The counting of dyskinetic movements of the limbs or trunk was not attempted because of the great variability in frequency and amplitude of these movements from minute to minute. The counting of oral movements is a rather simple and highly objective method for assessing the effects of drugs in tardive dyskinesia. Counts of oral movements made by the nonblind psychiatrist were almost identical with those made independently by the blind psychiatrist. Furthermore, the measured changes appeared clinically to parallel similar changes in the other manifestations of tardive dyskinesia.

As noted in the introduction, the relationship of tardive dyskinesia to dopaminergic activity in the basal ganglia is inferrable, but not proved. A recent post-mortem study by Christensen *et al.* (18) showed cell degeneration in the substantia nigra as well as in the gliosis in the brain stem and midbrain in most patients with tardive dyskinesia. This again suggests damage in the extrapyramidal system, but does not reveal anything about either dopamine levels or synaptic sensitivity to dopamine.

Since tetrabenazine is known to deplete brain dopamine (29,30), and has efficacy in the treatment of psychosis (35–39) and chorea (40–42), the findings of the present study are compatible with the hypothesis that reducing brain dopamine suppresses abnormal movements in tardive dyskinesia. The study also confirms smaller studies by Brandrup (43) and MacCullum (44), which yielded similar findings. Reports that reserpine has similar action on tardive dyskinesia (45) as does a presumed dopamine-blocking agent, thiopropazate (46), all support the hypothesis that overactive dopaminergic neurons are causal in tardive dyskinesia. Clinical observations that tardive dyskinesia may appear for the first time after neuroleptic drugs are stopped or reduced in dosage (6,47) are also relevant. It is interesting to note that, in the present study, tetrabenazine suppressed abnormal movements without producing any concomitant rise in extrapyramidal symptoms. The ability of phenothiazines to suppress dyskinetic movements has been attributed to the production of mild parkinsonian rigidity (6). Tetrabenazine appears to block the movements at a dose which causes no discernible increase in parkinsonian symptoms.

However, tetrabenazine and reserpine also reduce brain levels of other biogenic amines, so the evidence of this study cannot be considered as definitively establishing the role of dopamine in tardive dyskinesia. One could also argue that 6 patients in this study were unchanged after 2 weeks on 150 mg of tetrabenazine a day. Either some patients' abnormal movements are unaffected by dopamine depletion, or the maximum dosage of tetrabenazine used in the present study was too low for some patients to show an effect. One patient in Brandrup's study (43) required up to 300 mg of tetrabenazine a day. That patient had arteriosclerotic dementia, while the refractory patients in the present study were all chronic schizophrenics.

The present study only demonstrates a short-term effect of tetrabenazine in gradually rising dosage on the abnormal movements of tardive dyskinesia. The optimal dose for movement suppression in some patients caused undesirable fatigue in a few patients. Probably the effective dosage for any single patient would have to be clinically determined. On the basis of the present data it is impossible to determine whether or not prolonged tetrabenazine administration is an effective long-term approach to the treatment of tardive dyskinesia.

SHORT-TERM EFFICACY OF DOPAMINE-BLOCKING AGENTS HALOPERIDOL AND THIOPROPAZATE (48)

The first study of the dopamine-depleting agent tetrabenazine showed that this drug was effective in suppressing oral dyskinesia, a finding consistent with our hypothesis. Having demonstrated short-term efficacy in movement suppression with a dopamine-depleting agent, we then planned the study of two presumed dopamine-blocking agents, haloperidol (Haldol) and thio-propazate dihydrochloride (Dartal). Haloperidol has been alleged to be the most potent dopamine-blocking agent on a milligram per kilogram basis among the larger group of neuroleptics studies (49,50). Thiopropazate had been reported by Roxburch (46) to have specific antidyskinetic efficacy in the treatment of tardive dyskinesia.

Subjects and Method

Subjects. Twenty patients were selected for the study. They were all long-term inpatients at Boston State Hospital, manifesting typical bucco-linguo-masticatory oral dyskinesia associated with prolonged neuroleptic medication. All of them have been the subjects of a previous tetrabenazine study (28). Detailed neurological examinations of all patients were carried out by a neurologist prior to the tetrabenazine study to eliminate borderline cases showing questionable involuntary movements. These 20 patients included 11 males and 9 females, ranging in age from 44 to 70 years, with an average age of 56.9 years. The length of hospitalization of this group ranged from 14 to 52 years, with an average of 31.6 years. The diagnoses were as follows: chronic schizophrenia (15), chronic brain syndrome (3), and mental retardation (2).

Treatment Design. Before beginning this study, all patients had received tetrabenazine (50 to 150 mg daily) for 6 weeks in the earlier study (28), and had then been placed on placebo medication for 4 weeks. At the end of placebo period, all 20 patients were randomly divided into two groups, Group A and

Group B. Group A (11 patients) were then placed on haloperidol medication, while Group B (9 patients) received thiopropazate for 4 weeks, according to the dosage schedule shown in Table 3. Haloperidol was started at 2 mg/day, and thiopropazate at 10 mg/day. The dosage of each drug was doubled weekly for the next 2 weeks. At the end of the third week, if a patient failed to show any improvement of dyskinesia and was free of major side effects, the dosage was increased up to the maximum study dosage (haloperidol, 16 mg/day and thiopropazate 80 mg/day) in the fourth week. If a patient showed marked suppression of dyskinesia or any side effects, the dosage in the fourth week was held at the level of the third week. Actually, only 2 patients in Group A and 4 in Group B received the maximum dosage of either drug. After 4 weeks of the study drug period, the patients were placed on placebo medication for the final 4 weeks.

Evaluation. Quantitative evaluation of oral dyskinesia utilizing a frequency count of mouth movements (28) was carried out every two weeks by a psychiatrist during both placebo periods, and every week during active drug periods, using a modified ''bilan extrapyramidal'' (44). This consists of 6 items, each of which has 4 scores (0, absent, to 3, severe), and total score ranges from 0 (no symptoms) to 18 (the most severe symptomatology). The Nurses' Observation Scale for Inpatient Evaluation was completed by the ward nurses (who were blind to the study design) to assess changes of behavior of the patients in the ward during the study.

Results

During the 4-week predrug placebo period, all patients manifested very clear and constant oral dyskinesia. The average frequency of oral dyskinesia was 28.2 movements per minute in Group A and 32.3 in Group B. Reversible extrapyramidal symptom scores ranged from 1 to 6, with an average of 2.63 in

Table 3
Medication Schedule

Weeks	1–4	5	6	7	8	9–12
			Haloperidol			
Group A (n = 11)	Placebo	2 mg	4 mg	8 mg	8–16 mg*	Placebo
			Thiopropazate			
Group B (n = 9)	Placebo	10 mg	20 mg	40 mg	40–80 mg*	Placebo

*See text

Group A, while scores ranged from 1 to 5, with an average of 3.00 in Group B. In Group A, 2 of the initial 11 patients were dropped from the study. One male patient complained of general malaise while showing enhanced parkinsonism. A female patient obstinately refused to take medication by mouth. Nine patients completed a 4-week regimen of haloperidol. At the end of the second week (4 mg/day), oral dyskinesia had disappeared completely in 2 patients, and was markedly reduced to less than half of the predrug frequency in 3 other patients. The mean frequency of oral dyskinesia per minute was reduced to 44.8% of that of the predrug period, as shown in Table 4. At the end of the third week, oral dyskinesia had disappeared in 3 patients and was markedly reduced in 5 others. The final results obtained at the end of the fourth week were as follows: complete disappearance, 6; marked reduction, 1; almost no changes, 1; and slight worsening, 1. At the end of the fourth week, mean frequency of oral dyskinesia showed a slight increase over the level at the third week, although this increase was not statistically significant. Detailed scrutiny of data revealed that this increase was mainly attributable to reincrease in rates of oral movements in 2 of the 9 patients.

In Group B, no patient had to be dropped from the study. At the end of the first week, oral dyskinesia disappeared in 1 patient and was markedly reduced in 4 others. The average frequency of oral dyskinetic movements per minute was reduced from 32.3 to 15.3. The movement frequency then stayed at almost the same level for the following 2 weeks. A tendency toward a slight increase in the average frequency was also observed at the end of the fourth week, although it was not statistically significant. The final result at the end of the fourth week was as follows: complete disappearance, 2; markedly reduced, 2; slightly reduced, 4; and slight worsening, 1.

The changes in mean oral dyskinesia frequency are illustrated in Figures 3 and 4, together with the changes in reversible extrapyramidal symptom scores.

Table 4
Clinical Efficacy of Haloperidol and Thiopropazate on Tardive Dyskinesia as Compared to Placebo

Reduction Rate of Dyskinesia	Haloperidol		Thiopropazate	
	2 weeks (4 mg/day)	4 weeks (8–16 mg/(day)	2 weeks (20 mg/day)	4 weeks (40–80 mg/day)
100% disappearance	2	6	0	2
50%–99% reduction	3	1	4	2
0%–49% reduction	5	1	4	4
Worsening	1	1	1	1
Dropout	0	2	0	0
Total	11	11	9	9

After the fourth week, replacement of either haloperidol or thiopropazate by a matched placebo resulted in rapid reappearance of oral dyskinesia, the frequency rising essentially to the predrug level in all patients. In the haloperidol group, reversible extrapyramidal symptoms appeared to have reverse correlation with the oral movements ($r = -0.9436$, $p<.01$). However, this reciprocal relationship was less evident in thiopropazate group ($r = -0.4114$, $p<.2$). Comparison of different treatment conditions on oral dyskinesia and reversible extrapyramidal symptoms by paired t-test is shown in Table 5.

Nurses' ratings on the NOSIE were analyzed for pre-post differences on the 6 factors and on the total patient assets score. In the haloperidol group, ratings were available on 8 of the 9 patients who completed the 4-week study. Significant increases in the factor of social competence and personal neatness were observed at 4 weeks in the haloperidol group. The positive change in personal neatness was still present at 8 weeks after 4 weeks of placebo treatment. Changes in a similar direction were observed with thiopropazate, although these did not reach even the relaxed 10% level of statistical significance (Table 6).

Clinical responsiveness of the dyskinetic movements to haloperidol and thiopropazate was compared with the results observed in the tetrabenazine study. Most of those patients who had responded satisfactorily to tetrabenazine also responded well to haloperidol or thiopropazate, although there were a few patients who showed a different type of clinical response. Five refractory patients responded to neither the dopamine-depleting drug nor to a dopamine-blocking drug (Table 7).

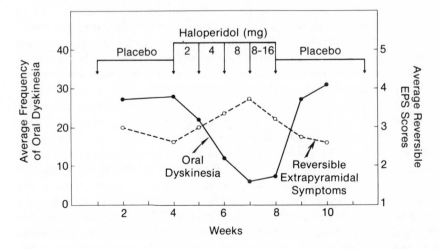

Figure 3. Changes of Oral Dyskinesia and Reversible Extrapyramidal Symptoms (EPS) with Haloperidol

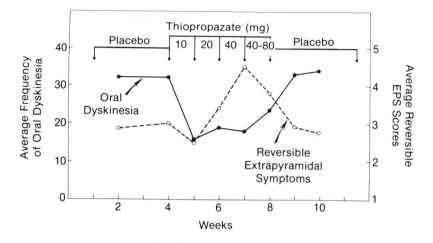

Figure 4. Changes of Oral Dyskinesia and Reversible Extrapyramidal Symptoms (EPS) with Thiopropazate

Comment

The results reported above show a clear effect of each of two antipsychotic drugs in the suppression of oral movements associated with tardive dykinesia. Haloperidol generally had a more striking effect upon these movements than did thiopropazate. Both drugs also caused a significant increase in reversible extrapyramidal symptoms. However, except for one patient receiving haloperidol, these effects were not intense enough to warrant the use of antiparkinsonian medication or the withdrawal of the patient from the study.

Since both haloperidol and thiopropazate are presumed to act by a blocking action at dopaminergic synapsis (51,52), and since haloperidol in animal studies has shown to be especially potent in blocking dopaminergic synapsis (49,50), the results of this small study are quite compatible with the hypothesis that the symptoms of tardive dyskinesia are caused by overstimulation of dopaminergic synapsis. Since we had obtained similar findings with the dopamine-depleting agent tetrabenazine, the two studies together lend considerable weight to the general assumption that dopamine is involved in the production of the tardive dyskinesia syndrome. Obviously, if the etiology of the condition is chronic dopamine blockade, then long-term treatment of the condition with a dopamine-blocking agent is, at its worst, likely to worsen the condition, and is at best unethical. Klawans et al. (27) have recently suggested that such chronic blockade could result in rebound hypersensitivity of receptors to dopamine, and have compared this hypersensitivity with that seen following denervation. Their theory is that chronic blockade of dopaminergic synapses results in a state of chronic chemical denervation of the synapses.

Table 5
Comparison of Different Treatment Conditions on Oral Dyskinesia and Reversible Extrapyramidal Symptoms (EPS)

Comparison	Oral Dyskinesia Mean Frequency	t	Reversible EPS Mean Score	t
	Haloperidol (n = 11)			
Predrug placebo vs.	28.2		2.63	
vs.		3.0201*	vs.	2.2290†
haloperidol 2 wk	12.5		3.36	
Predrug placebo vs.	28.2		2.63	
vs.		3.3695‡	vs.	3.0740*
haloperidol 4 wk	7.4		3.22	
Predrug placebo vs.	28.2		2.63	
vs.		0.4600	vs.	0.3217
postdrug placebo	27.2		2.73	
	Thiopropazate (n = 9)			
Predrug placebo vs.	32.3		3.00	
vs.		3.7080‡	vs.	1.5120*
thiopropazate 2 wk	18.8		3.44	
Predrug placebo vs.	32.3		3.00	
vs.		2.6853†	vs.	2.4010†
thiopropazate 4 wk	23.6		3.78	
Predrug placebo vs.	32.3		3.00	
vs.		0.1694‡	vs.	0.4264
postdrug placebo	33.3		2.89	

*$p < .02$ by paired t-test   †$p < .05$ by paired t-test   ‡$p < .01$ by paired t-test

The antidyskinetic efficacy of both haloperidol and thiopropazate shown in the present study could be explained if one assumes that these dopamine-blocking agents would suppress this hypersensitivity of dopaminergic receptors. Haloperidol is known to have a clinical effect on various hyperkinetic disorders such as Huntington's chorea (22,53,54) or Gille de la Tourette's disease (23,55,56), and thiopropazate is also reported to be effective for the symptomatic control of choreic syndrome (57–61). These antichoreic effects seem compatible with the results of the present study, since a similar abnormality of dopaminergic activity in the basal ganglia is also presumed as a pathogenetic mechanism underlying these conditions.

Reversible extrapyramidal symptom scores showed an inverse relationship with oral dyskinesia symptomatology during haloperidol medication. It appears that the antidyskinetic effect of haloperidol might be attributable to increased rigidity or akinesia. However, such an inverse relationship was less

Table 6
Changes of Nosie Scores

Factors	Weeks	Mean Scores 0	4	8	Mean Difference Scores* 0–4	0–8
				Haloperidol (n = 8)		
Social Competence		10.88	12.88	12.38	+2.00†	+1.50
Social Interest		2.75	2.25	2.50	−0.50	−0.25
Personal Neatness		6.75	7.63	7.38	+0.88‡	+0.63‡
Irritability		4.88	4.13	4.75	+0.75	+0.13
Manifest Psychosis		2.88	3.13	3.25	−0.25	−0.37
Retardation		5.25	5.00	5.38	+0.25	−0.13
Total Patient Assets		54.12	57.25	55.50	+3.13	+1.38
				Thiopropazate (n = 9)		
Social Competence		9.00	10.89	9.22	+1.89	+0.22
Social Interest		3.44	3.22	3.56	−0.22	+0.12
Personal·Neatness		8.22	8.67	8.44	+0.45	+0.22
Irritability		3.56	3.44	3.56	−0.12	0.00
Manifest Psychosis		3.22	3.00	3.22	+0.22	0.00
Retardation		4.67	4.44	4.67	+0.23	0.00
Total Patient Assets		57.22	60.66	58.00	+3.44	+0.88

*Difference score is score at week X-O week score (for factors 1,2,3, and 7), and O week score is score at week X (for factors 4,5, and 6). Therefore, + is improvement and − is worsening.
†p<.01 by paired t-test
‡p<.05 by paired t-test

Table 7
Correlation of Antidyskinetic Efficacy
Between Tetrabenazine and Haloperidol or Thiopropazate

Tetrabenazine	Haloperidol (n = 9)* Effective	No Effect	Thiopropazate (n = 9) Effective	No Effect
Effective†	7	0	3	1
No Effect	1	1	1	4

*Two dropout patients are not included
†Effective means disapperance of dyskinesia or reduction to less than 50% of predrug frequency.

evident in the case of thiopropazate, and was not observed with tetrabenazine in the previous study (28). Further detailed studies are needed to explore this somewhat complicated correlation between reversible extrapyramidal symptoms and oral dyskinesia.

The findings of both the present study and the earlier tetrabenazine study suggest that at least some patients show a tendency to increase the frequency of dyskinetic mouth movements on a stable or increasing dose of antipsychotic agents. Therefore, clinical practicability of these drugs over a longer period remains unestablished.

The use of thiopropazate in this study was occasioned by the favorable results obtained with this agent in a study carried by Roxburch (46). His study implies that thiopropazate may have some special utility in the treatment of tardive dyskinesia. The results of the previous tetrabenazine study and the present study would suggest that the ability to suppress dyskinetic movements may be shared by a fairly wide range of the neuroleptic agents, including both those with dopamine-blocking action and those with dopamine-depleting action.

CLINICAL EFFICACY OF A DOPAMINE-COMPETING AGENT, METHYLDOPA (62)

We have demonstrated in previous studies (28,48,63) that tardive dyskinesia responded significantly to the dopamine-blocking agents (haloperidol and thiopropazate hydrochloride) and to a dopamine-depleting agent (tetrabenazine). To further our exploration of the dopamine hypothesis, a dopamine-competing agent, methyldopa, was used in this study. Methyldopa (α-methyl-3, 4-dihydroxyphenyl-phenylalanine, Aldomet) is a commonly used, safe antihypertensive drug. Sourkes (64) has shown in an in vitro study that this compound is a competitive inhibitor of dopa decarboxylase, the enzyme which transforms dopa into dopamine. On the other hand, methyldopa itself is also known to be decarboxylated by aromatic amino acid decarboxylase to form methyldopamine (65). The latter compound displaces dopamine from storage granules in dopaminergic neurons, and acts as a false neurotransmitter when released at the synapse (66–69).

If the hypothesis is true that tardive dyskinesia is related to the hyperactivity of the dopamine receptor, then the dual action of methyldopa on the dopamine receptor can be expected, theoretically, to result in somewhat ambivalent response.

Since methyldopa differed significantly from both tetrabenazine and more potent antipsychotics in presumed modes of action, its effect on dyskinetic movements was deemed worthy of study.

Subjects and Method

Subjects. Nine patients—7 men and 2 women—were selected for this study. They were all chronic schizophrenic inpatients at Boston State Hospital, manifesting very clear bucco-linguo-masticatory oral dyskinesia, presumably associated with long-term neuroleptic medication. All of them had also been subjects in our earlier studies (28,48,63) on the treatment of tardive dyskinesia and had no physical diseases which would contra-indicate the use of methyldopa. The age of the patients ranged from 46 to 61 years, with an average age of 57, and the length of psychiatric hospitalization was from 15 to 43 years, with a mean of 29 years.

Treatment Design. Before administration of methyldopa, all neuroleptic and antiparkinsonian drugs were completely withdrawn for 4 weeks. Other medications, such as anticonvulsants, were continued unchanged. Daily dosage of methyldopa was started at 250 mg for the first 2 weeks. Then the dosage was doubled to 500 mg for the next 2 weeks, and again to 1,000 mg for the last 2 weeks. After 6 weeks of methyldopa medication, all patients remained off neuroleptic drugs for another 2 weeks. In case of either marked psychotic exacerbation or undesirable side effects during the study, methyldopa was immediately discontinued.

Clinical Evaluation. Oral dyskinesia was evaluated by taking frequency counts of mouth movements, the same technique was used in our earlier studies (28,48,63). These counts were made by a rater blind to the study design, and the mean frequency of oral dyskinetic movement per minute was obtained at each evaluation. The rater was a well-trained research assistant; before beginning the present study, it had been confirmed that his countings were consistent with those obtained by one of us who did several ratings on all patients independently. In addition to the frequency of counts of oral movements, judgments of the severity and types of dyskinesia were also made by utilizing a rating scale which is shown in Table 8. Reversible extrapyramidal symptoms were rated using a modified "bilan extrapyramidal" (31). The latter two ratings were carried out nonblindly. All evaluations were performed once a week during the study period at almost the same time on the same weekday on the patients' ward. The mental or physical status of the study patients was carefully determined at each evaluation. Sitting blood pressure in the right arm was recorded every week.

Results

Eight of 9 patients completed the study. Methyldopa had to be discontinued on a male patient in the first week because of acute psychotic symptoms described below. No other patient reactions requiring discontinuation of

Table 8
Rating Scale for Tardive Dyskinesia

1. Lingual movements
   0. None
   1. Slow lateral or torsion movements of tongue within oral cavity, only visible through lips and cheeks
   2. Lateral movements of tongue with occasional partial protrusion
   3. Lateral movements of tongue with complete protrusion

2. Bucco-mandibular movements
   0. None
   1. Slight lip movements without masticatory movements
   2. Masticatory movements of smaller amplitude, usually not accompanied by movements of elbows and arms
   3. Masticatory movements of bigger amplitude accompanied by mouth opening

3. Involuntary movements of extremities
   0. None
   1. Irregular or rhythmical movements of fingers and/or wrists, not accompanied by movements of elbows and arms
   2. Irregular choreic movements of arms
   3. Irregular choreic movements of both arms and legs

4. Involuntary movements of trunk
   0. None
   1. Occasional rocking movements of trunk
   2. Continuous rocking movements of trunk with smaller amplitude
   3. Continuous rocking movements of trunk with bigger amplitude

5. Other involuntary movements (eye, respiratory, etc.)
   0. None
   1. Slight
   2. Moderate
   3. Severe

methyldopa occurred during the study period. Table 9 presents the average values on each criterion measure obtained at each assessment.

Frequency of Oral Movements. The average frequency of oral movements decreased very slightly during methyldopa medication, being lower after the first week on each dose of methyldopa and returning toward baseline on the second week. However, compared with the counts obtained during the no-medication period, the changes reached a relaxed 10% level of statistical significance when analyzed by paired t-test only after one week of methyldopa 1,000 mg. However, after the second week on methyldopa 1,000 mg, the average frequency increased again. Discontinuance of methyldopa at the seventh week resulted in a rapid return of oral dyskinesia counts to essentially the premethyldopa level in all patients.

Table 9
Average of Ratings During the Study

Week	0	1	2	3	4	5	6	7	8
Daily Dosage of Methyldopa (mg)	0	250	250	500	500	1,000	1,000	0	0
Mean Frequency of Oral Movements	36.0	30.0	36.0	30.5	38.0	26.9*	31.4	35.9	37.6
Mean Reversible EPS Scores	1.5	1.8	1.5	1.3	1.6	1.5	1.4	1.5	1.4
Mean Scores of Dyskinesia Rating Scale	4.6	4.1	3.9	3.8	4.6	4.6	4.8	4.4	4.6
Mean Blood Pressure—Systolic/Diastolic	124/71	120/75	120/77	117/79	119/76	109†/69	113†/75	124/81	125/78

*p 0.1
†p 0.02

Severity and Symptom Areas of Dyskinesia. Slight changes in dyskinetic movements, i.e., amplitude reduction of masticatory movements or decrease of tongue protrusion, were observed in 2 patients during the first 2 weeks of methyldopa. However, after the third week, these changes were no longer found. No statistically significant differences between the average scores of the rating scale at baseline and those taken during methyldopa therapy were observed during the study.

Reversible Extrapyramidal Symptoms. None of the patients showed any noticeable change in reversible extrapyramidal symptoms, such as rigidity, tremor, or dystonia, during the study.

Behavioral Changes. Two patients showed increased psychotic behavior during methyldopa administration. A male schizophrenic, who had not manifested acute psychotic symptoms for several years, suddenly became agitated after 3 days of methyldopa at a daily dosage of 250 mg. He paced around in the ward all day and night talking loudly and incoherently to himself. Discontinuance of methyldopa and prescription of chlorpromazine (400 mg/day) resulted in quick disappearance of this psychotic behavior. In another male patient, continuous mumbling and giggling to himself appeared at the third week of methyldopa at a daily dosage of 500 mg, and persisted unchanged during the remaining 3 weeks of methyldopa administration. These symptoms disappeared soon after discontinuance of methyldopa without reinstitution of antipsychotic drugs. No clear behavioral changes were observed in the other seven patients.

Blood Pressure. Blood pressure could not be determined weekly in one female patient because of her psychotic negativism. The mean systolic pressure of the remaining 7 patients showed a significant decrease in the fifth and sixth week of methyldopa at a daily dosage of 1,000 mg ($p < 0.02$). Inspection of data from individual patients shows that methyldopa tended to reduce systolic blood pressure only in those patients with higher initial blood pressure.

Comment

Under the dosages and time periods used in this study, methyldopa clearly has at best a barely perceptible effect on the abnormal movements of patients with tardive dyskinesia at almost the same dosage used by Villineuve et al. (45), who found some benefit in 2 of 3 patients in an open study at a daily dosage ranging from 750 mg to 1,000 mg. The dosage is lower than that used by Sourkes et al. (70) in the improvement of the symptoms of Huntington's chorea (1,500 to 2,000 mg/day). Cotzias also saw some improvement in 2 such patients (20) at a dosage of 3,750 mg/day. Markham et al. (71) and Klawans (27) reported no success in treating Huntington's chorea with this drug.

Reports of the efficacy of methyldopa in parkinsonism are similarly very contradictory. Barbeau *et al.* (72) found that oral administration of 250 mg of methyldopa causes worsening of tremor and rigidity; Grodon (73) and Peaston (74) have reported independently the appearance of parkinsonism in hypertensive patients treated with methyldopa. Markham *et al.* (71) did not find any therapeutic effect of methyldopa in parkinsonism. On the contrary, Marsch *et al.* (75) observed that 1,000 to 2,000 mg/day of methyldopa decreased parkinsonian tremor when compared with placebo. Sweet *et al.* (76) administered methyldopa in doses from 125 to 750 mg/day, together with regular levodopa therapy, to 22 patients with parkinsonism, and they reported some improvement of parkinsonism symptoms in 16 patients. However, they also observed that combined use of methyldopa and levodopa produced worsening of levodopa-induced dyskinesia in 14 patients, and produced psychotic agitation in 6 patients. All of these studies were nonblind, uncontrolled ones, and the clinical results in this area are inconsistent and equivocal.

The suggestion in the study by Sweet *et al.* (76) that methyldopa might have produced psychotic agitation in parkinsonian patients when combined with levodopa reinforces our observation that methyldopa caused a clear exacerbation of psychotic behavior in 2 of 9 patients in this study. The fact that the psychotic behavior ceased after methyldopa was stopped without phenothiazine medication being required supports the possibility that methyldopa was directly responsible for the abnormal behavior.

Obviously, methyldopa is not of clinical utility as a treatment for tardive dyskinesia. From our data and our literature review, methyldopa appears to have quite a variable set of effects in both dyskinesia and parkinsonian symptoms. Perhaps these inconsistent effects are attributable to its dual effects on dopaminergic systems; its dopamine-decreasing effects may act at cross purposes with its false transmitter properties. It is, of course, possible that the drug has complex effects on other biogenic amines or on other brain systems.

In this study, the daily maximal dosage of methyldopa was limited to 1,000 mg. This is the usually recommended dosage in the treatment of hypertension, but less than the dosage used by Cotzias *et al.* (20) or Sourkes *et al.* (70), who obtained some beneficial effect on choreic disorders with this drug. Therefore, one cannot deny the possibility that more favorable results would have been obtained if we had administered a higher dosage. However, judging from its dual action, probably one cannot expect too much from this drug.

Worsening of the psychotic symptoms were observed in 2 patients during methyldopa administration. In one patient who had to be dropped from the study, we were unable to determine whether this psychotic exacerbation was due to methyldopa or due to discontinuation of neuroleptic drugs the patient had been receiving, since we gave an antipsychotic drug concurrently with the discontinuance of methyldopa and did not try to reproduce psychotic symptoms by readministration of methyldopa. However, this patient had experienced 3, four-week placebo periods in our earlier studies without any psychotic exacerbation. This fact may lead us to suppose that this psychotic episode might be attributable to methyldopa. In another patient, it seemed quite likely that psychotic changes were mainly due to methyldopa, since discontinuance of this drug produced rapid and complete disappearence of psychotic symptoms without any addition of antipsychotic drugs. Methyldopa is, chemically, levodopa with a methyl group on the α-carbon of the side chain. Levodopa has been reported to induce occasional agitation in patients with parkinsonism (19,77,78,79) or schizophrenia (80). If methyldopamine, which is derived from methyldopa, acts as a false transmitter in dopaminergic neurones, and if this compound has a somewhat similar effect as dopamine, methyldopa may well provoke psychotic changes similar to those seen with levodopa. This finding may also argue against clinical use of methyldopa in psychotic patients with tardive dyskinesia.

LONG-TERM TREATMENT OF TARDIVE DYSKINESIA WITH HALOPERIDOL AND TETRABENAZINE (63)

The purposes of the study were twofold. First, we wished to learn whether drugs that showed effective short-term suppression of dyskinetic movements would continue to manifest this effect when administered as maintenance therapy. Careful inspection of the data from our earlier studies left the impression that the stepwise dosage increases used may have served to maintain the suppression of dyskinetic movements that otherwise would have escaped from drug control. There is a widely held clinical belief that dyskinetic movements break through rather rapidly when they are suppressed by antipsychotic drugs. Second, we wished to determine whether the suppression of dyskinetic movements over a period of several months led to any appreciable exacerbation of the movements when the suppressant drug was discontinued.

SUBJECTS AND METHOD

Thirteen patients were selected for this study. They were all chronic psychotic inpatients at Boston State Hospital who manifested typical bucco-linguo-masticatory oral dyskinesia associated with long-term neuroleptic medication. All of them had been subjects in our previous studies (28,63); detailed physical and neurological examinations had been completed prior to the initiation of the previous studies. There were eight men and five women, ranging in age from 41 to 63 years, with an average age of 55.8 years. The length of psychiatric hospitalization ranged from 15 to 41 years, with an average of 29.3 years. Ten

454   TARDIVE DYSKINESIA

patients were diagnosed as chronic schizophrenics, 2 as mentally deficient, and 1 as having a chronic brain syndrome.

The 13 patients were divided randomly into 2 groups. In the initial phase, all neuroleptic and antiparkinsonian drugs were completely withdrawn and were replaced by placebo for the first 4 weeks. Other medications, such as antidiabetic or anticonvulsant drugs, were continued unchanged.

Seven patients received 4 mg of haloperidol twice a day, and 6 patients received 50 mg of tetrabenazine twice a day. These dosages were determined on the basis of the findings in our previous studies, which indicated that the majority of the patients with oral dyskinesia responded favorably to either 8 mg per day of haloperidol or 100 mg per day of tetrabenazine. It was originally planned that these dosages would be held constant for 24 weeks. However, by the twelfth week of the study, it became obvious that the marked reduction in abnormal movements observed during the first several weeks had not persisted for the majority of the patients; this was especially true for the patients receiving haloperidol.

A frequency count of mouth movements (28), done by a psychiatrist blind to the study design, was used to assess oral dyskinesia. The mean frequency of oral dyskinetic movements per minute was obtained at each evaluation. Evaluation was carried out weekly for the first 4 weeks of drug administration in the study, and biweekly for the rest of the study period. Reversible extrapyramidal symptoms were rated biweekly using a modified "bilan extrapyramidal" (31). The NOSIE-30 was completed every 6 weeks by the ward nurses, who were also blind to the study design, to assess the ward adjustment of the patients.

Results

PreDrug Placebo Period. During the 4 weeks of the predrug placebo period, all the patients manifested typical bucco-linguo-masticatory dyskinesia. The average frequency of oral dyskinetic movements per minute was 34.9 in the haloperidol group and 25.7 in the tetrabenazine group. Little change occurred in either oral movements or reversible extrapyramidal symptom scores during the 4-week predrug placebo period.

Clinical Efficacy of Haloperidol. Seven patients were given haloperidol at the daily dosage of 8 mg. At the end of the second week, oral dyskinetic movements had completely disappeared in 5 out of 7 patients and were markedly reduced in the other 2 patients. The average frequency of oral movements was 2.4 per minute. At the end of the fourth week, complete suppression of oral dyskinesia was still observed in 4 patients. In the other 3 patients, however, the frequency of oral dyskinesia had returned almost to the levels observed prior to administration of haloperidol. The average frequency of oral movements for all 7 patients was 18.0 per minute.

At the end of the eighth week, although complete disappearance of dyskinesia was still observed in 2 patients, marked suppression of dyskinesia was no longer seen in the other 5 patients. The average frequency of oral movements was 24.1 per minute. At the end of the twelfth week on haloperidol, all the patients manifested oral dyskinesias, even though the average frequency of oral movements was still significantly lower than that observed during the predrug placebo period (21.8 versus 34.9, p<.01).

Starting at the fifteenth week, the daily dosage of haloperidol was doubled to 16 mg. Two weeks after the increase in dosage, 3 patients showed considerable reduction in the frequency of oral dyskinesia. Two other patients, however, developed severe malaise and appeared not to be able to tolerate 16 mg of haloperidol; the drug was discontinued. The remaining 2 patients did not show any improvement in oral dyskinesia. Replacement of haloperidol by a matched placebo in the nineteenth week resulted in a rapid reappearance of oral dyskinesia, with the frequency rising to approximately the predrug level in all patients.

Table 10 depicts the clinical efficacy of haloperidol in treating oral dyskinesia, and Figure 5 illustrates the changes in frequency of both oral dyskinesia and reversible extrapyramidal symptoms. Comparison of each treatment period with the baseline period by paired t-test revealed that haloperidol administration was associated with a statistically significant reduction in the frequency of oral dyskinesia, even though its antidyskinetic efficacy was most

Table 10
Comparison of the Clinical Efficacy of Haloperidol and Tetrabenazine in Treating Oral Dyskinesia

Rate of Reduction of Oral Dyskinesia	Week*								
	2	4	6	8	10	12	14	16	18
Haloperidol Group (n = 7)									
100% disappearance	5	4	3	3	0	0	0	0	2
50–99% disappearance	2	0	1	0	3	2	2	3	0
0–49% disappearance	0	1	3	2	2	5	5	3	2
Worsening	0	2	1	3	2	0	0	1	1
Dropout	0	0	0	0	0	0	0	0	2
Tetrabenazine Group (n = 6)									
100% disappearance	2	2	2	2	1	2	2	2	2
50–99% disappearance	0	2	1	1	2	1	0	1	0
0–49% disappearance	3	2	2	2	2	2	3	3	3
Worsening	1	0	1	1	1	1	1	0	1

*The dosage for weeks 2–14 was 8 mg of haloperidol or 100 mg of tetrabenazine; for weeks 16 and 18, it was 16 mg or 200 mg, respectively.

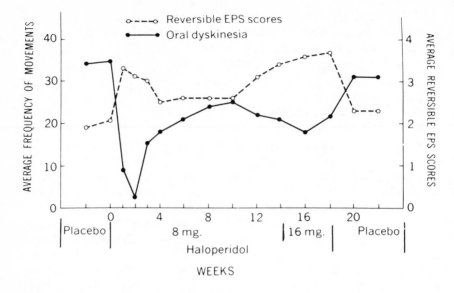

Figure 5.   Changes in Frequency of Oral Dyskinetic Movements and Reversible Extrapyramidal Symptoms During Administration of Haloperidol (n = 7)

striking during the first 2 weeks. Reversible extrapyramidal symptoms appeared to be negatively correlated with the changes in frequency of oral dyskinesia (r = .6292, p<.02).

Clinical Efficacy of Tetrabenazine

There were no dropouts among the 6 patients who received tetrabenazine. At the end of the second week, oral dyskinesia had completely disappeared in 2 patients and was unchanged in the other 4 patients. As shown in Table 10, this split remained almost constant throughout the 14 weeks during which the patients were receiving 100 mg per day of tetrabenazine. The average frequency of oral movements was reduced from 25.7 to 12.8 at the end of the second week, then increased to 16.8 at the end of the sixth week, and stayed at almost this same level until the 15th week (see Fig. 6).

The dosage increase of tetrabenazine to 200 mg per day at the fifteenth week produced a slight reduction in average frequency of oral dyskinesia. This effect, however, appeared to be a transient one, since an increase in oral dyskinesia was observed at the eighteenth week, i.e., 4 weeks after the dosage increase. The replacement of tetrabenazine by a matched placebo resulted in a rapid return of oral dyskinesia to the levels observed during the initial placebo

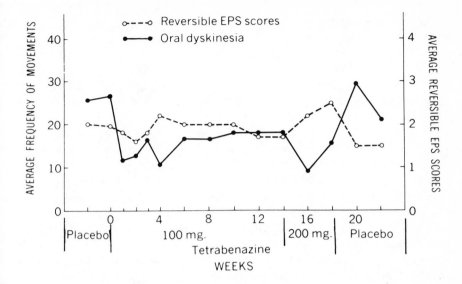

Figure 6. Changes in Frequency of Oral Dyskinetic Movements and Reversible Extrapyramidal Symptoms During Administration of Tetrabenazine (n = 6)

period. During the 18 weeks of tetrabenazine medication, no significant side effects were observed.

The comparison of each treatment period with the baseline period by paired t-test revealed that tetrabenazine administration was associated with a statistically significant reduction in the frequency of oral dyskinesia. The correlation between oral dyskinesia and reversible extrapyramidal symptoms was less clear than in the haloperidol group (r = .4149, p<.20).

Changes in Ward Behavior

NOSIE ratings were available for 6 out of 7 patients in the haloperidol group, and for all 6 patients in the tetrabenazine group. Although some slight changes in the patients' ward behavior occurred during the course of the study, there was neither clear deterioration nor clear improvement in either treatment group.

Comment

Studies of drug treatments for tardive dyskinesia involve serious ethical issues. The only kinds of drugs known to suppress dyskinesia reliably are either neuroleptic drugs (e.g., phenothiazines, butyrophenones) or amine-depleting agents (e.g., reserpine, tetrabenazine). In the present study, the aim was to determine whether drugs we had previously shown to suppress dyskinetic movements (haloperidol, tetrabenazine) would be as effective over an 18-week period as they had been over an 8-week period. Haloperidol has been claimed to cause tardive dyskinesia (4,81,82). Tetrabenazine has not been so implicated, though reserpine has (5).

Since 8-week studies had not led to any worsening in the dyskinesia of the study patients, and the need for a safe and reliable drug to suppress dyskinesia was clear, our ethics committee felt comfortable in approving an 18-week study if it was followed by a placebo period in which adverse effects on the abnormal movements could be determined. Since tardive dyskinesia usually appears after years of neuroleptic drug treatment, it seemed safe to assume that 18 additional weeks of such treatment would not cause any significant change in the underlying disorder.

As the results show, the two treatments did not, in fact, harm the patients. Unfortunately, neither did the treatments prove to be particularly useful in suppressing abnormal movements over an 18-week period. The initial suppression achieved did not persist, and even a doubling of the dosage in the latter phases of the study did not result in optimal suppression. Haloperidol was more effective than tetrabenazine early in the study.

At the present state of knowledge, no specific therapy for tardive dyskinesia can be recommended, although the withholding of all antipsychotic medications for prolonged periods (or the use of such agents in the smallest amounts that will prevent major exacerbations in the patient's psychosis) appears to be the wisest strategy.

Eighteen-Month Follow-up of Tardive Dyskinesia Treated with Various Catecholamine-Related Agents (83)

As described in the previous series of 4 studies, various pharmacological agents clearly known for their action on catecholamine were administered for different durations over a one-year period. Six months after the completion of the studies, a follow-up was made on the original cohort group in order to determine the clinical status of their tardive dyskinesia.

SUMMARY OF FIFTY-EIGHT WEEK STUDY

A group of 24 patients with tardive dyskinesia was recruited for the initial study from Boston State Hospital. The average age was 55. The average length of stay in the hospital was 29 years. All patients received various neuroleptic medication for more than 10 years prior to the study.

All or part of these 24 patients participated in the following series of studies using different categories of medication: (1) catecholamine-depleting agent—tetrabenazine, (2) catecholamine-blocking agents—haloperidol and thiopropazate, and (3) dopamine-competing agent—methyldopa. Each of the above three studies was preceded and followed by a 4-week placebo period. There were short-term (4–6 weeks) and long-term (18 weeks) studies with haloperidol and tetrabenazine. For methyldopa, the study period was 6 weeks. The total length of time required to complete the aforementioned studies was 58 weeks. Evaluation of the dyskinetic movement was focused on the frequency of bucco-linguo-masticatory movements only. Every movement in the oral region, such as chewing, licking, puffing, pursing of lips, and rolling or protrusion of tongue, was counted for 3 separate 1-minute periods. The mean frequency of dyskinetic movements per minute was calculated at 2-week intervals. The results indicate that catecholamine-depleting and -blocking agents diminished dyskinetic movements significantly (17,28,48), while the dopamine-competing agent showed equivocal effects (62). A worsening of psychiatric symptoms was also observed during the use of methyldopa. When the patient was switched to placebo from an active compound, the dyskinetic movement immediately returned to the prestudy placebo level.

Results at the End of Eighteen Months

After the completion of the 58-week study, 22 of the original 24 patients remained in the hospital and were placed on doctor's choice medication. Two evaluations of their dyskinetic symptoms were made, once at the seventieth to seventy-second week with doctor's choice medication (various neuroleptics), and once at the seventy-sixth to seventy-eighth week without any medication. Oral-movement counting method as used in the previous studies was used for these two evaluations. The group's average mouth movements were strikingly similar, 31/minute on each occasion. The degree of dyskinetic symptoms was the same as that of the first 8 weeks and without placebo (see Fig. 7).

The findings implied to us that despite such a prolonged period of the usage of different drugs which affected catecholamine, particularly with the 18-week usage of Haldol, the dyskinetic symptoms did not show any significant deterioration and practically remained the same, both clinically and statistically, as the status at the very beginning of this long-term study, which took place 18 months ago. The finding is somewhat assuring to the clinician that in the event that a patient's psychotic symptoms become life-threatening or dangerous to society, resumption of antipsychotic drugs can be considered with relatively little risk to provoke the previously existent tardive dyskinesia. After all, administration of any therapeutic agent to the patient is based on the benefit-risk ratio. Our 18-month follow-up findings can provide some information regarding the possible degree of risk, which was negligible in our study, for

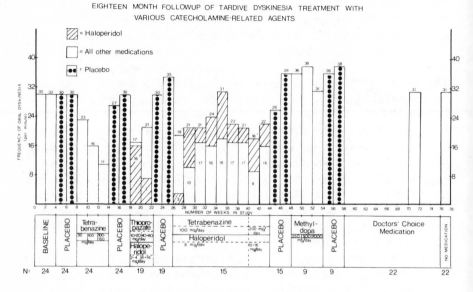

Figure 7. Eighteen-Month Follow-up of Tardive Dyskinesia Treatment with
Various Catecholamine-Related Agents

those clinicians who have to use antipsychotic drugs for psychotic dyskinetic
patients with justifiable clinical indication.

EFFICACIES OF AGENTS RELATED TO GABA (SODIUM VALPROATE), DOPAMINE (OXYPERTINE), AND ACETYLCHOLINE (DEANOL) (84)

This study took place at Albany Medical College, in New York, with a
twofold purpose: (1) to test the hypothesis that tardive dyskinesia (TD) can be
affected by several neurotransmitters; therefore, manipulation of neurotransmitters such as GABA, dopamine, and acetylcholine by sodium valproate (a
GABA potentiator), by oxypertine (a dopamine-depleting agent), and by
deanol (a precursor of acetylcholine) may result in a change in intensity and
frequency of dyskinetic movements; and (2) to compare these three drugs'
relative efficacies in the clinical management of TD.

Pharmacological rationale. To date, dopamine receptor hypersensitivity
or dopaminergic hyperactivity is by far the most popular hypothesis regarding
the etiology of TD. Direct manipulation of dopamine by oxypertine, a
dopamine-depleting agent, should result in the diminution or disappearance of

TD. It is also known that acetylcholine and GABA maintain a balance with dopamine at the synaptic site. Therefore, deanol, a precursor of acetylcholine, or solium valproate, a GABA potentiator through its inhibition of GABA transaminase, should, theoretically, diminish dopaminergic activity, thus resulting in the improvement of TD. Whether a change in the GABA-ergic and cholinergic activities affects TD directly or indirectly is not known and cannot be established by this study.

Subjects. Twenty dyskinetic outpatients of the Capital District Psychiatric Center of the Albany Medical College complex were selected for study. All study patients manifested persistent dyskinesia while on neuroleptics. They were not a transient TD group who usually reveals symptoms upon discontinuation of neuroleptics. All subjects had a long history of neuroleptic therapy, but at the time of study, 15 were receiving antipsychotic drugs, 1 was receiving antianxiety agents alone, and 1 was receiving a combination of antidepressants and antianxiety drugs.

Seventeen completed the study, while 3 dropped out for reasons unrelated to study procedures. The mean age of the 17 S's was 46.6 years; 7 were male and 10 were female; mean duration of psychiatric illness was 19.9 years; and all but one carried a clinical diagnosis of schizophrenia.

Instruments. The Abnormal Involuntary Movement Scale (AIMS), developed by the National Institute of Mental Health, was employed to assess TD movements. Two scores were derived from this scale: (1) the sum of the scores for 7 discrete body areas, assessed by the first 7 times of the AIMS (SUM), and (2) Global Rating (GR), a 5-point global severity rating called for in Item 8 of the AIMS. The interrater reliability coefficient for the SUM is .84 and .79 for the GR. A 7-point TD improvement rating (TDI) was also made. A psychologist and a nurse performed all ratings concurrently but independently at 1-week intervals without knowledge of the patient's drug assignment or of whether the patient was receiving active drug or placebo. Additionally, piezoelectric recordings were done for those who had significant bucco-linguo-masticatory movement (85,86).

Procedure. The subjects were randomly assigned to either sodium valproate, oxypertine, or deanol, and were treated for 3 weeks on active drug, either followed or preceded by 3 weeks on placebo. All active medication and placebo were prepared in identically appearing capsules. The prescribing physician did not contribute to the data collected. The number of subjects in each group and the starting and maximum daily dosages and number of capsules prescribed are depicted in Table 2. The dosage range of the three drugs in the design were adopted from the reported therapeutic dosage in the previous literature. All patients were treated for 2 weeks at maximum dosage.

All subjects tolerated the medication remarkably well without any noticeable side effects.

Data Analysis. The data was analyzed by nonparametric statistical techni-

Table 11

	Sodium Valproate (n = 5)	Oxypertine (n = 5)	Deanol (n = 7)	Placebo (n = 17)
Dose/Capsule	400 mg	40 mg	400 mg	—
Starting Daily Dose Week 1	1200 mg	120 mg	1200 mg	—
Number Caps/Day Week 1	3	3	3	3
Ending Daily Dosage Week 3	1600 mg	160 mg	1600 mg	—
Number Caps/Day Week 3	4	4	4	4

ques because of the small number of subjects in each group: Interdrug comparisons were done employing the Mann-Whitney U test, and within-group comparisons were made using the Wilcoxon matched-pairs signed rank test.

Results. Although interdrug comparison did not reveal any statistically significant differences, comparison within each group of subjects between active drug and placebo revealed different patterns among the three drugs. Oxypertine was significantly superior to placebo in SUM and GR. Sodium valproate showed superiority to placebo in GR but not in SUM, while deanol showed no difference from placebo by either measure (see Table 12).

Clinician's judgments of improvement in TD symptoms for each drug group can be seen in Table 13. Oxypertine shows the highest percentage of much to very much improved, sodium valproate shows the highest percentage of minimally improved, while 86% of deanol patients are rated as having no change or as having worsened.

Piezoelectric Recordings. Piezoelectric recordings also show some qualitative differences in the response to the three different drugs. The quantitative analysis of these recordings was not performed due to the relatively few *S*'s who volunteered for recording. However, the graphs are generally consistent with the data obtained from the double-blind study.

Discussion. The findings of the investigators seem to indicate that oxypertine ranks first, sodium valproate second, and deanol last in their therapeutic efficacy on TD. This seems to suggest that direct manipulation of dopamine results in more significant changes in TD than manipulating GABA-ergic and cholinergic neurotransmitters. The lack of therapeutic efficacy of deanol in this study cannot rule out the cholinergic role of TD. Davis *et al.* (86) demonstrated that the physostigmine responders responded well to choline hydrochloride, another precursor of acetylcholine, when the latter drug was used in the management of involuntary movement of TD and Huntington's

Table 12
Efficacy of Drugs on Tardive Dyskinesia
(By Aims and Global Ratings)

Drug	Placebo Sum	Placebo Global	Active Drug Sum	Active Drug Global	Superiority over Placebo p Value Sum	Superiority over Placebo p Value Global
Oxypertine	10.3	3.0	8.6	2.3	0.03*	0.02*
Sodium Valproate	7.0	2.3	6.3	1.5	0.17	0.05*
Deanol	8.1	2.2	7.9	2.1	0.37	0.37

*Statistically significant, by Wilcoxon matched-pairs signed ranks test.

Table 13
Improvement of Tardive Dyskinesia by
7-Point Improvement Scale

Drug	Oxypertine n	Oxypertine %	Sodium Valproate n	Sodium Valproate %	Deanol n	Deanol %
Improvement						
Much to Very Much Improved	2	40	0	0	1	14
Minimally Improved	2	40	3	60	0	0
No Change to Very Much Worse	1	20	2	40	6	86

chorea, a syndrome considered to share the same neurochemical mechanism with TD at the synaptic site.

The efficacy of sodium valproate on TD as reported by Linnoila et al. (87) was confirmed by the present study.

ACKNOWLEDGMENTS

Portions of the data used in this chapter are from "Treatment of tardive dyskinesia (I): clinical efficacy of a dopamine-depleting agent, haloperidol and thiopropazate," Archives of General Psychiatry, 27, pp. 95–99, July 1972; "Treatment of tardive dyskinesia (II): short-term efficacy of dopamine-blocking agents, haloperidol and thiopropazate," Archives of Gen-

FIGURE 8

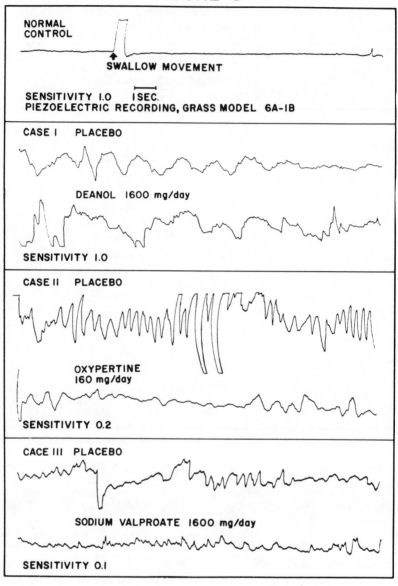

Figure 8. Effects of Deanol and Oxypertine on Tardive Dyskinesia
Symptoms Measured by Piezoelectric Recording Techniques

eral Psychiatry, 27, pp. 100–103, *July 1972; "Treatment of tardive dyskinesia (III): clinical efficacy of a dopamine agent, methyldopa," Archives of General Psychiatry, 27*, pp. 824–827, *December 1972; "Therapeutic approaches to tardive dyskinesia– a review of the literature," Archives of General Psychiatry, 27*, pp. 491–499, October 1972. Copyright © 1972, American Medical Association, *American Journal of Psychiatry*, vol. 130, pp. 479–483, 1974. Copyright 1974, the American Psychiatric Association. Reprinted by permission.

REFERENCES

1. Sigwald, J., Bouttier, D., Courvoisier, S. Les accidents neurologiques des medications neuroleptiques. *Rev. Neurol., 100*:553–595, 1959.
2. Sigwald, J., Bouttier, D., Raymondeaud, C., Piot, C. Quatre cas de dyskinesie facio-bucco-linguo-masticatrice a evolution prolongee secondaire a un traitement par les neuroleptiques. *Rev. Neurol., 100*:751–755, 1959.
3. Schönecker, M. Ein eigentumliches Syndrom im oralen Bereich bei Megaphen Applikation. *Nervenarzt, 28*:35, 1957.
4. Faurbye, A., Rasch, P.J., Petersen, P.B., Branborg, F., Pakkenberg, H. Neurological symptoms in pharmacotherapy of psychoses. *Acta Psychiatr. Scand., 40*:10–27, 1964.
5. Uhrbrand, L., Faurbye, A. Reversible and irreversible dyskinesia after treatment with perphenazine, chlorpromazine, reserpine and electroconvulsive therapy. *Psychopharmacologia, 1*:408–418, 1960.
6. Degkwitz, R., Luxemburger, O. Das terminale extrapyramidale Insuffizienzbzw. Defektsyndrom infolge chronischer Anwendung von Neuroleptika. *Nervenarzt, 36*:173–175, 1965.
7. Degkwitz, R., Wenzel, W., Binsack, K.F., Herkert, H., Luxemberger, O. Zum Probleme der terminalen extrapyramidalen Hyperkinesen an Han von 1600 langfristig mit Neuroleptica Behandelten. *Arzneim. Forsch., 16*:276–278, 1966.
8. Hunter, R., Earl, C.J., Janz, D. A syndrome of abnormal movements and dementia in leucotomized patients treated with phenothiazines. *J. Neurol. Neurosurg. Psychiatry, 27*:219–223, 1964.
9. Hunter, R., Earl, C.J., Thornicroft, S. An apparently irreversible syndrome of abnormal movements following phenothiazine medication. *Proc. R. Soc. Med., 57*:758–762, 1964.
10. Crane, G.E., Paulson, G. Involuntary movements in a sample of chronic mental patients and their relation to the treatment with neuroleptics. *Int. J. Neuropsychiat., 3*:286–291, 1967.
11. Crane, G.E., Ruiz, P.M., Kernoham, W.J. Effects of drug manipulation on tardive dyskinesia. Read at the 123rd annual meeting of the American Psychiatric Association, Detroit, Mich., May 8-12, 1967.
12. Crane, G.E. Tardive dyskinesia in patients treated with major neuroleptics: a review of the literature. *Am. J. Psychiatry, 124*:8, 40–48, Suppl., Feb. 1968.
13. Kline, N.S. On the rarity of "irreversible" oral dyskinesias following phenothiazines. *Am. J. Psychiatry, 124*:8, 48–54, Suppl. Feb. 1968.
14. Chien, C.P., Jung, K., Ross-Townsend, A., Stearns, B. The measurement of tardive dyskinesia by piezoelectric recording and clinical rating scales. *Psychopharmacol. Bull.*, 1977.

15. Crane, G.E. Tardive dyskinesia in schizophrenic patients treated with psychotropic drugs. 2nd International Symposium on Action Mechanism and Metabolism of Psychoactive Drugs Derived from Phenothiazine and Structurally Related Compounds. Paris, 17, 18, 19, October, 1967. *Agressologie, 9*:2, 209–218, 1968.

16. Jacobson, G., Baldessarini, R.J., Manschreck, T. Tardive and withdrawal dyskinesia associated with haloperidol. *Am. J. Psychiat., 131*:8, 910–913, 1974.

17. Kazamatsuri, H., Chien, C.P., Cole, J. Therapeutic approaches to tardive dyskinesia—a review of the literature *Arch. Gen. Psychiatry, 27,* 1972

18. Christensen, E., Moller, J.E., Faurbye, A. Neuropathological investigation of 28 brains from patients with dyskinesia. *Acta Psychiatr. Scand., 46*:14–23, 1970.

19. Yahr, M.D., Duvoisin, R.C., Shear, M.J., Barret, R.E., Hoehn, M.M. Treatment of parkinsonism with levodopa. *Arch. Neurol., 21*:343–354, 1969.

20. Cotzias, G.C., Papavasiliou, P.P., Gellene, R. Modification of parkinsonism: chronic treatment with L-dopa. *N. Engl. J. Med., 280*:337–345, 1969.

21. Barbeau, A. L-dopa therapy in parkinson's disease: a critical review of nine years' experience. *Can. Med. Assoc. J., 101*:791–800, 1969.

22. Nayac, P., Arnott, G., Milbred, G. Chorea de Huntington, trouble de l'humeur d'expression maniaque, effects benefiques de l'haloperidol, absence de syndrome akineto-hypertonique. *Encephale, 53*:225–227, 1964.

23. Lucas, A.R., Gilles de las Tourette's disease in children: treatment with haloperidol. *Am. J. Psychiatry, 124*:243–245, 1967.

24. Klawans, H.L., Ilahi, M.M., Shenker, D. Theoretical implications of the use of L-dopa in parkinsonism. *Acta Neurol. Scand., 46*:409–441, 1970.

25. Klawans, H.L. A pharmacologic analysis of Huntington's chorea. *Eur. Neurol., 4*:148–163, 1970.

26. Carlsson, A. Biochemical implications of dopa-induced action on the central nervous system with particular reference to abnormal movements. In *L-Dopa and Parkinsonism*, Barbeau, A., McDowell, F.H. (eds.) Philadelphia: Davis, pp. 205–212, 1970.

27. Prange, A.J., Sisk, J.L., Wilson, A.C., Balance, permission and discrimination among amines: a theoretical consideration of the actions of L-tryptophan in disorders of movement and affect. In *Proceedings of the NIMH Serotonin Conference*, Palo Alto, Calif.: Government Printing Office, pp. 966–1489, 1972.

28. Kazamatsuri, H., Chien, C.P., Cole, J.O. Treatment of tardive dyskinesia: I. Clinical efficacy of a dopamine-depleting agent, tetrabenazine. *Arch. Gen. Psychiatry, 27*:95–99, 1972.

29. Pletcher, A., Shore, P.A., Brodie, B.B. Benzoquinolidin, eine neue Körperklasse mit Wirkung auf den 5-Hydroxytryptamin und Noradrenalin Stoffwechsel des Gehirns. *Arch. Exp. Path. Pharmacol., 232*:499–505, 1958.

30. Leusen, I., Lacrois, E., Demeester, G. Quelques propriétés pharmacodynamiques de la Tétrabenazine, substance liberatrice de sérotonine. *Arch. Int. Pharmacodyn. Ther., 119*:225–231, 1959.

31. Bordeau, J.M., Albert, J.M., Hillel, J. Medication antiparkinsonnienne et bilan extrapyramidal, étude de trihexyphenidyl. *Can. Psychiatr. Assoc. J., 12*:588–595, 1967.

32. Honingfield, G., Klett, G.J. The NOSIE-30; a treatment sensitive ward behavior scale. *Psychol. Rep., 19*:180–182, 1966.

33. Crane, G.E., cited by Kurland, A.A. *Antipsychotic Drugs and Their Extrapyramidal Complications.* Orange, NJ: Knoll Pharmaceutical, p. 41, 1968.

34. Crane, G.E., Ruiz, P., Kernohan, W.J., Effects of drug withdrawal on tardive dyskinesia. *Activ. Nerv. Suppl., 11*:30–35, 1969.

35. Wright, R.L.D., Kine W.P. A clinical and experimental comparison of four anti-schizophrenic drugs. *Psychopharmacologia, 1*:437–449, 1960.

36. Stockhausen, F.G. Clinical studies with tetrabenazine (Ro I 9569). *Dis. Nerv. Syst.*, *21*(Suppl. 3):115–117, 1960.
37. Lende, N. Psychosedative effects of tetrabenazine (Ro I 9569) on hyperactive and disturbed mentally retarded patients. *Dis. Nerv. Syst.*, *21* (Suppl. 3):118–119, 1960.
38. Smith, M.E. Clinical comparison of tetrabenazine (Ro I 9569) and placebo in chronic schizophrenics. *Dis. Nerv. Syst.*, *21* (Suppl. 3):120–123, 1960.
39. Lingjaarde, O. Tetrabenazine (Nitoman) in the treatment of psychosis, with a discussion on the central mode of action of tetrabenazine and reserpine. *Acta Psychiatr. Scand.*, (Suppl. 170); 1–105, 1963.
40. Sattes, H. Die Behandlung der Chorea major mit dem Monoamin-Freisetzer Nitoman. *Psychiat. Neurol.*, *140*:13–19, 1960.
41. Delby, M.A. Effect of tetrabenazine on extrapyramidal movement disorders.*Br. Med. J.*, *1*:422–423, 1969.
42. Möller-Christensen, A.B., Videbech, T. Behandling af chorea Huntington med Tetrabenazin (Nitoman). *Ugeskr Laeger*, *125*:207–209, 1963.
43. Brandrup, E. Tetrabenazine treatment in persisting dyskinesia caused by psychopharmaca. *Am. J. Psychiatry*, *118*:551–552, 1961.
44. MacCullum, W.A.G. Tetrabenazine for extrapyramidal movement disorders. *Br. Med. J.*, *1*:760, 1970.
45. Villineuve, A., Böszörményi, Z., Dechambault, M. Tentative de traitment de dyskinésia postneuroléptique de type permanent. *Laval Med.*, *41*:923–933, 1970.
46. Roxburch, P.A. Treatment of phenothiazine-induced oral dyskinesia. *Br. J. Psychiatry*, *116*:227–280, 1970.
47. Kennedy, P.F. Chorea and phenothiazines. *Br. J. Psychiatry*, *115*:103–104, 1969.
48. Kazamatsuri, H., Chien, C.P., Cole, J.O. Treatment of tardive dyskinesia: II. Short-term efficacy of dopamine blocking agents, haloperidol and thiopropazate. *Arch. Gen. Psychiatry*, 27:100–103, 1972.
49. Nybäck, H., Borzecky, Z., Sedvall, G. Accumulation and disappearance of catecholamine formed from tyrosine 14-c in mouse brain: effect of some psychotropic drugs. *Eur. J. Pharmacol.*, *4*:395–403, 1968.
50. Laverty, R., Sherman, D.F. Modification by drugs of the metabolism of 3, 4-dihydroxy-phenylalanine and 5-hydroxytryptamine in the brain. *Br. J. Pharmacol.*, *24*:759–772, 1965.
51. Pletscher, A. Pharmacological and biochemical basis of some somatic side effects of psychotropic drugs. In *Neuropsychopharmacology*, Brill, H. (eds.). Amsterdam: Excerpta Medica Foundation, 1966.
52. Janssen, P.A.J. The pharmacology of haloperidol. *Int. J. Neuropsychiat.*, *3*(Suppl. 1):10–18, 1967.
53. Gilbert, M.M. Haloperidol in severe facial dyskinesia. *Dis. Nerv. Syst.*, *30*:481–482, 1969.
54. Siegel, G.J., Mones, R.J. Modification of choreiform activity by haloperidol. *JAMA*, *216*:675–676, 1971.
55. Challes, G., Chapel, J.L., Jenkins, R.L. Tourette's disease: control of symptoms and its clinical course. *Int. J. Neuropsychiat.*, *3*(Suppl. 1):95–109, 1967.
56. Shapiro, A.K., Shapiro, A. Treatment of Gille de la Tourette's syndrome with haloperidol. *Br. J. Psychiatry*, *114*:345–350, 1968.
57. Mathews, F.P. Dartal, a clinical appraisal. *Am. J. Psychiatry*, *114*:1034–1037, 1958.
58. Souder, G.L.R. Treatment of Huntington's chorea with thiopropazate dihydrochloride. *Del. Med. J.*, *31*:249–250, 1958.
59. Lyon, R.I. Drug treatment of Huntington's chorea, a trial with thiopropazate.*Br. Med. J.*, *1*:1308–1310, 1962.

60. Bruyn, G.W. Thiopropazate dihydrochloride (Dartal) in the treatment of Huntington's chorea *Psychiat. Neurol. Neurochirum, 65*:430-438, 1962.

61. Versberg, M., Saunders, J.C. Treatment of dyskinesias including Huntington's chorea with thiopropazate and R 1625. *Dis. Nerv. Syst., 24*:499, 1963.

62. Kazamatsuri, H., Chien, C.P., Cole, J.O. Treatment of tardive dyskinesia. II. Clinical efficacy of a dopamine competing agent, methyldopa. *Arch. Gen. Psychiatry, 27*:824–827, 1972.

63. Kazamatsuri, H., Chien, C.P., Cole, J.O. Long-term treatment of tardive dyskinesia with haloperidol and tetrabenazine. *Am. J. Psychiatry, 130*:4, 479–483, 1973.

64. Sourkes, T.C. Inhibition of dihydroxyphenylalanine decarboxylase by derivatives of phenylalanine. *Arch. Biochem. Biophys., 51*:444–456, 1954.

65. Carlsson, A., Lindqvist, M. In vivo decarboxylation of α-methyl-dopa and α-methyl metatyrosine. *Acta Physiol. Scand., 54*:87–94, 1962.

66. Day, M.D., Rand, M.J. Some observations on the pharmacology of α-methyldopa. *Br. J. Pharmacol., 27*:72–86, 1964.

67. Holtz, P., Palm, D. On the pharmacology of alpha-methylated catecholamines and the mechanism of the antihypertensive effect of α-methyldopa. *Life Sci., 6*:1847–1857, 1967.

68. Sourkes, T.L., The action of some alpha-methyl and other amino acids on cerebral catecholamines. *J. Neurochem., 8*:109–115, 1961.

69. Undenfriend, S., Zaltzman-Nirenberg, P. On the mechanism of the norepinephrine release produced by α-methyl-meta-tyrosine. *J. Pharmacol. Exp. Ther., 138*:194–199, 1962.

70. Sourkes, T.L. A clinical and metabolic study of dopa and methyldopa in Huntington's chorea. *Psychiatr. Neurol., 149*:7–27, 1965.

71. Markham, C.H., Clark, W.G., Winters, W.D. Effect of alpha-methyldopa and reserpine in Huntington's chorea, Parkinson's disease and other movement disorders. *Life Sci., 2*:697–705, 1963.

72. Barbeau, A., Sourkes, T.L., Murphy, G.F. Les catecholamines dans la maladie de parkinson. In Monoamines et systeme nerveaux central, de Ajuriaguerra (ed)., Paris: Masson, 247, 1962.

73. Grodon, M.D. Parkinsonism occurring with methyldopa treatment. *Br. Med. J., 1*:1001, 1963.

74. Peaston, M.J.T. Parkinsonism associated with α-methyldopa therapy. *Br. Med. J., 2*:687, 1964.

75. Marsch, D.O., Schneider, H., Marshall, J. A controlled trial of methyldopa in parkinsonian tremor. *J. Neurol. Neurosurg. Psychiatry, 26*:505, 1963.

76. Sweet, R.D., Lee, J.E., McDowell, F.H. Methyldopa as an adjunct to levodopa treatment of Parkinson's disease. *Clin. Pharmacol. Ther., 13*:24–27, 1962.

77. Celesie, G.G., Barr, A.N. Psychosis and other psychiatric manifestations of levodopa therapy. *Arch. Neurol., 23*:193–200, 1970.

78. McDowell, F.H. Changes in behavior and mentation. In *L-dopa and Parkinsonism*, Barbeau, A., McDowell, F.F. (eds.). Philadelphia: Davis, pp. 321–325, 1970.

79. McDowell, F.H. Treatment of Parkinson's syndrome with levodopa. *Ann. Intern. Med., 72*:29–35, 1970.

80. Yaryura-Tobias, J.A., Diamond, B., Merlis, S. The action of L-dopa on schizophrenic patients: a preliminary report. *Curr. Ther. Res., 12*:528–531, 1970.

81. Degkwitz, R., Binsack, K.F., Herkert, H. Zum Problem der persistierenden extrapyramidalen Hyperkinesen nach langfristiger Anwendung von Neuroleptika. *Nervenarzt, 38*:170–174, 1967.

82. Degkwitz, R. Uber die Ursachen der persisteirenden extrapyramidalen Hyperkinesen nach langfristiger Anwendung von Neuroleptika. *Act. Nerv. Super., 9*:389–400, 1967.

83. Chien, C.P., Cole, J.O. Eighteen-months follow-up of tardive dyskinesia treated with various catecholamine-related agents. *Psychopharmacol. Bull., 9*: 1973.

84. Chien, C.P., Jung, K., Ross-Townsend, A. Efficacies of agents related to GABA, dopamine and acetylcholine in tardive dyskinesia. (In press, *Psychopharmacol. Bull.,* 1977.)

85. Casey, E.D., Denney, D. Deanol in the treatment of tardive dyskinesia. *Am. J. Psychiatry, 132*:(8):864–867, 1975.

86. Davis, K.L., Hollister, L.E., Barchas, J.D., Berger, P.A. Choline in tardive dyskinesia and Huntington's disease. *Life Sci., 19*:1507–1516, 1976.

87. Linnoila, M., Viukari, M., Hietala, O. Effect of sodium valproate on tardive dyskinesia. *Br. J. Psychiatry, 129*:114–9, 1976.

41

Clinical Application of Receptor Modification Treatment

MURRAY ALPERT
and ARNOLD J. FRIEDHOFF

We are studying a novel treatment approach to tardive dyskinesia (TD) based on the assumption of an underlying pathogenic dopamine-receptor supersensitivity. The approach involves an attempt to reduce this hypothesized supersensitivity by temporarily increasing transmitter levels. It is expected that improvement will persist if normal sensitivity is reestablished and transmitter levels are permitted to return to their usual levels. Friedhoff, Rosengarten, and Bonnet have presented the rationale and basic animal data for this approach elsewhere in this volume. We are currently conducting studies to determine optimal parameters of the approach and can report at this time only impressions from the first 7 patients we have treated in open trials.

Patients are admitted to study only if they show at least mildly severe involvement of at least 3 of the facial and oral items on the Abnormal Involuntary Movement Scale (AIMS) after having been off neuroleptic medication for 3 months. This extended drug washout period is indicated because we have observed that a majority of patients (9 out of 12) who meet this criteria while receiving medication will show regression of dyskinetic signs within 6 weeks of drug discontinuation. Most patients show some transient worsening within a week or two of drug discontinuation. Sedatives are permitted as needed during the washout and treatment periods.

We are investigating the minimal dose and duration of treatment that is effective. We have had a good response with a dose of 6g per day administered over a 2-month period. With one patient, we found only partial improvement with a ten-day trial at 2g per day. A second trial with this patient at 3g per day for 2 weeks produced an excellent response.

L-dopa may produce some worsening in the patient's psychiatric condition, although we have found that this can be managed if the dose ranging proceeds very gradually. Some patients may actually show improvement in their psychiatric condition while on L-dopa (1). This is most likely to appear as a reduction in deficit symptoms in markedly asocial patients. Also it is not uncommon to find patients whose TD is mixed with parkinsonism. These patients may show improvement in the latter condition with the introduction of L-dopa.

Of the 7 patients treated thus far, 2 had to be discontinued because of side effects. One patient developed an allergic reaction involving flushing and rash to a mixture of L-dopa and carbidopa, and one patient had a grand mal seizure. The latter patient had a history of epilepsy, and a relationship between the seizure and the treatment could not be confirmed. For two other patients, administrative matters curtailed the treatment period. It was possible to continue at the maximal dose for only one week; they did not show signs of adaptation to the L-dopa during this period. When the L-dopa was withdrawn, their schizophrenia and their TD were as equally severe as at baseline. Of the other 3 patients, one showed a good, and two an excellent, response to the treatment.

Both of the patients with excellent reversal of TD have been followed, off-drug, for over 2 years without the return of TD signs. We have been fortunate in being able to manage these patients clinically without neuroleptic drugs during the follow-up period. All of the patients we have treated carry a primary diagnosis of schizophrenia, although it is our impression that they show an increased incidence of depressive signs, either by history or currently.

The use of L-dopa in schizophrenic patients is controversial, and we have addressed that issue in separate studies (1). In brief, we have noted that a group of schizophrenic patients do not appear to show much increase in schizophrenic signs, even at 6g per day of L-dopa, if that dose is achieved gradually. Where there is an increase in pathology, it is diffusely expressed; and it appears that schizophrenics may be vulnerable to psychotoxic effects of the treatment.

We also have questions as to the specificity of the relationship between oral dyskinesia and late-appearing drug withdrawal phenomena. We have noted a range of extrapyramidal changes following withdrawal from neuroleptic and anticholinergic drugs and feel that TD may be part of a spectrum of late-appearing phenomena. Using a sensitive quantitative measure of digital tremor, we have found, in a study of a homogeneous group of young female schizophrenics, a correlation between the amount of prior exposure to neuroleptic drugs and their amplitude of low-frequency tremor (2). These patients did not demonstrate oral dyskinesia. An increase in low-frequency tremor is a regular accompaniment of TD.

Tremographic evidence of withdrawal phenomena from anticholinergic drugs has also been noted (3). We have explored cholinergic pharmacologic manipulations in TD and have found that physostigmine can produce significant, transient improvement. The improvement did not appear attributable to the sedative or to other side effects of physostigmine. However, we were not able to demonstrate exacerbation of dyskinetic signs with anticholinergics (4).

In summary, there is considerable evidence that prolonged exposure to neuroleptic drugs can produce dopamine-receptor supersensitivity. Patients with TD show evidence of supersensitivity. In at least some cases of TD, attempts to reduce receptor supersensitivity have been associated with improvement.

However, the temporary salutory effect of physostigmine does not appear to be mediated via alteration of receptor supersensitivity, nor does the usual concept of a reciprocal interaction between dopaminergic and cholinergic processes (5) appear pertinent, at least in relation to the action of anticholinergic drugs.

In addition, there is a further observation which does not easily fit the supersensitivity model. While we have observed that L-dopa can exacerbate the profile of dyskinetic symptoms, it does not appear to produce a progression to new symptom involvement. A mildly dyskinetic patient on high doses of L-dopa need not develop the full oral-facial picture of the most severe patients with TD. In short, dopamine-receptor supersensitivity appears to be a necessary, but not a sufficient, prerequisite for TD.

REFERENCES

1. Alpert, M., Friedhoff, A.J., Marcos, L., Diamond, F. Paradoxical reaction to L-dopa in schizophrenics. *Am. J. Psychiatry,* (In press.)
2. Alpert, M. Tremography as a measure of extrapyramidal function in study of the dopamine hypothesis. In *Catecholamines and Behavior*, vol. 1, Friedhoff, A.J. (ed.). New York: Plenum Press, ch. 6, 1975.
3. Alpert, M., Diamond, F., Laski, E.M. Anticholinergic exacerbation of phenothiazine-induced extrapyramidal syndrome. *Am. J. Psychiatry, 133(9)*:1073–1075, 1976.
4. Alpert, M., Diamond, F., Friedhoff, A.J. Cholinergic mechanisms in tardive dyskinesia. *Biol. Psychiatry.* (In press.) Paper presented at annual meeting of Society of Biological Psychiatry, May 3-7, 1978.
5. Friedhoff, A.J., Alpert, M. A dopaminergic-cholinergic mechanism in production of psychotic symptoms. *Biol. Psychiatry, 6*(2): 165–169, 1973.

42

Clozapine in the Treatment of Tardive Dyskinesia: an Interim Report

LOU GERBINO
BARON SHOPSIN
and **MARIA COLLORA**

INTRODUCTION

Tardive dyskinesia has been one of the most persistent concerns in neuroleptic drug treatment because of its potential irreversibility; no *consistently* effective treatment for the syndrome has been found to date. Reviews of the current clinical information on the subject have been published (1–8).

Clozapine is a drug of the dibenzoxazepine group, whose chemical structure is given below in Figure 1.

It has been widely marketed throughout the world under the trade name of Leponex. It has a unique clinical profile in that it is a potent antipsychotic agent, although extrapyramidal reactions are nonexistent or rare (9–11). Animal studies also indicate that it does not meet the classic screening criteria for so-called neuroleptic drugs (12–14).

There have been anecdotal reports suggesting efficacy for clozapine in the treatment of tardive dyskinesia and intractable extrapyramidal symptoms. The present investigation was undertaken precisely to determine the effectiveness of this agent in the treatment of tardive dyskinesia, using a flexible dose schedule in an open study design.

MATERIALS AND METHODS

The study was divided into an inpatient phase of variable duration, but with

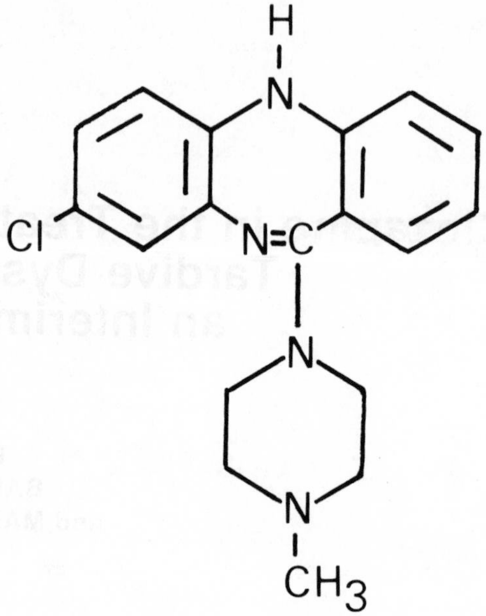

CLOZAPINE

Figure 1.

a minimum of one month of hospital treatment. The purpose of this phase was stabilization on medication. This was followed by an outpatient maintenance phase in those cases showing a satisfactory stabilization in hospital. Patients in this phase were required to continue for a total of at least one year to be considered as having completed the study.

Inpatient Phase

Thirty patients (15 male, 15 female), who had signed written informed consents, were admitted to the psychopharmacology inpatient unit where they were entered into the study. Twenty-five of these individuals carried the diagnosis of schizophrenia of various subtypes, and 5 were given the diagnosis of depressive neurosis. (Diagnoses were on the basis of DMS-II criteria). All but 2 patients demonstrated the classical abnormal involuntary movements of tardive dyskinesia. These consisted of facial grimacing, bucco-linguo-masticatory movements, athetoid movements of the neck, trunk, and extremities, or diaphragmatic dyskinesia. The remaining 2 patients were suffering from acute extrapyramidal symptoms refractory to antiparkinsonian agents. Patients ranged in age from 19 to 64, and most had been treated with neuroleptics for many years prior to entering the study. Also, some of the patients had been largely refractory to neuroleptic regimes in the past (Table 1). Patients with a history of seizures, drug or alcohol abuse, or debilitating physical illness were excluded, as were patients who had received ECT within the previous 6 months prior to the study. Patients who had been on psychotropic drugs were given a 14-day washout period prior to being entered into the study, and this period was extended to 6 weeks in cases where long-acting psychotropics had been used.

Prestudy laboratory criteria required that CBC, SMA-6, SMA-12, UA, and EKG all be within normal limits. An exception was made in the case of patient 17 (see Results).

After all inclusion criteria were met, each patient was started on clozapine tablets in divided doses, with a maximum of 900 mg daily permitted by the investigational protocol. In 3 patients this dose was exceeded, because in these cases the possible therapeutic benefits outweighed the potential risks. Dose adjustments were made at the discretion of the investigator based on clinical response and/or the occurrence of adverse effects. Tablets were all supplied by Sandoz Corporation in dosage strengths of 5, 10, 25, 50, 75, 100, and 150 mg. Although the dose schedule was flexible at our discretion, we devised a general modus operandi, as outlined in Table 2. No other psychoactive drugs were given. Patients were evaluated at baseline using an Abnormal Involuntary Movement Scale (AIMS), and a neurological rating scale for extrapyramidal symptoms. The AIMS was repeated at weekly intervals during this phase until the patient was stabilized. The neurological rating scales are completed monthly. Physical examinations were also performed at monthly intervals. Blood chemistries were repeated monthly, and CBCs were done twice a week. The patient's psychiatric status was assessed daily by the treating physician.

In order to be continued in the outpatient phase of the study, the patient's psychiatric status had to improve to the point where discharge and outpatient follow-up could be attained. Dischargeability on our unit depended on a variety of factors, including ability to care for oneself, reliability in compliance with medication regimes, ability to manage one's own money, and reliability in returning for follow-up.

Outpatient Phase

All patients who completed the inpatient phase were entered into the maintenance phase of the study. The purpose of this phase was to determine the continued efficacy and safety of the drug. In those cases showing total remission, dose reductions were attempted in order to establish minimum effective doses. To complete this phase, patients were required to maintain remission while being treated with clozapine as an out-patient, and to return for scheduled follow-up evaluations. Those who completed this phase were offered the option of continuing in treatment indefinitely.

RESULTS

Inpatient Phase

Of the 30 patients entered into the study, 6 patients (patients 2, 5, 9, 21, 23, and 30; see Table 1) did not complete the stabilization period. In 4 of these (9, 21, 23, 30; Table 1) the patient's psychiatric status did not improve to the point of dischargeability. One patient (2) was dropped because of the development of a toxic confusional state which precluded achieving effective dose levels. One patient (5) refused to cooperate with the treatment protocol. All 6 individuals who dropped out showed significant remission of dyskinetic symptoms as evidenced by at least a 75% reduction in total score on the AIMS; 4 of these patients experienced 100% remission.

Of the 24 patients who completed this phase, 2 (8 and 10) had their total daily dose raised beyond the 900 mg maximum permitted by the protocol. In both patients, a total body dyskinesia had been present for many years and was unremitting. At 1600 mg daily, patient 10 had a grand mal seizure, necessitating dose reduction to 1200 mg daily. He subsequently stabilized at this dose with a 75% reduction in dyskinetic movements, as measured by the AIMS. Patient 8 was increased to 1400 mg daily. She too suffered a grand mal seizure, and the dose was lowered to 1200 mg daily. At this dose the patient underwent a 95% remission of dyskinesia (AIMS) with no further adverse effects.

Patients 7, 15, 24 (Table 1) developed toxic confusional states at doses of 300 to 400 mg daily. These reactions responded to i.v. physostigmine, and disappeared with dose reduction. When the dose was raised more slowly, the confusional states did not recur despite the fact that total dose eventually exceeded the dose that had originally produced the reactions. Patient 15 began to display ataxia at a dose of 800 mg daily. He also began to manifest organic mental symptoms, e.g., memory loss and perceptual motor deficits, which had been masked by his psychiatric illness. Neurological consultations and computerized axial tomography were obtained, revealing the presence of a degenerative brain disease. The ataxia disappeared when the dose of clozapine was lowered to 700 mg daily, but approximately 10% of the dyskinetic movements were persistent at discharge. Patient 17, a 64-year-old woman, had suffered from disabling dyskinesia of the trunk and all four extremities. She had been treated for several years with fluphenazine decanoate. Prestudy examination revealed evidence of an old myocardial infarct and hypertension of 180/120. This patient was included in the study since it was felt that the benefits would outweigh the potential risks in her case. Her hypertension was treated with hydrodiuril 50 mg and Aldomet 250 mg t.i.d., concomitantly with clozapine 50 mg t.i.d. She underwent a complete remission of her psychiatric, neurologic, and hypertensive illness, and attempts to withdraw the clozapine led to a return of hypertension, which did not respond to an increase in the Aldomet dosage to 2g daily. It was therefore decided to keep her on the clozapine, and she was discharged on the above regime for follow-up.

The average dosage for all patients during the inpatient phase was 550–750 mg daily.

Outpatient Phase

Of the original 30 patients entered into the inpatient phase, 24 continued on to the outpatient, or maintenance, phase of the study. Seven such patients did not complete this part of the study; 3 (patients 3, 28, 29; Table 1) failed to return for clinic visits and were lost to follow-up. At the time of termination, they had all experienced a 100% remission of dyskinetic symptoms (AIMS). Two patients (19 and 20; Table 1) were terminated for administrative reasons; both had experienced an 80% to 90% remission of dyskinesia at the time that medication was withdrawn. One of these (20) remains free of abnormal movements at the time of this writing, 6 months after discontinuation of clozapine. One patient (16) dropped out voluntarily and was lost to follow-up; at the time of terminations, she had attained a 75% remission in dyskinetic symptoms (AIMS). One patient (18) experienced agranulocytoses (see Side-Effects section below).

Of the 17 patients who remained in the study, 3 patients (7, 25, 26; Table 1) are no longer in treatment; all 3 completed a year of treatment and were withdrawn from the clozapine with no recurrence or neurological symptomatology. They remain in remission at the time of writing, i.e., 3–6 months after discontinuation of clozapine. None of the 3 are presently on neuroleptic medication.

The remaining 14 patients remain under treatment with the drug. Dosage in each patient has been reduced to a mean 50%–60% of the maximum they had required with no recurrence of symptoms. Remission of dyskinetic symptoms in this group of patients remains at about 90%, as measured by the AIMS. It should also be noted that all these patients, with the sole exception of case 24, had suffered from psychotic symptomatology at baseline, which was ameliorated or reversed under clozapine treatment. They have achieved a significantly

Table 1

Patient	Sex	Age	Neurologic Diagnosis	Psychiatric Diagnosis	Previous Drug Treatment	Length of Previous Drug Treatment
1–GF	M	38	TD	schiz. CUT	neuroleptics	15 yrs
*2–JD	M	27	TD	schiz. CUT	neuroleptics	7 yrs
3–JM	M	41	TD	schiz. CUT	neuroleptics	15 yrs
4–MB	F	64	TD	schiz. CUT	neuroleptics	25 yrs
*5–RH	M	51	TD	schiz. simple	neuroleptics	22 yrs
6–DF	M	38	eps	schiz. para-noid type	neuroleptics	8 yrs
*7–CJ	F	64	TD	depressive neurosis	neuroleptics ECT	3 yrs
8–MK	F	30	TD	schiz., para-noid type	neuroleptics tricyclics	8 yrs
*9–JR	M	19	eps	schiz., para-noid type	neuroleptics	5 yrs
10–SR	M	25	TD	schiz., para-noid type	neuroleptics	6 yrs
11–EF	M	22	TD	schiz., CUT	neuroleptics	2 yrs
12–AP	F	40	TD	depressive neurosis	neuroleptics	1 yr
13–NF	F	34	TD	borderline syndrome	neuroleptics	6 mos
14–MBg	F	34	TD	schiz., schizo-affective	neuroleptics	4 yrs
15–DL	M	53	TD Alzheimers	OBS	neuroleptics ECT	2 yrs

*16–DW	F	58	TD	depressive neurosis	neuroleptics, amphetamines	10 yrs
17–JK	F	64	TD	schiz. CUT	neuroleptics	27 yrs
*18–ML	F	59	TD	schiz. CUT	neuroleptics	18 yrs
19–AM	M	33	TD	schiz. CUT	neuroleptics	8 yrs
*20–TR	F	53	TD	schiz. CUT	neuroleptics	10 yrs
*21–CE	M	27	TD	schiz. CUT	neuroleptics	9 yrs
22–CM	M	27	TD	schiz. CUT	neuroleptics	6 yrs
*23–ER	M	51	TD	schiz. CUT	neuroleptics, diazepam	16 yrs
24–HS	M	62	TD	depression	neuroleptics	8 mos
†25–CR	F	44	TD	depressive neurosis	tricyclics	2 yrs
*26–EH	F	63	TD	schiz. CUT	neuroleptics	4 yrs
27–IR	F	54	TD	schiz. CUT	neuroleptics	14 yrs
*28–MB	M	51	TD	schiz. CUT	neuroleptics ECT	2 yrs
*29–JM	F	47	TD	schiz., paranoid	neuroleptics	6 yrs
*30–MM	F	30	TD	schiz. CUT	neuroleptics	10 yrs

TD = Tardive Dyskinesia
OBS = Organic Brain Syndrome
Schiz. = Schizophrenic
CUT = Chronic undifferentiated subtype

Table 2
Dosage Schedule of Clozapine Used in the Study

Day	Dose
1	5 mg t.i.d.
2	10 mg t.i.d.
3	15 mg q.i.d.
4	20 mg q.i.d.
6	25 mg q.i.d.
8	50 mg t.i.d.
12	100 mg t.i.d.
13	100 mg q.i.d.
16	150 mg t.i.d.
18	200 mg t.i.d.
20	250 mg t.i.d.
22	300 mg t.i.d.

*This schedule should not be rigidly adhered to , but must be flexible and individually tailored to each patient's response. The maximum of 900 mg may not be required. We found that it was necessary to raise the dose rather aggressively to prevent the dyskinesia from breaking through early on in treatment. Although 900 mg per day was the maximum permitted by the protocol, we found that a maximum of 1200 mg daily could be used safely with added benefit and no increased risk of side effects.

higher level of functioning and general psychiatric well-being than under any previous therapy. Several patients have been able to return to work or school for the first time in years, and their object relations have become more satisfying and productive to the point of normality. A summary of final outcomes appears in Table 5.

SIDE EFFECTS

A summary of side effects appears in Table 3. All 30 patients complained of nocturnal salivation at some time during the study. Several patients found their pillows saturated upon waking in the morning, and some patients complained of being awakened gagging on their own saliva. This reaction did not occur in any patient during waking hours. The reaction tended to diminish over a period of months, but persisted to some degree in all the patients who remained on the drug. Dry mouth during daytime (awake) hours occurred in 3 patients. Transient sedation occurred in several patients, and postural hypotension occurred in 2 patients. These effects could be avoided by beginning at low doses (15–30 mg daily) and increasing at 10–20 mg increments every other day until a daily dose of 100–200 mg was reached. At that point, more aggressive increases could be made (50–100 mg daily) with no further incidence of sedation or hypotension. Toxic confusional states occurred in 5 patients. These reactions included confusion, disorientation, visual hallucinations, and incoherence, and were responsive to i.v. physostigmine. One patient (2) had to be dropped from the study because it proved impossible to raise his dose above 30 mg daily because of side effects. At this dose, the patient's dyskinesia had largely remitted, but his schizophrenic symptoms required intervention with neuroleptics. In the other 4 patients, the reactions disappeared with a dose reduction. When the dose was raised more slowly, the confusional states did not recur, despite the fact that total daily dosage eventually exceeded the dose level that had originally produced the reaction. Blurred vision occurred in 3 patients. These reactions were transient and mild (see Discussion). Two patients experienced grand mal seizures. In both cases the dose of clozapine had been raised above 1200 mg daily (1400 mg in patient 8, 1600 mg in patient 10). The dose was reduced to 1200 mg in each case with no further seizure activity, and both patients have continued on 1200 mg for one year with good control of both dyskinetic and psychotic symptomatology. Ataxia occurred in one patient at a dose of 800 mg daily. This patient was later found to have a degenerative brain disease which predated his entry into the study. On CAT scan, cerebellar atrophy was prominent. Reduction in dose to 700 mg daily resulted in complete remission of gait disturbance.

Tachycardia of 120 to 140 beats per minute occurred in 5 patients. In 4 of these the reaction was transient, remitting in 2 to 3 weeks; in one patient (1) the tachycardia persisted at 100 beats/min for 4 months, then gradually disappeared.

Agranulocytosis occurred in one patient. This was during the third month of treatment, after the patient had been stabilized in a dose of 600 mg daily for one month. This reaction occurred suddenly and was detected by one of the routine biweekly CBCs, which were performed as part of the study protocol. Clozapine was discontinued and the patient was admitted to the medical service where CBC and bone marrow biopsies revealed a complete absence of granulocytes and their precursors. The patient was kept in protective isolation on antibiotic coverage. She began manufacturing granulocytes again 8 days after the reaction was discovered, and was discharged on the tenth day, completely recovered. This patient had been off all psychoactive drugs for 4 months at the time of this writing, and has had no return of either dyskinetic or psychotic symptomatology. This case will be reported in detail elsewhere. All 30 patients showed transient leukocytosis. This reaction occurred at the beginning of treatment and at each subsequent dose increase. The increase was in the neutrophil count, which reached 70%–80%, with total WBC count as high as 22,000. Blood counts would return to normal in 4 to 6 weeks after no further dose increases were made. These data will be reported in a separate publication.

Table 3
Summary of Outcomes

Patient	Outcome (Inpatient phase)		Outcome (Outpatient phase)		Final Status
	Neurological	Psychiatric	Neurological	Psychiatric	
1	75% remission	50% remission	100% remission	100% remission	still in treatment
2	75% remission	deterioration	—	—	terminated during inpt phase
3	100% remission	75% remission	—	—	terminated—lost to follow-up
4	100% remission	75% remission	100% remission	90% remission	still in treatment
5	75% remission	no change	—	—	terminated voluntarily inpt; still in treatment
6	100% remission	80% remission	100% remission	100% remission	still in treatment
7	75% remission	no change	95% remission	no change	terminated without recurrence
8	75% remission	75% remission	90% remission	75% remission	still in treatment
9	100% remission	50% remission	—	—	terminated in inpt phase
10	100% remission	50% remission	50% remission	100% remission	terminated inpt phase
11	75% remission	100% remission	100% remission	100% remission	still in treatment
12	75% remission	100% remission	90% remission	100% remission	still in treatment
13	100% remission	75% remission	100% remission	90% remission	still in treatment
14	100% remission	75% remission	100% remission	90% remission	still in treatment
15	50% remission	unchanged	90% remission	unchanged	still in treatment
16	50% remission	unchanged	—	—	dropped out—lost to follow-up
17	75% remission	75% remission	100% remission	90% remission	still in treatment
18	75% remission	50% remission	100% remission	90% remission	dropped 2° agranulocytosis

					Outcome
19	75% remission	75% remission	90% remission	75% remission	terminated with recurrence of TD
20	75% remission	50% remission	90% remission	75% remission	terminated without recurrence
21	100% remission	no change	—	—	terminated—no recurrence of TD
22	100% remission	50% remission	100% remission	90% remission	still in treatment
23	75% remission	75% remission	—	—	terminated
24	50% remission	no change	75% remission	no change	still in treatment
25	75% remission	no change	100% remission	no change	terminated without recurrence
26	75% remission	50% remission	100% remission	90% remission	still in treatment
27	50% remission	50% remission	80% remission	90% remission	still in treatment
28	50% remission	50% remission	—	—	terminated—lost to follow-up
29	90% remission	50% remission	90% remission	75% remission	terminated—lost to follow-up
30	90% remission	25% remission	—	—	terminated—lost to follow-up

Table 4
Side Effects of Clozapine

Side Effect	Number of Patients Experiencing Side Effect	Outcome
Nocturnal salivation	30	Persisted moderately to severely, with some decrease after 6–8 months
Toxic confusional state	5	Reversed with i.v. physostigmine— disappeared with lowering of dose followed by slower dose increases— 1 patient terminated as a result
Dry Mouth	15	Transient
Blurred Vision	3	Transient
Sedation	5	Transient
Orthostatic Hypotension	3	Transient
Grand mal seizures	2	Disappeared with dose reduction
Agranulocytosis	1	Reversed when drug discontinued—pt. dropped from study
Leukocytosis	30	Transient, occurring at initiation of Rx and at each dose increase
Ataxia	1	Disappeared with dose reduction
Tachycardia	5	Transient

DISCUSSION

In the present population, and in the dose range used, clozapine proved to be a highly effective agent, significantly ameliorating the symptoms of psychosis and tardive dyskinesia. Some patients show a total remission—i.e., a total disappearance of TD symptoms. After the inpatient stabilization phase, patients were able to be maintained on clozapine over an extended period of time (up to 2 years, at the time of writing). The patients maintained on clozapine during this outpatient phase were able to have their dose reduced by up to 60% of the original inpatient dose without clinical deterioration or reemergence of TD symptoms, and some patients have been weaned off the drug without reappearance of TD. Clinical indications which were used for reducing dosage in the maintenance of the study were the side effects of daytime drowsiness and inability to awaken in the morning.

The best results in controlling the dyskinesia were obtained by a gradual but steady build-up of clozapine dosage so that the patient could develop tolerance to the side effects. This regimen is necessary to prevent breakthrough of symptoms; we have seen this breakthrough occur if the dosage is increased too slowly and/or if the dosage is plateaued too long at the dose at which a partial initial psychiatric symptomatic response is first seen. In summary, we have found that a steady dose increment during the initial treatment phase with clozapine is critical to assure a successful stabilization and reversal of TD symptoms.

As in two previous studies from this unit (15,16), clozapine continued to show excellent antipsychotic efficacy. Some of the patients treated with clozapine in this study were previously regarded as "treatment-resistant" to standard neuroleptics, and many of these patients also showed enhanced ability to function, improved object relationships, and increased socialization on the maintenance clozapine regimen.

Although previous studies (15,16) suggested that the inconvenient side effects of daytime drowsiness and sedation occurred with clozapine treatment, in the present study we saw relatively few instances of these symptoms. There was an equally low incidence of hypotension. The soporific effects of clozapine as a nighttime sedative were sustained, when h.s. loading doses were employed. The frequent occurrence of the side effect of excessive salivation during hours of sleep, with the pillow saturated on awakening in the morning, was found in the current study as it had been found in our prior series.

Previous studies examining the efficacy of drug treatment of tardive dyskinesia have been largely unrewarding. Even when a drug has shown some efficacy in reducing or abolishing TD symptoms in the first few weeks, continued use has usually not resulted in sustained improvement, and the patient's dyskinetic symptoms have often recurred. Considering the postulated mechanisms involved in causation of TD suggested by current theories, treatment of TD with traditional neuroleptic medication may be a treatment of "no return"; it would be predicted that ever-increasing doses of neuroleptics or amines depleters (such as reserpine or tetrabenazine) might be required to block or deplete dopamine at receptors each time dyskinetic symptoms break through again (17–26). The present study with clozapine, on the other hand, suggests that this drug is not only able to ameliorate it, but in many cases it totally reverses any clinical evidence of tardive dyskinesia. The fact that some patients have been totally weaned off of clozapine after a period of maintenance treatment without the recurrence of tardive dyskinesia symptoms suggests the possibility that clozapine may actually have a "curative," rather than only a suppresant, effect on TD. This could occur through a "renormalization" of the pathological, structural, or neurochemical changes in the CNS, induced by chronic treatment with traditional neuroleptics.

Clozapine appears clinically and pharmacologically unique as an antipsychotic in several respects. Unlike most other antipsychotic drugs, clozapine does not produce extrapyramidal symptoms, although it is an effective antipsychotic agent. It is also an effective treatment for tardive dyskinesia that is unresponsive to other remedial forms of treatment. It also appears that in some cases, if the patient's psychosis remits, clozapine may be withdrawn without TD symptoms recurring. In animal screening profiles, clozapine also differs from other antipsychotic drugs (12–14). Although it is markedly anticholinergic, clozapine produces excessive and profuse salivation during hours of sleep. Clozapine also appears to differ from other antipsychotic drugs in its antidopaminergic properties in certain regions of the brain. Although most other effective neuroleptics have dopamine-blocking properties in the tubuloinfundibular system in man, which results in a rise in serum prolactin when the drugs are given to humans, clozapine has not been shown to substantially or consistently raise serum prolactin levels in man (27,28).

The initial report presented in this chapter has discussed some of the results of an open study using a flexible dose schedule by a research team having extensive clinical experience with clozapine. This interim report will be followed by a more comprehensive and detailed analysis of the drug's effects, using standardized test scales from PRB-NIMH rating instruments. More extensive data relating to side effects will also be reported. However, we have felt the need to report these preliminary results at this time because of the implications of our findings for the treatment of an otherwise potentially irreversible neurological disorder which can result with long-term treatment with traditional neuroleptics.

ACKNOWLEDGMENTS

This work was supported by PHS–NIMH grant # MH029540–01. Reprint requests should be addressed to Dr. Shopsin.

REFERENCES

1. Kobayash, R.M. Drug therapy of tardive dyskinesia. *N. Engl. J. Med.*, *296*:5, 257–260, 1977.
2. Crane, G.E. The prevention of tardive dyskinesia. *Am. J. Psychiatry*, *134*:7, 756–759, 1977.
3. Fann, W.E., Stafford, J.R., Malone, R.L., Frost, J.D., Richman, B.W. Clinical research techniques in tardive dyskinesia. *Am. J. Psychiatry*, *134*:7, 759–763, 1977.
4. Smith, R.C., Tamminga, C.A., Haraszti, J., Chanshyam, N., Davis, J.M. Effects of dopamine agonists on tardive dyskinesia. *Am. J. Psychiatry*, *134*:7, 763–769, 1977.
5. Tamminga, C.A., Smith, R.C., Ericksen, S.E., Chang, S., Davis, J.M. Cholinergic influences on tardive dyskinesia. *Am. J. Psychiatry*, *134*:7, 769–775, 1977.
6. Crayton, J.W., Smith, R.G., Klass, D., Chang, S., Ericksen, S.E. Electrophysiological (H-reflex) studies of patients with tardive dyskinesia. *Am. J. Psychiatry*, *134*:7, 775–781, 1977.
7. Gerlach, J. The relationship between parkinsonism and tardive dyskinesia. *Am. J. Psychiatry*, *134*:7, 781–785, 1977.
8. Carroll, B.J., Curtiss, C.G., Kokmen, E. Paradoxical response to dopamine agonists in tardive dyskinesia. *Am. J. Psychiatry*, *134*:7, 785–790, 1977.
9. Angst, J., Bente, D., Berner, P. Das Klinische Wirkungsbild von Clozapin: Vatersuchung mit dem AMP-System. *Pharmakopsychiatr. Neuropsychopharmakol.*, *4*:201–211, 1971.

10. Gerlach, J., Koppelhus, P., Helweg, E. Clozapine and haloperidol in a single-blind crossover trial: therapeutic and biochemical aspects in the treatment of schizophrenia. *Acta Psychiatr. Scand.*, *50*:410–424, 1974.

11. Ayd, F.J. Clozapine: a unique new neuroleptic. *Int. Drug Ther. Newslett.*, *9*:5–12, 1974.

12. Burki, H.R., Eichenberger, E., Sayers, A.C., White, T.G. Clozapine and the dopamine hypothesis of schizophrenia, a critical appraisal. *Pharmakopsychiatr. Neuropsychopharmakol.*, *8*:115–121, 1975.

13. Wilk, S., Watson, E., Stanley, M.E. Differential sensitivity of 2 dopaminergic structures in rat brain to haloperidol and to clozapine. *J. Pharmacol. Exp. Ther.*, *195*(2):265–270, 1975.

14. Anden, N.E., Stock, G. Effect of clozapine on the turnover of dopamine in the corpus striatum and the limbic system. *J. Pharm. Pharmacol.*, *25*:346–348, 1973.

15. Matz, R., Rick, W., Oh, D., Thompson, H., Gershon, S. Clozapine—a potential antipsychotic agent without extrapyramidal manifestations. *Curr. Ther. Res.*, *16*:687–695, 194.

16. Shopsin, B., Klein, H. A double-blind controlled study of clozapine vs. chlorpromazine in schizophrenic inpatients. *Psychopharmacol. Bull.*, (In press).

17. Kazamatsuri, H., Chien, C.P., Cole, J.O. Long-term treatment of tardive dyskinesia with haloperidol and tetrabenazine. *Am. J. Psychiatry*, *130*(4):479–483, 1973.

18. Kazamatsuri, H., Chien, C.P., Cole, J.O. Treatment of tardive dyskinesia—clinical efficacy of a dopamine depleting agent, tetrabenazine. *Arch. Gen. Psychiatry*, *27*:95–99, 1972.

19. Claveria, L.E., Teychenne, P.F., Calne, D.B. Tardive dyskinesia treated with pimozinde. *J. Neurol. Sci.*, *24*:393–401, 1975.

20. Curran, D.J., Nagaswami, S., Mohan, K.J. Treatment of phenothiazine-induced bulbar persistent tardive dyskinesia with deanol acetamidobenzoate. *Dis. Nerv. Syst.*, *36*(2):71–73, 1975.

21. Fann, W.E., Lake, C.R., Gerber, C.J., McKenzie, G.M. Cholinergic suppression of tardive dyskinesia. *Psychopharmacologia (Berl.)*, *37*:101–107, 1974.

22. Linnoila, M., Viukari, M., Hietala, O. Effect of sodium valproate on tardive dyskinesia. *Br. J. Psychiatry*, *129*:114–119, 1976.

23. Gerlach, J., Thorsen, K., Munkvad, I. Effect of lithium on neuroleptic-induced tardive dyskinesia compared with placebo in a double-blind cross-over trial. *Pharmakopsychiatr. Neuropsychopharmakol.*, *8*:51–56, 1975.

24. Fann, W.E., Davis, J.M., Wilson, I.C. Methylphenidate in tardive dyskinesia. *Am. J. Psychiatry*, *130*:8, 922–924, 1973.

25. Curran, J.P. Management of tardive dyskinesia with thiopropazate. *Am. J. Psychiatry*, *130*:8, 925–927, 1973.

26. Klawans, H.L., McKendall, R.R. Observations on the effect of levodopa on tardive lingual-facial-buccal dyskinesia. *J. Neurol. Sci.*, *14*:189–192, 1971.

27. Gruen, P., Sachar, E., Langer, G., Prolactin response to neuroleptics in normals and schizophrenics. *Arch. Gen. Psychiatry*, (In press.)

28. Akkenheil, M., Matussek, N., Hippius, H., International Group for the Study of Affective Disorders, Munich, June 24, 1976.

43

Clozapine and Tardive Dyskinesia

GEORGE SIMPSON

INTRODUCTION

Clozapine is a dibenzodiazepine with the structure shown in Figure 1. It was one of a group of drugs discovered by Wander Laboratories in the early 1960's. Included in this group are antidepressants and conventional neuroleptics (1). However, clozapine differs from the other members of this group in a variety of ways. It depresses spontaneous activity in the mouse, rat and cat, but does not block apomorphine-induced gnawing in the rat (2). In this respect, it is similar to thioridazine but differs from it, having weak or absent cataleptic effects in the rat (2). In addition, it has a powerful anticholinergic effect (2). The ability to produce catalepsy and to block apomorphine are generally associated with neuroleptic activity. Further studies on clozapine revealed that there was no difference in regard to turnover of noradrenalin in the brain stem and dopamine in the corpus striatum as compared to other neuroleptics (3). However, clozapine increased HVA content in the corpus striatum (4), but selectively more so in the limbic system (5). When given apomorphine, rats, with a unilateral lesion in the striatum, indulged in circling behavior, which can be completely suppressed by classical neuroleptics (3). Clozapine has very little effect on this circling. Moreover, clozapine was able to block this effect when produced by haloperidol (3). Another interesting property of clozapine is that despite its powerful anticholinergic effect, it produces hypersalivation in animals and in humans (2,6). In these it also shows marked sedation, tachycardia and lowering of blood pressure (2,7). Delirium has also been reported to occur in humans when administered clozapine (8).

The above effects may be related to the surprising claims that clozapine had an antipsychotic effect but did not produce any extrapyramidal effects (7,8,9).

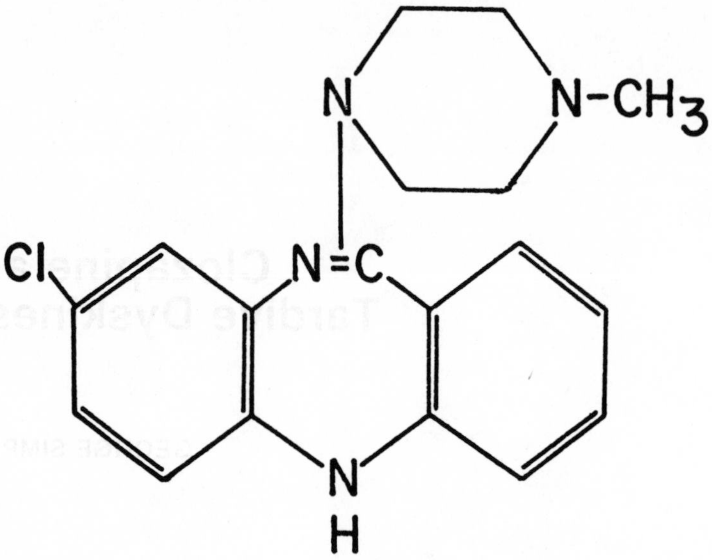

Figure 1.

This unique property of the drug immediately called into question the animal models and the conventional ideas of what was a "neuroleptic" (10). It is still unclear why or how the decision was made to test the drug in schizophrenic patients. It is also unclear as to why a drug, developed as early as 1962, had no reports on its activity published until 1966 (8). Indeed, a few more years were to pass before substantial reports were available to confirm these claims (5,7,11,12,13,14). Thereafter, claims appeared for its use in a variety of conditions, e.g., insomnia, depression, mania and psychopathy (15). In all of the studies carried out, the absence of EPS was consistently reported.

CLOZAPINE AND EXTRAPYRAMIDAL SYMPTOMS

In 1974 a thorough evaluation of the potential for producing EPS was carried out in a group of chronic schizophrenic patients who received slowly increasing dosages of clozapine (16). The patients received placebo followed by treatment period, and then a 4-week placebo period in a single blind trial. Included in the evaluation was a neurological rating scale for signs of parkinsonism (17) and an evaluation of handwriting samples. It was confirmed that clozapine had antipsychotic activity, whereas the rating scale for extrapyramidal side effects showed the presence of a nonspecific tremor and increased salivation. Handwriting changes and rigidity, routinely found during neuroleptic administration, were absent. Two patients included in the study had tardive dyskinesia during the placebo period, which disappeared when they received clozapine and showed a rebound when the patients were withdrawn (16). This exacerbation or rebound phenomenon was associated with clouding of consciousness, which disappeared rapidly (i.e., within 2 weeks). The dyskinesias, which were exaggerated during this time, also remitted to their baseline level. In that same year, Ruther also commented on the ability of clozapine to suppress tardive dyskinesia (18). Gerlach et al, in a comparison of clozapine and haloperidol, claimed clozapine, in a contrast to haloperidol, did not induce the so-called extrapyramidal side effects "hypokinesia, rigidity, akathisia, tremor and tardive dyskinesia" (13). However, one year later these same authors, in a study of eight schizophrenic patients, claimed that clozapine had no definite effect on tardive dyskinesia in any patient (14). On the basis of the biochemical effects, namely the effect of clozapine on HVA and 5HIAA in the CSF, the authors did claim that clozapine would not produce tardive dyskinesia (14). However, it should be noted that this study lasted for 20 days only, and the upper limit of clozapine was 225 mg (13). In a second study we selected 12 hospitalized patients with moderate tardive dyskinesia. Each patient had both facial involvement and choreoathetoid movements of the limbs. Only 7 patients completed the study (19). These patients were evaluated using two rating scales for tardive dyskinesia (20,21) as well as a rating scale for extrapyramidal side effects (17). Twenty weeks of clozapine treatment was preceded and followed by 2 weeks of placebo administration. A starting dose of 10 mg b.i.d. was increased at weekly intervals to a final dose range of 900 mg; the actual dose ranged from 20 mg to 900 mg. The results showed considerable fluctuation over the trial but with a downward trend in all ratings, particularly pronounced in the second half of the trial, and with a marked rebound during the final 2-week placebo period (Fig. 2). During the placebo withdrawal period, the symptoms of tardive dyskinesia became worse, in some cases worse even than during the baseline period in some patients associated with a toxic confusional reaction. After 2 weeks, the patients again reached baseline conditions. It was noted that improvement in general began when dosages reached 300 to 400 mg daily. The results, while convincing, were not impressive, but the subjects were chronically hospitalized patients who had received large amounts of neuroleptics, who had well-marked tardive dyskinesia at the baseline period, and who may indeed take a long time to improve, if ever.

Unfortunately, reports of clozapine-produced agranulocytosis in Finland led to curtailment of its use (22). A report of similar findings in the United States led to a very limited use. At the time of writing it is to all intents and purposes no longer in the United States. A number of investigators who specifically studied the effects of clozapine on tardive dyskinesia in the United States reported positive results in general. Small (23), in a study that included 10 patients with abnormal movements, found that in all cases clozapine was

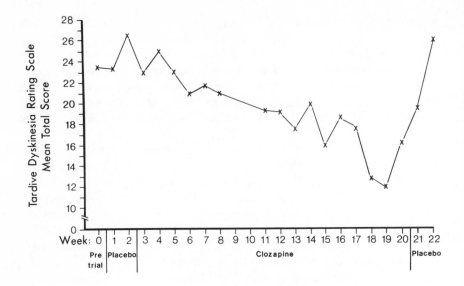

Figure 2. Effect of clozapine on T.D. (n=7)

associated with a marked reduction or disappearance of the dyskinesias. When clozapine was stopped the motor disturbance recurred. Cole (24) treated 25 patients with tardive dyskinesia and reported that in general, the drug had a mild to moderate effect in reducing dyskinesias. The best effects occurred in patients who had been on the treatment for more than 3 months, 2 of which showed complete remission. Several other investigators who used clozapine in patients suffering from tardive dyskinesia reported that in most cases it was beneficial and in no case was there a worsening.

DISCUSSION

The slow appearance and rapid eclipse of clozapine as an antipsychotic agent is in many ways as startling as its unique properties. On the basis of numerous reports, including controlled studies, it is an active antipsychotic agent that produces no parkinsonian rigidity. This latter has also been shown in open and double-blind, controlled studies. Because of biochemical effects of reduced HVA and 5HIAA concentrations in the CSF and failure to produce a withdrawal dyskinesia, it was postulated that clozapine would not cause tardive dyskinesia. Equally important would be the suppression of tardive dyskinesia.

Many agents have been claimed to benefit tardive dyskinesia in open studies and yet failed to stand up to a controlled trial. The number of patients treated with clozapine, the length of time treated, and the severity of the tardive dyskinesia treated support the claim that it has a beneficial effect on tardive dyskinesia.

Thus, there are several open studies and anecdotal reports concerning the efficacy of clozapine in reducing or eliminating tardive dyskinesia. Although almost all of the reports were positive, there were some slight discrepancies in the findings. The heterogeneity of patients treated, dosages, and length of trial make this understandable. Gerlach's study (14), which reported negative findings, used a small dose for a short period of time. The studies of Simpson and Cole suggest that higher dosages and longer time periods would be necessary to demonstrate efficacy. Neither of these authors reported more than a modest effect of clozapine on tardive dyskinesia. However, even this would be a remarkable advance in treating schizophrenia and tardive dyskinesia. It is therefore unfortunate that no rigorously controlled trial against placebo or a conventional neuroleptic is available to demonstrate convincingly whether clozapine does or does not suppress, cure, or even cause tardive dyskinesia.

Clozapine is a unique antipsychotic agent that no doubt will be the forerunner of many similar types of agents. Despite the difficulties produced by agranulocytosis, many investigators feel that it should be available and has a place for the selective treatment of patients who are very sensitive to conventional neuroleptics or for young people who show dyskinetic symptoms on conventional neuroleptics. The evidence that clozapine has a beneficial effect on tardive dyskinesia is, to this writer, quite convincing.

REFERENCES

1. Bente, D., Engelmeier, M.-P., Heinrich, K., Hippius, H., and Schmitt, W. Clinical studies on a new group of tricyclic neuroleptics. *CINP Neuro-Psycho-Pharmacol.* 5th, Washington, D.C. 1966. pp. 977–983, 1967.

2. Stille, G., Lauener, H., Eichenberger, E. The pharmacology of 8-cholro-11-(4-methyl-1-piperazinyl) 5H-dibenzo (b,e) (1,4) diazepine (clozapine). *Farmaco*, Ed. prat *26*, 603–625, 1971.

3. Honigfeld, Gilbert, Ph.D., Sandoz. Clozapine. International perspectives on a new psychotropic drug. New Jersey, March 1, 1977.

4. Bartholini, G., Haefely, W., Jalfre, M., Keller, H.H., Pletscher, A. Effects of clozapine on cerebral catecholaminergic neurone systems. *Br. J. Pharmacol.*, *46*:736–741, 1972.

5. Anden, N.E., Stock, G. Effect of clozapine on the turnover of dopamine in the corpus striatum and in the limbic system. *J. Pharm. Pharamacol.*, *25*: 346–348, 1973.

6. Gross, H., Langner, E. The neuroleptic 100-129/HF-1854 (clozapine) in psychiatry. *Int. Pharmacopsychiatry*, 1974.

7. Berzewski, H., Helmchen, H., Hippius, H., Hoffmann, H., Kanowski, S. The clinical spectrum of activity of a new dibenzodiazepine derivative. *Arzneim.-Forsch.* (Drug Res), *19*:495–496, 1969.

8. Gross, H., Langner, E. The activity profile of a novel broad-spectrum neuroleptic of the benzodiazepine group. *Wien. Med. Wochenschr.*, *40*:814–816, 1966.

9. Gross, H., Langner, E. Clinical evaluation of a neuroleptic from the benzodiazepine series: 9-chloro-11-(4'methyl)-piperazino-5-dibenzo (b.e.) (1,4) diazepine, W 108/HF 1854. *Arzneim.-Forsch.* (Drug Res.), *19*:496–498, 1969.

10. Stile, G., Hippius, H. A critical assessment of the concept of neuroleptics. *Pharmakopsychiatr., Neuropschopharmakol., 4:*182-191, 1971.

11. Angst, J., Bente, D., Berner, P., Helmann, H., Helmchen, H., Hippius, H. Das klinische wirkungsbild von clozapin. *Pharmakopsychiatr., Neuropsychopharmakol., 4:* 201–211, 1971.

12. Angst, J., Jaenicke, U., Padrutt, A., Scharfetter, C. Ergebnisse eines doppelblindversuchs von clozapin (8-chlor-11-(4-methyl-1-piperazinyl) -5 H-dibenzo (b,e) (1,4) diazephin) im vergleich zu levomepromazin. *Pharmakopsychiatr. Neuropsychopharmakol., 4:* 192–200, 1971.

13. Gerlach, J., Koppelhus, P., Helweg, E., Monrad, A.V. Clozapine and haloperidol in a single-blind cross-over trial: therapeutic and biochemical aspects in the treatment of schizophrenia. *Acta Psychiatr. Scand., 50:*410–424, 1974.

14. Gerlach, J., Thorsen, U., Fog, R. Extrapyramidal reactions and amine metabolites in cerebrospinal fluid during haloperidol and clozapine treatment of schizophrenic patients. *Psychopharmacologia* (Berl.), *40:*341–350, 1975.

15. Ayd, F.J., (ed.). Clozapine: a unique new neuroleptic. In *International Drug Therapy Newsletter*, 9 (2 and 3), 1974.

16. Simpson, G.M., Varga, E. Clozapine—a new antipsychotic agent. *Current Ther. Res., 16, 7,* July 1974.

17. Simpson, G.M., Angus, J.W.S. A rating scale for extrapyramidal side effects. *Acta Psychiatr. Scand.* [Suppl.], 212: 1970.

18. Rüther, E. Leponex-Rundtischgespräch. *Psychiatrische Klinik der FU Berlin, 14:* 12, 1974.

19. Simpson, G.M., Lee, J.H. Shrivastava, R.K. Clozapine in tardive dyskinesia. *Psychopharmacology, 56:*75–80, 1978.

20. National Institute of Mental Health, Psychopharmacology Research Branch: Development of a dyskinetic movement scale. *ECDEU Intercom. 4, 1:*3–6, 1975.

21. Simpson, G.M., Lee, J.H., Zoubok, B., Cole, J., Gardos, G. A rating scale for tardive dyskinesia. (Submitted for publication, 1978.)

22. Idanpaan-Heikkila, J., Alhava, E., Olkinoura, M., Ilmari, P. Clozapine and agranulocytosis. *Lancet,* September 27, p. 611, 1975.

23. Small, Joyce G., M.D. (Personal communication, 1978.)

24. Cole, Jonathan, M.D. (In press, 1978).

44

Effect of Haloperidol, Haloperidol + Biperiden, Thioridazine, Clozapine, Alpha-Methyl-P-Tyrosine, and Baclofen on Tardive Dyskinesia

J. GERLACH
P. KRISTJANSEN
and T. RYE

In the study of neurological side effects related to the neuroleptic treatment of psychiatric patients, some important problems are still unsolved and demand further investigation.

1. Are some neuroleptic drugs more likely than others to induce tardive dyskinesia?

2. Will an anticholinergic treatment (either inherent in the neuroleptic drug or given as a concomitant anti-Parkinson drug) inhibit or facilitate the development or the intensity of tardive dyskinesia after withdrawal of the combined neuroleptic-anticholinergic treatment?

3. Do antidopaminergic drugs with a presynaptic action influence hyperkinetic movements and psychotic symptoms in another way than traditional receptor-blocking neuroleptics?

We have tried to elucidate these problems in clinical pharmacological studies of receptor-blocking neuroleptics biperiden, alfa-methyl-p-tyrosine, and baclofen.

HALOPERIDOL, HALOPERIDOL + BIPERIDEN, THIORIDAZINE, AND CLOZAPINE

In a crossover trial, 16 psychiatric patients (10 females and 6 males, ages

497

between 66 and 90 years, median 74) with tardive dyskinesia were treated with haloperidol, haloperidol + biperiden, thioridazine, and clozapine (1). On account of the cardiovascular state of several of these elderly patients, only 7 were included in the clozapine part of the trial.

The trial was so arranged that each patient would first be treated with thioridazine for 3 months. After 4 weeks without medicine, the patients were submitted to 4 further different types of neuroleptic treatments, all of 4 weeks' duration and all interrupted by 4 weeks without medicine. The patients received haloperidol or haloperidol + biperiden in randomized sequence, then the alternative treatment, then thioridazine, and finally clozapine. The median doses were 5.25 mg of haloperidol, in one period supplemented with 6 mg of biperiden. The median dose of thioridazine was 225 mg, and of clozapine 75 mg. When a higher dose of clozapine was attempted, the patients became markedly sedated.

The tardive dyskinesia syndrome and the parkinsonism were studied weekly during the whole study by means of videotape recordings from which the results were later blindly evaluated.

Antihyperkinetic effect. Figure 1 shows the total hyperkinesia score during the whole study. Compared with the respective pretreatment values, the mean hyperkinesia score was significantly reduced during treatment with haloperidol, haloperidol + biperiden, and thioridazine. The score during treatment with haloperidol was lower than during treatment with both haloperidol + biperiden and thioridazine, but the score during thioridazine was lower than during haloperidol + biperiden. It should be noted that the hyperkinesia score at the end of the initial thioridazine period was significantly lower than at the end of the later thioridazine period. However, the continuing decline of the curve during the second thioridazine period might suggest that the hyperkinesia score would have further decreased if the treatment had continued.

Treatment with clozapine slightly reduced the hyperkinesia score in 5 of the 7 patients included in this part of the study. In spite of slight sedation, the effect of clozapine was less than the effect obtained by other treatments. Only in one patient was the hyperkinesia score clearly reduced, but this patient showed marked sedation on clozapine, 12.5 mg in the morning and 25 mg in the evening.

Effect of treatment withdrawal. The hyperkinesia score was significantly lower after the initial thioridazine period than after all the following periods of treatment. On the other hand, there was no significant difference between the withdrawal hyperkinesia after the second thioridazine period and after the two haloperidol periods. The increase in the withdrawal hyperkinesia from the first to the second thioridazine period might be related to the difference in the duration of the treatment periods (3 months versus 4 weeks). However, as the duration of neuroleptic treatment appears to be positively correlated to the

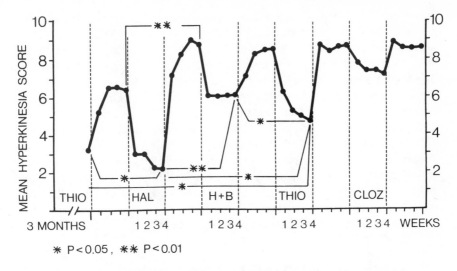

* P<0.05 , ** P<0.01

Figure 1. Mean hyperkinesia score of 16 patients with tardive dyskinesia at the end of treatment with thioridazine (THIO) for months, and during and following treatment with haloperidol (HAL), haloperidol + biperiden (H + B) (the last two mentioned in randomized sequence), thioridazine and clozapine (CLOZ), the last 4 treatment periods for 4 weeks, each interrupted by 4-week drug-free periods (see text).

Statistics: Wilcoxon's test for paired differences.

development of tardive dyskinesia (2,3), it is possible that the increase in the withdrawal hyperkinesia is due to a long-term effect of haloperidol, including the so-called dopaminergic receptor hypersensitivity. If this assumption can be confirmed in other studies, our observations might imply that haloperidol has a greater capacity to induce tardive dyskinesia than thioridazine. This is in accordance with animal studies, showing that the degree of dopaminergic hypersensitivity is related to the degree and the duration of dopamine receptor blockade (4,5), and that tardive dyskinesia in monkeys is related to earlier acute dystonia and parkinsonism (6).

Effect of anticholinergic drugs. During the combined treatment with haloperidol + biperiden, the hyperkinesia score was increased, compared to that of haloperidol alone. On the other hand, no significant difference was found in the intensity of the tardive dyskinesia after withdrawal of haloperidol and after withdrawal of haloperidol + biperiden. Eight patients scored less after haloperidol + biperiden than after haloperidol alone, while 3 patients scored less after haloperidol than after haloperidol + biperiden. If there is a real difference, much longer periods of investigation will undoubtedly be required in order to clarify this problem.

In animal studies, Smith and Davis (7) found that behavioral dopaminergic hypersensitivity after treatment for 7 weeks with haloperidol + benztropine was less than after haloperidol alone, while Sayers *et al.* (8) found a slightly accentuated dopaminergic hypersensitivity when haloperidol was combined with atropine for 6 days. Neither Tarsy and Baldessarini (9) nor Christensen and Møller Nielsen (5), however, found any difference between dopaminergic hypersensitivity after treatment with neuroleptics with or without concomitant anticholinergic drugs. This, together with our observations, suggests that anticholinergic drugs administered with neuroleptics do not involve any real risk of accentuating tardive dyskinesia *after termination* of treatment. Furthermore, there is an important practical aspect of the matter: By reducing possible parkinsonism, an anticholinergic treatment given as supplement to a neuroleptic therapy might improve our chances of uncovering tardive dyskinesia at an early stage, and thereby provide a better opportunity of preventing the development of irreversible tardive dyskinesia.

ALPHA-METHYL-P-TYROSINE AND BIPERIDEN

Tardive dyskinesia is mainly localized in the oral area as the so-called bucco-linguo-masticatory (BLM) syndrome (10). These oral dyskinesias may be described with respect to the following movements elements: frequency (or degree of hypermotility when frequency cannot be measured), amplitude, and duration of each separate tongue protrusion and/or mouth opening (11). The relationship among these elements differs from patient to patient. At times the tongue protrusions are rapid and rhythmic, and at times they are slow and prolonged.

These oral movement elements were studied in 24 psychiatric patients with tardive dyskinesia during treatment with alpha-methyl-p-tyrosine (AMPT, an inhibitor of the catecholamine synthesis), 4g daily for 3 days, and biperiden, 12 mg daily for 3 weeks (11). The study was carried out with crossover design and blind evaluation of the results with the help of video technique.

Frequency/hypermotility of the BLM syndrome. Figure 2 shows the results of the study. AMPT caused a clear (average 51%) reduction in frequency/hypermotility ($p < 0.01$). In general, the movements became slower, and in 7 cases stopped entirely. In contrast, biperiden significantly increased (average 93%) the hypermotility of the BLM syndrome ($p < 0.01$), the movements becoming rapid and frequent. In only 2 cases, which were treated with clozapine, 75 and 225 mg, respectively, did biperiden leave the dyskinesias unchanged.

Amplitude of the BLM syndrome. AMPT reduced the amplitude in 10 of the 24 patients. In one case only the reduction was total; otherwise, a slight tongue protrusion and/or mouth opening remained during the recordings. In 12 cases the amplitude remained unchanged, and in 2 others—the 2 youngest

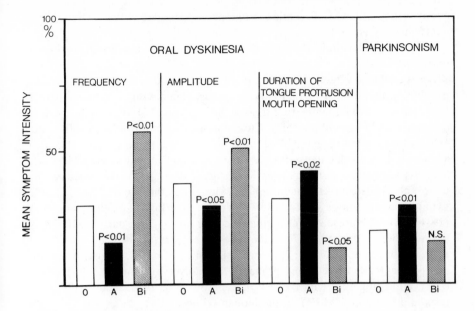

Figure 2. Oral dyskinesia and parkinsonism in 24 patients before treatment (0) and during treatment with AMPT (A) and biperiden (Bi).

Statistics: Wilcoxon's test for paired differences.

patients (21 and 26 years), treated with flupenthixol 8 mg daily, and haloperidol 12 mg daily, and penfluridol 80 mg weekly, respectively—it was increased by AMPT. In these two patients the syndrome was characterized by a clearly permanent, slight tongue protrusion, accompanied by a pronounced mouth opening; there were no evident signs of parkinsonism. Biperiden significantly ($p < 0.01$) increased the amplitude of the BLM syndrome.

Duration of tongue protrusion and mouth opening. AMPT increased the duration of each separate tongue protrusion and/or mouth opening in 7 cases; otherwise, the duration was unchanged. Nevertheless, in some cases the total protrusion time decreased because the total number of individual protrusions was reduced. Biperiden reduced the duration ($p < 0.05$) corresponding to the increased motility. In one case only was the duration increased.

Parkinsonism. Fifteen of 24 patients showed clear signs of parkinsonism. AMPT significantly increased the Parkinson score ($p < 0.01$). All the classical parkinsonian features (hypokinesia, rigidity, tremor, salivation) were either induced or aggravated. Three patients being treated with flupenthixol decanoate 100 mg weekly, perphenazine decanoate 150 mg weekly, and penfluridol 100 mg weekly, respectively (relatively high doses of specific antidopaminergic depot neuroleptics), showed the most intense reaction after the administration of AMPT, while the two patients treated with clozapine were unaffected by AMPT.

Biperiden had a clinically relevant, but in this sample not significant effect on the parkinsonism.

Antipsychotic effect. There is some indirect evidence suggesting certain psychoses, including schizophrenia, to be associated with a relative hyperactivity within some dopaminergic areas in the brain (12,13). If this hypothesis is correct, AMPT should diminish schizophrenic symptoms and potentiate the effect of dopamine-receptor blocking drugs. Several studies within this area are now indicating that in itself AMPT has no certain antipsychotic effect (14), and that added to a high neuroleptic dosage it does not further increase the antipsychotic effect of the neuroleptic (15); on the other hand, AMPT is able to potentiate the antipsychotic effect of a reduced dosage of a neuroleptic drug (16,17,18). The present three studies indicate that 2–3 mg daily AMPT may permit a 60%–70% reduction in the otherwise necessary dosage of different neuroleptic drugs. However, this potentiation also includes most, if not all, neurological side effects, and probably the tardive dyskinesia as well. This observation, together with the risk of nephrotoxicity (19), reduces the long-term application of AMPT in the human clinic.

BACLOFEN

Baclofen (Lioresal®), the parachloro-phenyl analogue of GABA, was originally thought to be a GABA-agonist. Thus it was shown that baclofen (1) inhibits the release of dopamine into the synaptic cleft, (2) increases the brain concentration of dopamine, and (3) counteracts the pimozid-induced increase in dopamine turnover (20). These biochemical effects correspond to the effect of GABA-agonists. Further studies, however, have shown that baclofen fails to act as a GABA-receptor agonist (21). Different hypotheses concerning the mechanism of action of baclofen have been proposed, but the exact mechanism of action of baclofen on the dopaminergic processes remains to be elucidated.

In a double-blind crossover study, 18 chronic psychiatric patients (ages 47–79 years, median 66) with tardive dyskinesia were treated in a randomized sequence with baclofen and placebo (22). Baclofen and placebo were each given for 3 weeks; effects were evaluated with the aid of videotape at the end of each phase.

The study showed that baclofen (20–120 mg/day, median 75 mg) had both antihyperkinetic and parkinsonism-eliciting effects. The antihyperkinetic effect, however, was only moderate (average 42%, p <0.05). Figure 3 shows the mean scores of the three movement elements of oral dyskinesia and parkinsonism. Frequency was reduced in 10 out of 18 patients, and unchanged in 8. Amplitude was reduced in 8 patients and was unchanged in 10. The duration of

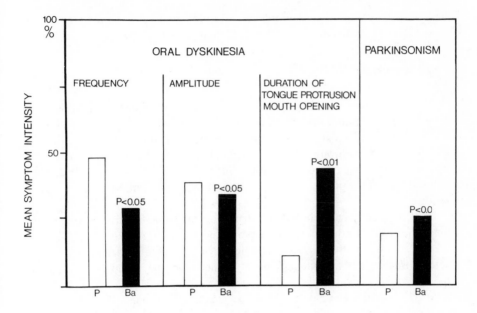

Figure 3. Oral dyskinesia and parkinsonism in 18 patients during treatment with baclofen (Ba) and placebo (P).

Statistics: Wilcoxon's test for paired differences.

each mouth opening was increased in 9 patients and unchanged in 9. Korsgaard (23) found a more pronounced antihyperkinetic effect of baclofen.

Two-thirds of the patients in our study showed obvious signs of parkinsonism together with tardive dyskinesia. Baclofen slightly but significantly increased parkinsonism; bradykinesia was aggravated in 4 patients, rigidity in 2, tremor in 5, and akathisia in 5.

In antihyperkinetic doses, baclofen, however, has considerable side effects. In this study, 50% of the patients showed signs of sedation, and 50% showed signs of confusion. Elderly patients were especially sensitive to these side effects, so that even modest increases in dosage could immobilize the patient for several days. Even though these side effects may be reduced a little by very slow increases in dosage, they are obviously limiting the practical usefulness of the drug in the treatment of elderly patients with tardive dyskinesia.

Antipsychotic effects. Originally, baclofen was found in combination with neuroleptics to have a marked antipsychotic effect in the treatment of schizophrenic patients (24). Later studies, however, have failed to confirm the antipsychotic effect of baclofen, whether administered alone (25,26) or given together with traditional neuroleptic drugs (27). In some cases the psychotic symptoms seem to aggravate during baclofen treatment (26). On the other hand Gulman *et al.* (27) in a double-blind randomized study found a significant anxiolytic effect of baclofen in the treatment of schizophrenic patients.

CONCLUSION

1. After withdrawal of thioridazine, the tardive dyskinesia syndrome was less than after withdrawal of haloperidol, with or without biperiden (see Fig. 1). This might suggest stronger dopamine-receptor-blocking neuroleptics to be more potent as producers of the pathophysiological alterations of tardive dyskinesia than weaker dopamine-receptor blockers. There are animal data supporting this assumption, but long-term studies with humans or monkeys are required.

2. Biperiden (an anticholinergic drug) increased the hypermotility and the amplitude of the tardive dyskinesia syndrome *during treatment* (Fig. 2), but 4 weeks' treatment with biperiden did not significantly influence the syndrome *after withdrawal* of treatment (Fig. 1). We need long-term studies on this point as well.

3. Haloperidol had a better antihyperkinetic effect than either haloperidol + biperiden or thioridazine, all for 4 weeks, but by prolonged treatment the antihyperkinetic effect of thioridazine (Fig. 1) might be further increased.

4. Clozapine has only a slight antihyperkinetic effect in patients with irreversible tardive dyskinesia, less than thioridazine, and this effect may be due to the sedative action of the drug. In certain cases clozapine may aggravate the syndrome.

5. AMPT (an inhibitor of the catecholamine synthesis) has a moderate antihyperkinetic effect, less than haloperidol. Furthermore, AMPT potentiates the antipsychotic and parkinsonism-eliciting effect of a reduced dosage of a traditional neuroleptic treatment. However, due to the potential nephrotoxic effect of AMPT in the doses necessary for therapeutic effect, AMPT should not be used for long-term therapy.

6. Baclofen has a slight (less than AMPT) antihyperkinetic effect, which—like the effect of AMPT—mainly becomes apparent when the patient is treated with a dopamine-receptor-blocking neuroleptic. However, the sedation, confusion, and muscular weakness provoked by baclofen is reducing its value in the treatment of aged patients with tardive dyskinesia.

REFERENCES

1. Gerlach, J., Simmelsgaard, H. Tardive dyskinesia during and following treatment with haloperidol, haloperidol + biperiden, thioridazine and clozapine. *Psychopharmacology*. (In press.)

2. Crane, G.E. Factors predisposing to drug-induced neurologic effects. In *The Phenothiazines and Structurally Related Drugs.* Forrest, C.J., Usdin, E. (eds.). New York: Raven Press, pp. 269–279, 1974.

3. Gardos, G., Cole, J.P., La Brie, R.A. Drug variables in the etiology of tardive dyskinesia application of discriminant function analysis. *Prog. Neuro-Psychopharmaco., 1*:147–154, 1977.

4. Hyttel, J. Changes in dopamine synthesis rate in the supersensitivity phase after treatment with a single dose of neuroleptics. *Psychopharmacology, 51*:205–207, 1977.

5. Christensen, A.V., Moller Nielsen, 1. On the supersensitivity of DA-receptors after single and repeated administration of neuroleptics. In *Tardive Dyskinesia* Fann, Smith, Davis, Domino (eds.). New York: Spectrum Publications, (this vol.).

6. Gunne, L.-M., Barany, S. Haloperidol-induced tardive dyskinesia in monkeys. *Psychopharmacology, 50*:237–240, 1976.

7. Smith, R.C., Davis, M.D. Behavioral supersensitivity to apomorphine and amphetamine after chronic high dose haloperidol treatment. *Psychopharmacol. Commun., 1*:285–293, 1975.

8. Sayers, A.C., Bürki, H.R., Ruch, W., Asper, H. Anticholinergic properties of antipsychotic drugs and their relation to extrapyramidal side-effects. *Psychopharmacology, 51*:15–22, 1976.

9. Tarsy, D., Baldessarini, R.J. Behavioral supersensitivity to apomorphine following chronic treatment with drugs which interfere with the synaptic function of catecholamines. *Neuropharmacology, 13*:927–940, 1974.

10. Gerlach, J. Relationship between tardive dyskinesia, L-DOPA-induced hyperkinesia and parkinsonism. *Psychopharmacology, 51*:259–263, 1977.

11. Gerlach, J., Thorsen, K. The movement pattern of oral tardive dyskinesia in relation to anticholinergic and antidopaminergic treatment. *Int. Pharmacopsychiatry, 11*:1–7, 1976.

12. Randrup, A., Munkvad, I. Evidence indicating an association between schizophrenia and dopaminergic hyperactivity in the brain. *Orthomolecular Psychiatry, 1*:2–7, 1972.

13. Synder, S.H. The dopamine hypothesis of schizophrenia: focus on the dopamine receptor. *Am. J. Psychiatry, 133*:197–202, 1976.

14. Gershon, S., Hekimian, L.J., Floyd, A., Hollister, L.E. α-Methyl-p-tyrosine (AMT) in schizophrenia. *Psychopharmacologia, 11*:189–194, 1967.

15. Nasrallah, H., Donnelly, E., Bigelow, L., Rivera-Calimlim, L., Rogol, A., Potkin, S., Rauscher, F.P., Wyatt, R.J., Gillin, J.C. Inhibition of dopamine synthesis in chronic schizophrenia. *Arch. Gen. Psychiatry, 34*:649–655, 1977.

16. Wålinder, J., Skott, A., Carlsson, A. Potentiation by metyrosine of thioridazine effects in chronic schizophrenia. *Arch. Gen. Psychiatry, 33*:501–505, 1976.

17. Carlsson, A., Persson, T., Roos, B.E., Walinder, J., Skott, A. Further studies on the mechanism of antipsychotic action: potentiation by α-methyltyrosine of thioridazine effects in chronic schizophrenia. *J. Neural Trans*., *34*:125–132, 1973.

18. Magelund, G., Gerlach, J. The neuroleptic-potentiating effect of α-methylparatyrosine and haloperidol in the treatment of schizophrenia. A double-blind cross-over study of antipsychotic effect and side-effect of two catecholamine antagonists, a synthesis inhibitor and receptor blocking agent. (In preparation.)

19. Moore, K., Wright, P., Bert, J. Toxicologic studies wtth α-methyltyrosine, an inhibitor of tyrosine hydroxylase. *J. Pharmacol. Exp. Ther., 155*:506–515, 1967.

20. Anden, N.E., Wachtel, H. Biochemical effects of baclofen (B-parachloropheny-GABA) on the dopamine and the noradrenaline in the rat brain. *Acta Pharmacol.*

22. Gerlach, J., Rye, T., Kristjansen, P. Effect of baclofen on tardive dyskinesia. *Psychopharmacology.* (In press.)

23. Korsgaard, S. Baclofen (Lioresal ®) in the treatment of neuroleptic-induced tardive dys-
     kinesia. *Acta. Psychiat. Scand.*, *54*:17–24, 1976.
24. Frederiksen, P. Baklofen vid behandling av schizofreni—ett preliminärt meddelande.
     Läkartidningen, *72*:456–458, 1975.
25. Simpson, G., Branchey, M., Shrivastava, R. Baclofen in schizophrenia. *Lancet*,
     i:967–968, 1976.
26. Davis, K., Hollister, L., Berger, P. Baclofen in schizophrenia. *Lancet*, *i*:1245, 1976.
27. Gulman, N., Bahr, B., Andersen, B., Eliassen, H.M.M. A double-blind trial of baclofen
     against placebo in the treatment of schizophrenia. *Acta. Psychiatr.*, *Scand.*, *54*:287–293,
     1976.

45

Combination Treatment of Choreiform and Dyskinetic Syndromes with Tetrabenazine and Pimozide

RASMUS FOG
and **H. PAKKENBERG**

The treatment of patients with choreiform syndromes (such as Huntington's chorea) is difficult. Neurosurgical procedures have been used but are not always successful, and have shown only temporary effect in other cases. Furthermore, they can not be applied to patients of higher age without great risk.

Pharmacological treatment has, however, shown to be of great value. This treatment is theoretically based upon the dopamine hypothesis of movement disorders (especially Parkinson's disease), which was developed by Carlsson and coworkers (1). They suggested that a relative excess of dopamine in the basal ganglia is accompanied by a hyperkinesia (e.g., Huntington's chorea, bucco-linguo-masticatory [BLM] syndrome), whereas a reduced amount of dopamine results in hypokinesia (e.g., Parkinson's disease). Hornykiewicz (2), however, found that the dopamine content in the substantia nigra and corpus striatum was normal in patients with Huntington's chorea. It has, therefore, later been suggested that the dopaminergic receptor cells have an increased excitability (or hypersensitivity) to a normal level of dopamine, or that the turnover of dopamine is increased (or any combination of these two mechanisms).

A great amount of new evidence concerning the interaction of the various transmitter substances in the brain (acetylcholine, gamma-aminobutyric acid, 5-hydroxytryptamine, glutamic acid a.o.) have shown that a single substance in a single brain area cannot be held responsible for all movement disorders.

Nevertheless, dopamine still seems to play a central role in the treatment, at least from a practical clinical point of view. This is underlined by the fact that patients with other hyperkinetic syndromes, such as tardive dyskinesias and Gilles de la Tourette syndrome, also benefit from a pharmacological antidopaminergic treatment (3,4).

In 1960 it was reported that tetrabenazine (Nitoman®,Roche) had effect on choreiform movements (5,6), but also on persisting dyskinesia caused by psychopharmaca (7). Tetrabenazine has also been useful in other forms of hyperkinesia, e.g., the BLM syndrome (8), but the effect of the drug often diminishes after weeks or months, and it can totally disappear.

Tetrabenazine is a neuroleptic drug with antipsychotic properties. Like reserpine, it has a presynaptic antidopamine effect because of its inhibiting effect upon dopamine storage in the nerve terminals. In clinical use tetrabenazine has fewer side effects than reserpine.

Most neuroleptic drugs have a postsynaptic antidopamine effect. Drugs such as chlorpromazine, perphenazine, and haloperidol have blocking effect on dopamine-sensitive receptors in the brain. These drugs have also been used in the treatment of hyperkinetic disorders. But again, the effect often diminishes after weeks or months and can totally disappear.

We, therefore, felt that a treatment with a combination of these two types of drugs with different antidopamine effect might have a more lasting effect upon hyperkinesia. We have chosen tetrabenazine in combination with pimozide (which is a neuroleptic drug related to haloperidol, but with very few side effects).

In 1969 we performed a study with this combination treatment. We investigated 12 patients with Huntington's chorea, and 4 with BLM syndrome. The results are seen from Table 1. The patients with an oral dyskinesia had the best effect of the treatment. This result was confirmed by our second study (9): In this investigation, we treated 16 patients suffering from spontaneous oral dyskinesia with tetrabenazine, pimozide, or both. The results are seen in Table 2. The treatment period was at least 3 months. Again, the effect was best on oral symptoms.

The effect of the combined treatment seems more permanently efficient than the effect of one drug alone. Normally one would be reluctant of using more than one drug for one disease. In this case, however, the two drugs have the same end effect upon dopamine but in different sites of action. An advantage of such a combination therapy can, therefore, be that it is possible to use lower dosages of both drugs resulting in diminishing of the side effects. In these investigations, the most common side effect was slight sedation. Some patients reacted with a hypokinetic syndrome, but this was clearly dose-related and disappeared upon dose reduction.

There is a substantial amount of evidence for the importance of other neurotransmitters for the various dyskinesias. GABA (gamma aminobutyric

Table 1
Effect of Treatment with a Combination of Tetrabenazine and Pimozide on Huntington's Chorea and Tardive Dyskinesia

Hyperkinesia	No. of Patients	Disappearance of Symptoms	Moderate Effect	Weak Effect
Huntington's Chorea	12	6	4	2
BLM Syndrome	4	3	1	0

Dose range of tetrabenazine was 3–6 mg/day.
Dose range of pimozide was 37.5–75 mg/day.
Treatment period was 2–7 months.
The age of the patients varied from 39 to 92 years.

Table 2
Effect of Treatment with Tetrabenazine or Tetrabenazine Plus Pimozide on Spontaneous Oral Dyskinesia

Type of Dyskinesia	No. of Patients	Treatment	No. of Patients	Immediate Effect	Effect After 3 Months
Oral	9	tetrabenazine	2	†††	†
		tetrabenazine + pimozide	7	†††	†††
Oral and Extremity	5	tetrabenazine	2	††	(*)
		tetrabenazine + pimozide	3	††	††
Oral and Truncal	1	tetrabenazine	1	(†)	
Extremity	1	tetrabenazine + pimozide	1	0	0

The dosage of tetrabenazine was 40–75 mg daily.
The dosage of pimozide was 2–3 mg daily.

*Effect only upon oral symptoms.
††† indicates disappearance of symptoms. †† decrease in dyskinesia, and † weak effect upon symptoms.

acid) has an inhibiting effect on dopamine, and should also be suggested in the treatment of hyperkinetic disorders. Such attempts of "pharmacological manipulation" may add to our knowledge of biological mechanisms of hyperkinetic syndromes.

REFERENCES

1. Carlsson, A., Lundquist, M., Magnusson, T. 3,4-dehydroxyphenalanine and 5-hydroxtryptophan as reserpine antagonists. *Nature* (Lond.), *180*:1200, 1967.
2. Hornykiewicz, O. Gegenwartiger Stand der biochemischpharmakologischen Erforschung des extrapyramidal-motorischen Systems. *Pharmakopsychiat 1*:6–17, 1968.
3. Gerlach, J. Relationship between tardive dyskinesia, L-DOPA induced hyperkinesia and parkinsonism. *Psychopharmacologia, 51*:259–263, 1977.
4. Sweet, R.D., Bruun, R.D., Shapiro, A.K., Shapiro, E. The pharmacology of Tourette's syndrome. In *Clinical Neuropharmacology*. H.L. Klawans (ed.). New York: Raven Press, pp. 81-105, 1976.
5. Sattes, H. Die Behandlung der Chorea maior mit dem Monoamine Freisetzer Nitoman. *Psych. Neurol., 140*:13–19, 1960.
6. Brandrup, E. Reserpin og tetrabenazin ved chorea Huntington. *Nord. Med., 64*:968–969, 1960.
7. Brandrup, E. Tetrabenazine treatment in persisting dyskinesia caused by psychopharmaca. *Amer. J. Psychiatry, 118*:551–552, 1961.
8. Pakkenberg, H., Fog, R. Spontaneous oral dyskinesia. Result of treatment with tetrabenazine, pimozide, or both. *Arch. Neurol.*, 1974.
9. Fog, R., Randrup, A., Pakkenberg, H. A dopaminergic mechanism in corpus striatum and amphetamine-induced stereotyped behavior. *Psychopharmacologia, (Berl.), 11*:179-183, 1967.
10. Pakkenberg, H. The effect of tetrabenazine in some hyperkinetic syndromes. *Acta Neurol. Scand., 44*:391–393, 1968.

46

Maintenance Antipsychotic Therapy and the Risks of Tardive Dyskinesia

CARYLE H. CHAN
JOHN M. DAVIS
ROBERT C. SMITH
and KEN REED

The increasing awareness of the risk of tardive dyskinesia in patients on long-term maintenance neuroleptics has raised questions about the rationale of such antipsychotic drug therapy. However, the risks of tardive dyskinesia must be considered in terms of the overall psychiatric benefits of maintenance versus the risks of relapse upon discontinuation of drug therapy.

This chapter will assess the advantages of antipsychotic maintenance therapy by reviewing the findings of 24 controlled studies (1–24), which compared the relapse rates of patients receiving neuroleptics with those maintained on placebo. We will then consider the clinical issues of long-term antipsychotic maintenance in schizophrenic patients in the light of the associated risks of tardive dyskinesia occurring with such therapy.

REVIEW OF CONTROLLED STUDIES

The discovery of chlorpromazine's antipsychotic action resulted in a plethora of uncontrolled studies reporting that maintenance medication decreased the frequency of clinical relapse. Although these early studies had a pioneering function in evolving more sophisticated methodologies, this chapter will only consider the more recent double-blind controlled studies. It should be noted, however, that the earlier uncontrolled reports and the later double-blind studies yield consistent results. The controlled studies of neuroleptic maintenance of schizophrenics are summarized in Table 1. It is noteworthy that these studies were carried out in a number of different settings, including public, private, and Veterans Administration hospitals; in both

TABLE 1
Summary of Controlled Studies of Antipsychotic Medication Versus Placebo

Study	Number of Patients			Relapsed Patients				Analysis of Relapse Rate	Significance
	Drug Group	Placebo Group	Total	Drug Group N	Percent	Placebo Group N	Percent		
Caffey and associates (4)	88	171	259	4	5	77	45	$\phi=.40$	$p=5 \times 10^{-13}$
Prien and Cole (18)	573	189	762	91	16	79	42	$\phi=.27$	$p=1 \times 10^{-12}$
Prien and associates (19)	218	107	325	44	20	60	56	$\phi=.35$	$p=1 \times 10^{-10}$
Schiele and associates (21)	60	20	80	2	3	12	60	$\phi=.61$	$p=1.5 \times 10^{-7}$
Adelson and Epstein (1)	191	90	281	93	49	81	90	$\phi=.39$	$p=2 \times 10^{-12}$
Morton (17)	20	20	40	5	25	14	70	$\phi=.40$	$p=5.2 \times 10^{-3}$
Baro and associates (2)	13	13	26	0		13	100	$\phi=.92$	$p=9.6 \times 10^{-8}$
Hershon and associates (11)	30	32	62	2	7	9	28	$\phi=.24$	$p=2.8 \times 10^{-2}$
Rassidakis and associates (20)	41	43	84	14	34	25	58	$\phi=.22$	$p=2.3 \times 10^{-2}$
Melynk and associates (16)	20	20	40	0		10	50	$\phi=.52$	$p=2.2 \times 10^{-4}$
Schawver and associates (22)	40	40	80	2	5	7	18	$\phi=.16$	$p=7.7 \times 10^{-2}$
Freeman and Alson (7)	44	42	86	6	14	13	31	$\phi=.18$	$p=4.6 \times 10^{-2}$
Whitaker and Hoy (24)	13	26	39	1	8	17	65	$\phi=.49$	$p=6.8 \times 10^{-4}$
Garfield and associates (8)	9	18	27	0		4	22	$\phi=.18$	$p=1.7 \times 10^{-1}$
Diamond and Marks (5)	20	20	40	5	25	14	70	$\phi=.40$	$p=5.2 \times 10^{-3}$
Blackburn and Allen (3)	25	28	53	6	24	15	54	$\phi=.26$	$p=2.7 \times 10^{-2}$
Gross and Reeves (10)	36	73	109	5	14	42	58	$\phi=.46$	$p=9.2 \times 10^{-6}$
Englehardt and associates (6)	152	142	294	23	15	42	30	$\phi=.20$	$p=2.2 \times 10^{-3}$
Leff and Wing (14)	18	12	30	6	33	10	83	$\phi=.42$	$p=9.2 \times 10^{-3}$
Hogarty and Goldberg (13)	187	174	361	57	30	117	67	$\phi=.36$	$p=1.1 \times 10^{-8}$
Troshinsky and associates (23)	24	19	43	1	4	12	63	$\phi=.59$	$p=1.7 \times 10^{-5}$
Hirsch and associates (12)	36	38	74	3	8	25	66	$\phi=.56$	$p=2.7 \times 10^{-7}$
Good and associates (9)*			112						
Marjer ison and associates (15)**	47	31	78						

*No overall statement was made in this study about the relapse rate of individual patients. At 6 months patients in the placebo group showed significant ($p<.01$) worsening of such schizophrenic symptoms as hallucinations plus delusions.

**No overall statement was made in this study about the relapse rate of individual patients. The antipsychotic drugs (chlorprothixene and trifluoperazine) were superior to placebo ($p=.004$; $p=.02$; $p=.03$).

outpatient and inpatient facilities; and also in both the United States and the United Kingdom.

All these studies randomly assigned patients to groups receiving an antipsychotic, usually chlorpromazine, or groups receiving (double-blind) placebo. The frequency of relapse was then measured. Since there are numerous studies, and many of them include large numbers of patients, it is possible to estimate the degree of drug prophylaxis as well as the statistical significance of this prophylactic effect.

The reviewed outpatient studies included schizophrenics who had had a partial or a total symptomatic remission while in the hospital for a time sufficient to allow their discharge back into the community. While still on maintenance therapy in the community, some patients remained in a stable psychiatric state, whereas others deteriorated or relapsed to an extent that often required rehospitalization. The inpatient studies involved, for the most part, partially remitted chronic schizophrenics. The relapse rates for these studies indicate whether the psychiatric status of these patients remained at the level of their initial psychiatric evaluation at the start of the study or had significantly worsened during the study period.

In all studies more patients relapsed on placebo than on drug. It is obvious that baseline relapse rates will depend on a particular study's relapse criteria, and that the relapse frequency will be higher in those studies that contain sicker patients with a more active disease. Because of these two points, the most relevant comparisons of relative drug and placebo relapse rate is by comparison within a given group. The number and percentage of relapsed patients is listed in Table 1.

The sample sizes in each study were large enough to allow quantitative estimates of the relationship between relapse frequency and the presence or absence of maintenance neuroleptics. Likewise, in the appropriately controlled studies an assessment of the statistical reliability of the prophylactic effect and the magnitude of the association between relapse rate and treatment can be determined. Every study except two (9,15) indicated how many patients relapsed or remained stable. These data can therefore be presented in a 2 × 2 contingency table, and the Fisher Exact Test can be applied to compute the probability for the statistical association. For each study the *Phi* correlation indicates the magnitude of the association between relapse rate and drug treatment. *Phi* is the equivalent of the product-moment correlation where the value 1 was assigned to a patient who relapsed and/or was on placebo, and the value 0 was assigned to the patient who did not relapse and/or was on a neuroleptic. A positive *Phi* coefficient would indicate that the drug treatment prevents relapse.

Table 1 gives the number and percentage of patients who did and did not relapse for each study, the statistical significance of the Fisher Exact Test, and the *Phi* coefficient. The *Phi* coefficients are positive in all the listed double-blind studies, implying a substantially greater relapse tendency on placebo than on neuroleptic. In most of the studies, the probability of the statistical association was significant. In those studies where statistical significance was not reached, the sample size was small. However, the difference was of the same order of magnitude.

All of the reported studies were designed to test the same hypothesis. Hence the results can be combined by the Fliess modification of the Cochran method (25) that allows the partitioning of the combined data from all the studies into two components. The similarity of the degree of the association between the different studies is reflected in the first component, whereas the second component reflects the magnitude of the association. Analysis of the first component shows a similar degree of association, and the second component gives a highly statistically significant magnitude of association; the probability that chance alone could account for the result was less than 10^{-7}. If one combines the probabilities for each of the 24 studies by the method of Winer (26) the p value is less than 10^{-80}. Thus, the statistical evidence is overwhelming that maintenance neuroleptic medication prevents relapse in schizophrenia.

Figure 1 illustrates the relapse of schizophrenia as a function of time for two typical studies (4,13) after the neuroleptic had been substituted by a placebo. It is important to note both for clinical purposes and for research considerations that most patients do not relapse within a few days or weeks after discontinuation of an active drug, but rather begin to do so after a few months. Therefore, in studies of relapse rates one must have a time period of a *minimum* of several months for any valid indication of the relapse rate after discontinuation of neuroleptic medication.

The risk of clinical relapse after discontinuation of medication is present for a considerable period of time, as was shown by Hogarty and Goldberg (13). The relapse rates did not begin to level off until 1 year after discontinuation of medication, and this leveling off was not completed even after 2 years. The leveling-off phenomenon seen after 1 year may mean that the majority of those who relapse will do so within a year of discontinuation of therapy, and that relapse risks after 1 year continue to decrease with time. On the other hand, this phenomenon may be a reflection of the fact that the relapse rate of the placebo group is so marked within the first year that too few placebo patients remain after 1 year for an appropriate statistical analysis. It is clinically important to be aware, however, that a relapse can first occur at any time during a period of up to 2 years, and possibly longer, after discontinuation of neuroleptics.

Rates of relapse for patients maintained on neuroleptics or placebo can be estimated from several of the studies. For example, Hogarty and Goldberg (13) found a relapse rate for patients receiving drug therapy of 3.5% per month while the rate for patients receiving placebo was 10.7% per month. Caffey *et*

Percent of Patients Not Relapsed on Maintenance Medication or Placebo in Two Studies (4, 13)

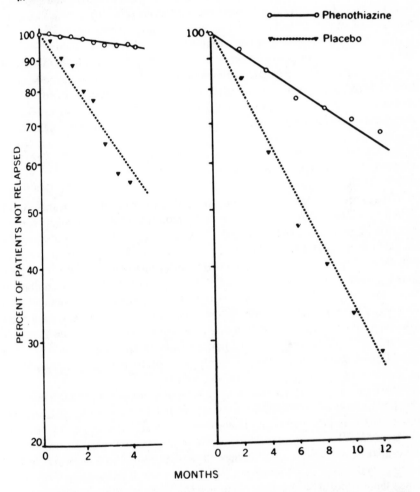

*The left-hand portion of the graph shows the percent of 259 patients who did not relapse on maintenance medication or placebo in a 4-month double-blind controlled study by Caffey and associates (4); the right-hand portion shows the percent of 43 patients who did not relapse on maintenance medication or placebo in a 12-month double-blind controlled study by Hogarty and Goldberg (13). In each case the data were fitted by the method of least squares to an exponential curve.

al. (4) found a relapse rate of 1.5% per month for patients on neuroleptics, and 15.7% for those on placebo treatment. An excellent fit ($r^2 = .96$) to the data will be found by applying a least-square regression to an appropriate exponential equation. By using an appropriate calculation, it can be shown that in the majority of studies (which generally ran from a few months to 18 months), the relapse potential is almost 3 times greater for the group maintained on placebo than for that maintained on neuroleptics. Moreover, several factors in the design of these studies mitigate against obtaining so large a difference between the drug and placebo patients, particularly in the later months of follow-up. Therefore, the degree of protection offered by neuroleptics against relapse may be even somewhat greater than is calculated from these studies.

CLINICAL ISSUES

The review presented in the preceding section has unequivocally established that antipsychotic medication does prevent relapse for many schizophrenic patients, and that a definite risk of deterioration occurs when the medication is discontinued. The risk of relapse after discontinuation is apparent after a few months and continues to be of clinical significance for greater than a 2-year period. Over the period of 2 years, the risk of relapse on placebo maintenance is almost 3 times greater than on neuroleptic maintenance therapy. The relapse of schizophrenia into a marked active psychosis can occur very rapidly and be preceded by few warning symptoms. For example, Hogarty and Goldberg (13) noted that patients can remain in a fairly stable condition of remission and then suddenly deteriorate markedly in psychological functioning.

Although long-term maintenance of schizophrenics with neuroleptics increases the risks of tardive dyskinesia, the decision to remove neuroleptics for this reason may prove an even greater overall threat to the patient by virtue of the increased chance of relapse into active psychosis. For patients under 45 to 50 years of age, most survey studies show a quite low rate of prevalence of tardive dyskinesia in patients maintained on neuroleptics, and most of the cases that do occur in this age group have mild or even doubtful symptoms. Indeed, even in the older age group, where the rate of tardive dyskinesia is higher, only a small percentage of patients develop dyskinetic symptoms that are severe or disabling. Therefore, the risks of psychiatric relapse and the accompanying repercussions, which in placebo maintenance can range from a rate of 11% to 15% per month, are quantitatively larger than the development of clinically significant symptoms of tardive dyskinesia.

The question still arises, however, as to whether or not there are any criteria that the clinician can use in making decisions about the benefits of maintenance neuroleptic therapy for specific patients, or any regimens he can use in order to reduce the risks of tardive dyskinesia. We will discuss below several issues relevant to these clinical questions.

Indications for Maintenance Therapy

Although maintenance therapy with neuroleptics clearly helps prevent relapses into active psychotic episodes, recent studies suggest that up to 20% of schizophrenic patients do not relapse on placebo treatment for as long as 2 years of follow-up. A few studies also suggest that certain of the reactive, or "good prognosis," schizophrenics (characterized by particular psychological and physiological factors) may do as well or better without neuroleptic medication as with the antipsychotic drug treatment. In view of the risks of tardive dyskinesia associated with neuroleptics, it would be ideal if one could clearly identify this subgroup of patients and choose, therefore, to treat them with other pharmacological agents or by psychological methods alone. Unfortunately, at the present time there is no easy or certain method that most clinicians could use routinely to identify this subgroup of schizophrenics. Furthermore, good prognosis patients have not been consistently shown to benefit any less from neuroleptic medication than the other subgroups of schizophrenia. For example, one less well controlled study by Leff and Wing (14) suggested that good prognosis schizophrenic patients benefited less from maintenance neuroleptics than patients with "middle prognosis" features. However, a more recent and better controlled study by Goldberg et al. (27) showed that schizophrenics with "good" signs, such as less psychopathology or less situational stress, benefited more from neuroleptic maintenance therapy than patients with "poor" signs (as defined by these variables). Goldstein (29) suggested that patients with good signs did not have the same beneficial response to antipsychotic medication as those with poor prognostic signs. Yet results of another study by Klein and Rosen (28) came to almost the opposite conclusion.

Thus, at the present time there is no simple way to detect that small group of patients who may not have a substantially increased risk of psychotic relapse if their maintenance neuroleptics are discontinued. Under these conditions of uncertainty it is the sociological as well as psychological consequences of a relapse to an active psychosis that become more primary clinical considerations. For many outpatients, the relapse, which as stated earlier may be both severe and acute in onset and have little warning, can have many disorganizing consequences over a broad social spectrum involving the patient, his family, his occupation, and his social network. For example, if the patient loses his job or if increased stress leads to divorce or marital separation, these events may have a markedly adverse effect on the patient's subsequent reentry into the community after the remission of the psychosis such that he cannot attain again his prerelapse level of social or occupational functioning. In such tenuous situations of sociological and psychological balance, a 2 or 3 times greater rate of relapse into a psychotic episode may be too high. These risks should be seriously considered, even when maintenance neuroleptics have resulted in the development of mild dyskinetic side effects.

On the other hand, in situations in which the social and psychological repercussions of a relapse are not so great, more consideration can be given to a trial period off of medication, even if this may precipitate a relapse. In the hospital setting the relapse into a more florid psychotic episode may not have the same disastrous consequences for the patient in terms of the social and psychological spectrum. Also, it is more likely that the onset of the psychiatric relapse will be recognized earlier than in the outpatient settings, and that a resumption of neuroleptic medication could be more quickly and easily implemented.

With this important assessment of the social and psychological consequences of relapse for a specific patient, a clinician might use some of the results from anecdotal reports or clinical studies discussed below to help make a decision as to whether there is any justification for not starting or continuing maintenance therapy with antipsychotic drugs:

A. Patients who have had a number of relapses when they self-discontinue their antipsychotic medication would be poor candidates for a drug-free maintenance program. On the other hand, patients who have had no or very infrequent relapses over a long time span would be better candidates for a drug-free therapy trial.

B. The dose of neuroleptics that a patient requires to achieve remission may be a good indicator of the need for drug therapy maintenance. Prien *et al.* (19) found that those patients who required higher doses of chlorpromazine to achieve remission of their psychotic symptoms had a relapse rate of 50% to 60% on placebo maintenance. This was higher than the 23% relapse rate for those who required low doses of neuroleptics to ameliorate the initial psychotic episode, and much higher than the 3% relapse rate for those patients who required no antipsychotic medication for remission of their psychotic illness (see Table 2).

C. Patients who have not shown a great deal of improvement with neuroleptic therapy in the past may warrant an extended trial of drug-free management.

D. Many long-term hospitalized chronic schizophrenics may benefit from a trial period of drug-free maintenance.

E. Some first-episode schizophrenic illnesses may be "reactive" schizophrenia or schizophreniform illness. One can consider giving some of these patients a short trial of treatment without neuroleptics, or a short-term period of treatment with antipsychotics followed by a longer drug-free maintenance period. Many of these reactive schizophrenics or schizophreniform psychoses have affective symptoms in their clinical presentation and history, and would be likely labeled as schizo-affective by research diagnostic criteria (RDC) or DSM III.

Dosage Considerations

Several studies reported in this volume indicate that higher dose administration of neuroleptics may be a more important risk factor in causing tardive dyskinesia than even the total amount of neuroleptics administered to a patient over a period of time. Therefore, patients should be treated with the lowest dosage of neuroleptics to maintain a remission of their psychotic symptoms, so that the risks of tardive dyskinesia would be reduced. Very low doses of neuroleptics in the range of 20–50 mg (CPZ eq.) per day may be ''homeopathic'' as regards their antipsychotic effects in schizophrenia, but most outpatients can be maintained on dosages which do not exceed 200–400 mg (CPZ eq.) per day. Patients over 60–65 years of age may require lower maintenance dosage because they may achieve higher plasma levels for a given oral dosage and may have slower metabolism of the neuroleptic. Clinical studies by George Crane suggest that although some long-term hospitalized chronic schizophrenic patients show periodic fluctuations in their psychoses, these variations are not substantially different when they are maintained on fairly low, as compared to standard or high doses, of neuroleptics.

Despite the problems associated with high doses of antipsychotic medication, there is certainly a role for a trial of high-dose treatment with neuroleptics for patients whose psychotic symptoms fail to respond to standard dosages. High-dose therapy may be particularly relevant for the acute or relapsing schizophrenic who has been shown to have low blood levels of neuroleptics when he is treated with standard oral dosage. However, these high-dose trials should be carried out only for a clearly defined time period and in a situation in which the patient's psychiatric status and the development of any movement disorders can be closely monitored. Unless the high-dose therapy produces a

Table 2

Relapses on Placebo by Prestudy
Dose Level of Chlorpromazine or Equivalent

Prestudy Dose Level	No. of Patients	Patients Relapsed	
		n	Percent
No medication	30	2	3
Under 300 mg	99	23	23
300 mg to 500 mg	91	47	52
500 mg	81	53	65

substantially greater degree of improvement compared to standard dose administration, it should not be continued indefinitely for many months or years.

Specific Neuroleptics and Risks of Tardive Dyskinesia

Tardive dyskinesia has been reported in patients receiving most of the neuroleptics currently in use in the United States, and at the present time there is no conclusive evidence that tardive dyskinesia is especially associated with a particular neuroleptic. The results of the three retrospective and one uncontrolled prospective study reported in other chapters of this volume suggest that fluphenazine, and especially depot fluphenazine, may have a higher association with tardive dyskinesia than some other neuroleptics. One should bear in mind, however, that the long-acting depot neuroleptics, such as fluphenazine, have been an important advance in the treatment of chronic schizophrenics to be maintained in the community and have avoided frequent or long-term hospitalizations due to drug discontinuation relapses. Before a clinical decision can be made that depot fluphenazine definitely poses too high a risk of tardive dyskinesia, a good controlled prospective study involving several dose levels of the drug is needed to provide stronger evidence of the association of depot neuroleptics and tardive dyskinesia. In a few reports thioridazine has been shown to have a slightly lower association with tardive dyskinesia, although some cases of tardive dyskinesia have been found in patients taking this neuroleptic.

Clozapine, a neuroleptic which has been used for several years in Europe, has not been reported to produce tardive dyskinesia. Furthermore, some recent clinical studies (see Chapters 42-44) indicate that clozapine may reduce or essentially reverse the symptoms of tardive dyskinesia while still maintaining an antipsychotic effect. However, in a small percentage of cases a side effect—a rapid onset of agranulocytosis—occurs with this drug, and this has lead Sandoz to discontinue clinical trials and marketing of the drug in the United States; some European countries are also decreasing or abandoning use of clozapine. A complete abandonment of the clinical use of clozapine may be unfortunate, however, since this drug does have definite advantages for selected schizophrenic patients. In situations where the hematological and other side effects can be monitored, clozapine would be quite helpful in the chronic schizophrenic with tardive dyskinesia symptoms whose psychiatric condition necessitates maintenance on neuroleptics.

The best solution for reducing the risks of tardive dyskinesia while maintaining the benefits of maintenance neuroleptics in the treatment of schizophrenia would be the development of new antipsychotic medications which meet the following criteria: (1) They have less pharmacological effects on striatial dopamine neurons or receptors, since these may be particularly related to the pathophysiology of tardive dyskinesia; (2) they nevertheless continue to have good antipsychotic potency; and (3) they do not have potential side effects which would prohibit their safe use for outpatients for whom monitoring is a problem. The continued progress in basic and clinical psychopharmacological research offers a good chance that drugs with these desirable properties will be developed in the next 5–10 years.

At the present time, however, the best guide for the clinician is careful attention to the dosage of the neuroleptics employed in long-term maintenance, and the judicious use of drug-free maintenance trials in carefully selected patients. For many schizophrenics, the overall spectrum of relapse complications, both psychological and sociological, which is frequently associated with discontinuation of neuroleptics, far outweighs the smaller risk of the tardive dyskinesia associated with maintenance of the currently available neuroleptics.

REFERENCES

1. Adelson, D., Epstein, L.A. A study of phenothiazines in male and female chronically ill schizophrenics. *J. Nerv. Ment. Dis., 134*:543–554, 1962.
2. Baro, F., Brugmans, J., Dom, R., *et al*. Maintenance therapy of chronic psychotic patients with a weekly oral dose of R 16341. *J. Clin. Pharmacol., 10*:330–341, 1970.
3. Blackburn, H., Allen, J. Behavioral effects of interrupting and resuming tranquilizing medication among schizophrenics. *J. Nerv. Ment. Dis., 133*:303–307, 1961.
4. Caffey, E.M., Diamond, L.S., Frank, T.V., *et al*. Discontinuation of reduction of chemotherapy in chronic schizophrenics. *J. Chronic Dis., 17*:347–358, 1964.
5. Diamond, L.S., Marks, J.B. Discontinuance of tranquilizers among chronic schizophrenic patients receiving maintenance dosage. *J. Nerv. Ment. Dis., 131*:247–251, 1960.
6. Englehardt, D.M., Rosen, B., Freedman, D., *et al*. Phenothiazines in the prevention of psychiatric hospitalization. *Arch. Gen. Psychiatry, 16*:98–99, 1967.
7. Freeman, L.S., Alson, E. Prolonged withdrawal of chlorpromazine in chronic patients. *Dis. Nerv. Syst., 23*:522–525, 1962.
8. Garfield, S., Gershon, S., Sletten, L., *et al*. Withdrawal of ataractic medication in schizophrenic patients. *Dis. Nerv. Syst., 27*:321–325, 1966.
9. Good, W.W., Sterling, M., Holtzman, W.H. Termination of chlorpromazine with schizophrenic patients. *Am. J. Psychiatry, 115*:443–448, 1958.
10. Gross, M., Reeves, W.P. Relapse after withdrawal of ataractic drugs. In *Mental Patients in Transition*, Greenblatt, M. (ed.). Springfield, Ill.: Charles C. Thomas, pp. 313–321, 1961.
11. Hershon, H.I., Kennedy, P.F., McGuire, R.J. Persistence of extrapyramidal disorders and psychiatric relapse after withdrawal of long-term phenothiazine therapy. *Br. J. Psychiatry, 120*:41–50, 1972.
12. Hirsch, S.R., Gaind, R., Rohde, P.D., *et al*. Outpatient maintenance of chronic schizophrenic patients with long-acting fluphenazine double-blind placebo trial. *Br. Med. J., 1*:633–637, 1973.
13. Hogarty, G.E., Goldberg, S.C. Drugs and sociotherapy in the aftercare of schizophrenic patients. One-year relapse rates. *Arch. Gen. Psychiatry, 28*:54–62, 1973.
14. Leff, J.P., Wing, J.K. Trial of maintenance therapy in schizophrenics. *Br. Med. J., 2*:599–604, 1971.

522   TARDIVE DYSKINESIA

15. Marjerrison, G., Irvine, D., Stewart, C.N., et al. Withdrawal of long term phenothiazines from chronically hospitalized psychiatric patients. Can. Psychiatr. Assoc. J., 9:290–298, 1964.
16. Melynk, W.T., Worthington, A.G., Laverty, S.G. Abrupt withdrawal of chlorpromazine and thioridazine from schizophrenic inpatients. Can. Psychiatr. Assoc. J., 11:410–413, 1966.
17. Morton, M.R. A study of withdrawal of chlorpromazine or trifluoperazine in chronic schizophrenia. Am. J. Psychiatry, 124:1585–1588, 1968.
18. Prien, R.F., Cole, J.O. High dose chlorpromazine therapy in chronic schizophrenia. Report of National Institute of Mental Health—Psychopharmacology Research Branch Collaborative Study Group. Arch. Gen. Psychiatry, 18:482–495, 1968.
19. Prien, R.F., Levine, J., Cole, J.O. High dose trifluoperazine therapy in chronic schizophrenia. Am. J. Psychiatry, 126:305–313, 1969.
20. Rassidakis, N.C., Kondakis, X., Papanastassiou, A., et al. Withdrawal of antipsychotic drugs from chronic patients. Bull. Menninger Clin., 34:216–222, 1970.
21. Schiele, B.C., Vestre, N.D., Stein, K.E. A comparison of thioridazine, trifluoperazine, chlorpromazine, and placebo: a double-blind controlled study on the treatment of chronic hospitalized schizophrenic patients. J. Clin. Exp. Psychopathol., 22:151–162, 1961.
22. Schawver, J., Gorhman, D.R., Leskin, L.W., et al. Comparison of chlorpromazine and reserpine in maintenance drug therapy. Dis. Nerv. Syst., 20:452–457, 1959.
23. Troshinsky, C.H., Aaronson, H.G., Stone, R.K. Maintenance phenothiazine in the aftercare of schizophrenic patients. Penn. Psychiatr. Quart., 2:11–15, 1962.
24. Whitaker, C.B., Hoy, R.M. Withdrawal of perphenazine in chronic schizophrenia. Br. J. Psychiatry, 109:422–427, 1963.
25. Fleiss, J.L. Statistical methods for rates and proportions. New York: Wiley, 1973.
26. Winer, G.J. Statistical principles in experimental design. New York: McGraw-Hill, 1971.
27. Goldberg, S.C., Schooler, N.R., Hogarty, G.E., Roer, M. Prediction of relapse in schizophrenic outpatients treated by drug and sociotherapy. Arch. Gen. Psychiatry, 34:171–184, 1977.
28. Klein, D.F., Rosen, B. Premorbid asocial adjustment and response to phenothiazine treatment among schizophrenic inpatients. Arch. Gen. Psychiatry, 29:480–485, 1973.
29. Goldstein, M.J. Premorbid adjustment, paranoid status and patterns of response to phenothiazine in acute schizophrenia. Schizo. Bull. (ext. issue No. 3) 24–37, 1970.

Index

523